Body Size in Early Modern Germany

STUDIES IN GERMAN HISTORY

Body Size in Early Modern Germany

HOLLY FLETCHER

OXFORD
UNIVERSITY PRESS

OXFORD
UNIVERSITY PRESS

Great Clarendon Street, Oxford, OX2 6DP,
United Kingdom

Oxford University Press is a department of the University of Oxford.
It furthers the University's objective of excellence in research, scholarship,
and education by publishing worldwide. Oxford is a registered trade mark of
Oxford University Press in the UK and in certain other countries.

Published in the United States of America by Oxford University Press
198 Madison Avenue, New York, NY 10016, United States of America

British Library Cataloguing in Publication Data
Data available

Library of Congress Control Number: 2025947849

ISBN 9780198972969

DOI: 10.1093/9780198972983.001.0001

Printed and bound by
CPI Group (UK) Ltd., Croydon, CR0 4YY

The manufacturer's authorized representative in the EU for product safety is
Oxford University Press España S.A. of Parque Empresarial San Fernando de Henares,
Avenida de Castilla, 2 – 28830 Madrid (www.oup.es/en or product.safety@oup.com).
OUP España S.A. also acts as importer into Spain of products made by the manufacturer.

FSC
www.fsc.org
MIX
Paper | Supporting responsible forestry
FSC® C013604

For Jack

Acknowledgements

I could not have written this book without the support of many friends, colleagues, and institutions to whom I am extremely grateful. The majority of research for the book was completed during my PhD at the University of Cambridge which was generously funded by the Cambridge Trust and Murray Edwards College. I thank the College, University, and History Faculty for their institutional and financial support. I have also received funding from the German History Society and the Pasold Research Fund which I gratefully acknowledge.

My utmost thanks go to Ulinka Rublack for her incredible guidance, enthusiasm, and belief in this project. It was a privilege to work with Ulinka and to be part of the community of students and researchers she brings together in Cambridge—I thank all fellow members of this group, and especially those ahead of me who generously shared their experiences, writing drafts, and career advice: Eleanor Barnett, Victoria Bartels, Katy Bond, Abigail Gomulkiewicz, Suzanna Ivanič, Laura Kounine, Regine Maritz, Sophie Pitman, and Valerio Zanetti. Over the course of the PhD, I benefited immensely from discussions and feedback from Joachim Whaley at Cambridge; Renate Dürr, Philip Hahn, Andreas Holzem, and Volker Leppin in Tübingen; and Melanie Braun and Jenny Tiramani at the School of Historical Dress in London. Further insights came from conversations with Benedikt Brunner, Joel Harrington, Michael Stolberg, Sarah Toulalan, Fernando Vidal, and Heide Wunder, as well as questions from the audiences of various workshops and conferences in Boston, Cambridge, Frankfurt, London, Oxford, Pisa, Sheffield, Stockholm, Vienna, and online. I also thank the Early Modern Work in Progress group for their thoughtful comments on chapter drafts, especially organizers Kat Hill, Hannah Murphy, Allie Stielau, and Róisín Watson. My examiners, Mary Laven and Lyndal Roper, were generous with their time and feedback, and offered many insightful suggestions to which I hope I have done justice.

Since Cambridge, I have found an amazingly supportive community of early modernists at the University of Manchester who have helped me to refine and persevere with this research. I am particularly grateful to Sasha Handley for allowing me time to work on the book alongside my role as a Research Associate on the project 'Sleeping Well in the Early Modern World'. The project's focus on entangled environmental and material histories has shaped the development of this book, as well as my approach to the past in general. I also thank Sasha, Rachel Winchcombe, and Ed Wouk for their extremely helpful comments on several chapters. Stephen Mossman helped with some particularly tricky translations.

Special thanks go to Stefan Hanß who read and commented on the full manuscript and has been the most supportive and enthusiastic mentor I could have wished for.

Jill Burke, Christine Ott, and I co-organized the conference 'Fat Bodies in Early Modern Europe' in 2022 and we have since co-edited a volume with the same title. I greatly appreciate their shared intellectual interest in early modern fatness (and thinness) which, when I first started this research, was still fairly unusual. I have learned a lot from all those involved in both the conference and edited collection.

I thank the editors of the series 'Studies in German History', especially Bridget Heal, and OUP editors Hannah Doyle and Jamie Mortimer, for their patience and guidance throughout the publication process. I am also grateful to the production team at OUP, especially Project Manager Dolarine Fonceca and copyeditor Jane Robson for their support and expertise. The anonymous reviewers offered thoughtful feedback which helped to streamline and consolidate the text.

I am very lucky to have the love and support of my family and friends. Finishing my PhD during lockdown in 2020 was made endurable thanks to the hospitality and entertainment provided by Sarah, William, Jack, Harry, Liv, and George. Sue and Barry have put me up in Manchester countless times over the last four years, and Becky, Sam, Imogen, and Jonah have provided the best distractions from work. My parents, Margaret and Peter, have always been my biggest cheerleaders and I thank them for their all-round, unconditional support. I met Jack, my husband, in the same year that I took my first undergraduate paper on early modern Germany—he has embraced my fascination ever since and has filled the intervening years with happiness and love.

Contents

List of Illustrations

Note on Translation

Translations are the author's own unless otherwise stated. Where original language is given in quotation marks, this has not been modernized but retains the spelling and grammar of the original source.

1

Introduction

Fatness, Thinness, and Germanness

Matthäus Schwarz cared about the size of his body. At the age of 29, the head accountant for the Fugger merchant company had become 'fat and wide'. He noted this above two watercolour paintings of his naked body which were completed in 1526 and included in his 'little book of clothes' (Figures 1.1 and 1.2).[1] Consisting of 137 images, this book was a celebration of Schwarz's wardrobe, recording the many outfits he had worn from infancy to the age of 63. Alongside the vivid colours and sensuous fabrics of Schwarz's clothing, the paintings of his

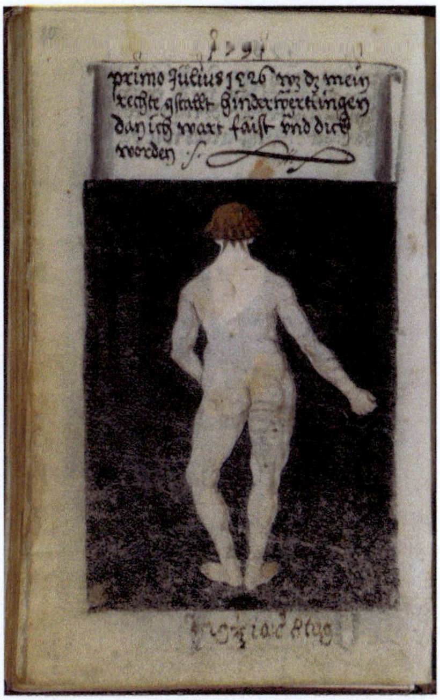

Figure 1.1 Matthäus Schwarz, Little Book of Clothes, Nude Portrait at 29 1/3 from behind, 1526. © bpk/Herzog Anton Ulrich Museum, Braunschweig.

[1] Ulinka Rublack and Maria Hayward (eds), *The First Book of Fashion: The Book of Clothes of Matthäus and Veit Konrad Schwarz of Augsburg* (London, 2015), 128–9. See also 288–9.

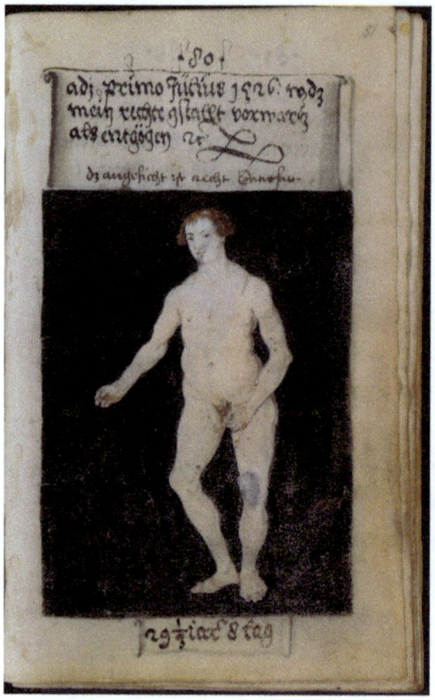

Figure 1.2 Matthäus Schwarz, Little Book of Clothes, Nude Portrait at 29 1/3 from front, 1526. © bpk/Herzog Anton Ulrich Museum, Braunschweig. Schwarz presented his naked body from the front and back and wrote that these images showed his 'real figure' which had become 'fat and wide'. The watercolours present a striking contrast to the 137 images of his dressed body contained in his 'little book of clothes'.

bare body offer a striking juxtaposition. In these images Matthäus revealed the fleshy curves of his new figure, released from the constraints of form-fitting dress. His body had been increasing in size for over a year; above a portrait of himself from 1525, he noted that this was the point at which he had started to grow fatter. This comment appears to have been written at a later date, as though Schwarz leafed back through the manuscript to identify the exact moment at which his slender body began to expand.[2]

This book is the first to examine the significance of body size—of fatness and thinness—in early modern Germany, and indeed, in early modern Europe. It uncovers what it meant to be fat or thin for early modern Germans like Matthäus Schwarz, in terms of both the cultural meanings attached to body size and personal perceptions and experiences of the body. It is often assumed that concern with body size is a modern phenomenon and that, if body size was considered at all in past societies, fatness was simply understood as a sign of wealth while thinness

[2] Ibid. 121 and 283.

represented poverty.[3] Scholars interested in historical accounts of fatness have thus tended to focus on the nineteenth and twentieth centuries as periods in which body size began to take on cultural significance.[4] This book firmly disrupts this narrative by uncovering the various ways in which body size was made to matter in early modern Germany. Body size held far richer meaning than merely the demonstration of lack or plenty in a time of food scarcity. Complex concepts of fatness and thinness were deeply embedded in the cultural landscape of early modern Germany, and they played vital roles in people's gendered identities and experiences of religious and social change.

Body size assumed new significance throughout Germany from the late fifteenth to the early seventeenth centuries. During these tumultuous years, perceptions and practices of body size shifted dramatically, as the size and shape of people's bodies attracted unprecedented attention. Medical advice on how to increase or decrease one's body size proliferated, as debates about the cause and effects of fatness and thinness intensified. With the development of print culture, early modern Germans had access to a growing range of instructions to alter their bodies through daily regimens relating to food and drink, sleep, bathing, and even emotional regulation. Body size thus became embedded in everyday habits and experiences as never before, as well as in interactions between the body and its material environment. Yet body size was not just a health concern. Bodily form increasingly became a subject of artistic and aesthetic interest. It also assumed new spiritual meanings as the Lutheran Reformation took hold across many parts of Germany. The Reformation elevated discussions concerning the flesh and the earthly appetites in connection to ideas about gluttony, fatness, and the belly, while the large figure of Reformation leader Martin Luther (1483–1546) embodied his rejection of Catholicism and its teachings concerning fasting and celibacy.[5] Moreover, this was a period in which clothing styles increasingly acted to mould bodies into idealized forms, with tailored and structured garments elevating people's awareness of personal body size. Such personal bodies were then compared with the bodies of 'others', as sixteenth-century global expansion meant Germans came into increasing contact with non-European bodies, whose size and fleshiness they rarely failed to mention. In what follows, I situate the growing significance of

[3] See e.g. Garabed Eknoyan, 'A History of Obesity, or How What was Good Became Ugly and Then Bad', *Advances in Chronic Kidney Disease* 13 (2006), 421–7, and Sylvia Tara, *The Secret Life of Fat* (New York, 2017).

[4] Studies focusing on modern historical accounts of fatness include Hillel Schwartz, *Never Satisfied: A Cultural History of Diets, Fantasies and Fat* (New York, 1986); Peter N. Stearns, *Fat History: Bodies and Beauty in the Modern West* (New York, 1997); Sander L. Gilman, *Fat: A Cultural History of Obesity* (Cambridge, 2008); Elena Levy-Navarro (ed.), *Historicizing Fat in Anglo-American Culture* (Columbus, OH, 2010).

[5] Lyndal Roper, 'Martin Luther's Body: The "Stout Doctor" and his Biographers', *American Historical Review* 115 (2010), 351–84.

body size in early modern Germany against the backdrop of profound social, religious, and political developments which characterize the Reformation era.

A distinctive culture of body size began to take shape in sixteenth-century Germany. Alongside the developments outlined above, a striking shift was occurring in the presentation of German men who were increasingly shown with bulky, expansive, and fleshy bodies from around 1500. While the presentation of masculine bulk was not unique to Germany (Henry VIII is a prominent example for the English context), the sheer number of portraits of elite and patrician German men who were presented with expansive bodies suggests it was an exceptionally popular silhouette among Germans in particular.[6] By 1525, extreme bulk

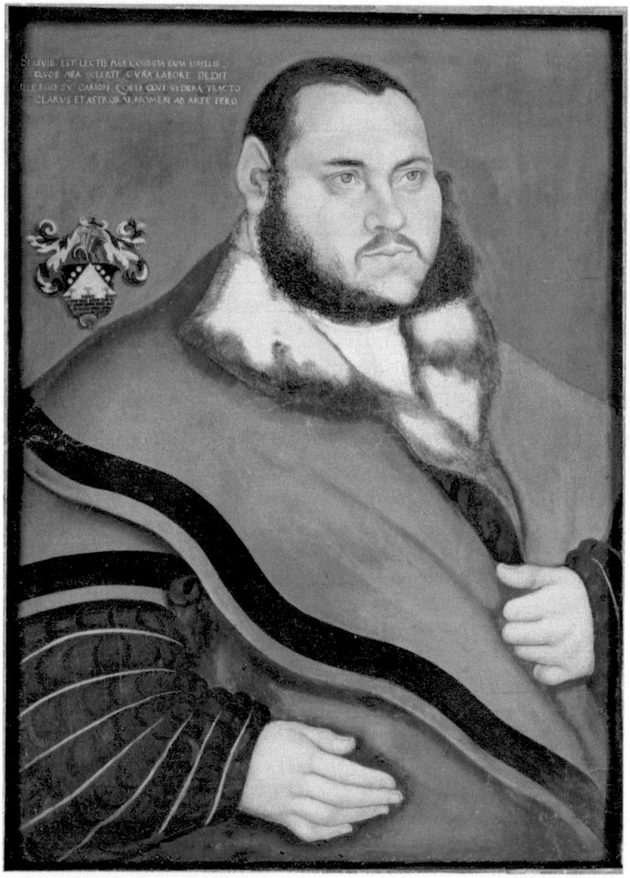

Figure 1.3 Lucas Cranach the Elder, Portrait of Johannes Carion, c.1530. Oil on beech, 52 × 37.3 cm. Staatsbibliothek zu Berlin. © bpk/Gemäldegalerie, SMB/Jörg P. Anders. Carion, court astrologer to Elector Joachim I Nestor of Brandenburg is shown around the age of 30. His bulky presentation exemplifies the German ideal for mature men in the early sixteenth century.

[6] On Henry VIII see Maria Hayward, *Dress at the Court of King Henry VIII* (Leeds, 2007), 3–6.

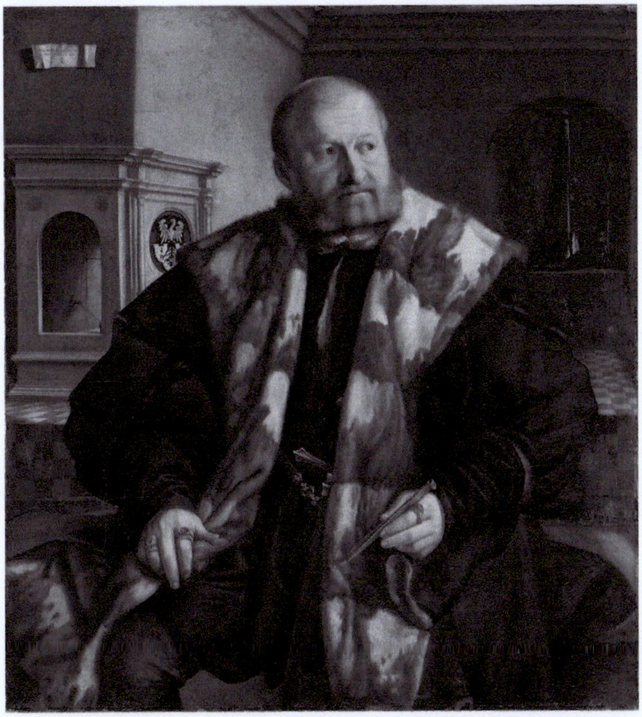

Figure 1.4 Georg Pencz, Portrait of Jörg Herz, 1545. Oil on panel, 109 × 98 cm. Staatliche Kunsthalle, Karlsruhe, public domain. Herz, Nuremberg's Master of the Mint, wears a voluminous, fur-lined gown which creates an imposing and bulky figure. Pencz may have been a student of Dürer's and produced several large-scale portraits of Nuremberg inhabitants which display similarly powerful corporeality.

characterized the presentation of mature German men, whose large size was accentuated through clothing such as wide-shouldered gowns, flat hats, and square-toed shoes (Figures 1.3 and 1.4).[7] Even beards were brushed and cut horizontally to create a sense of breadth and volume. Contemporaries were thus encouraged to invest in bodily appearances which foregrounded body size and shape in new ways, as physical heft came to represent masculine power, status, and honour.[8]

This was a dramatic transformation. Just decades earlier, it would have been almost unimaginable for these men to be presented with such massive bodies. In the late fifteenth century, German bodies were typically shown as notably thin. Throughout visual culture, the bodies of both men and women had been almost

[7] Aileen Ribeiro offers a brief outline of this development in *Dress and Morality* (London, 1986), 59.

[8] On the construction of appearances see Ulinka Rublack, 'Renaissance Dress, Cultures of Making, and the Period Eye', *West 86th: A Journal of Decorative Arts, Design History and Material Culture* 23 (2016), 6–34; Stefan Hanß, 'Face-Work: Making Hair Matter in Sixteenth-Century Europe', *Gender and History* 33 (2021), 314–45.

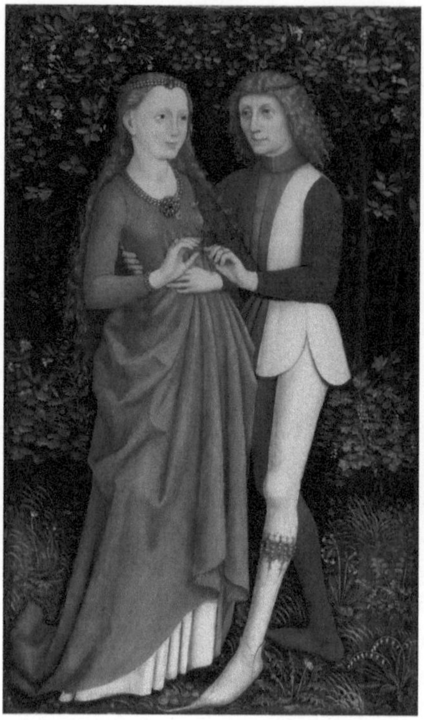

Figure 1.5 Anonymous (Swabian School) Bridal Couple, c.1470. Oil on panel, 62.3 × 36.5 cm. Cleveland Museum of Art, public domain. The male figure is shown with long slender legs which are further elongated through pointed shoes. This slenderness was typical of the gothic silhouette.

uniformly presented with narrow torsos and long slender limbs (Figure 1.5). Such slenderness typified the gothic silhouette, inspired by the artistic influence of the Burgundian court.[9] Aesthetic ideals involving body size were present in the late medieval period, yet prior to the sixteenth century explicit references to body size in health regimens, literary texts, and religious works were far fewer, while visual representations of bodies involved little consideration of diverse bodily forms.[10]

[9] See Angus Patterson, *Fashion and Armour in Renaissance Europe: Proud Lookes and Brave Attire* (London, 2009), 18. On the influence of the Burgundian court see Marina Belozerskaya, *Rethinking the Renaissance: Burgundian Arts across Europe* (Cambridge, 2002).

[10] See Theresa A. Vaughan, *Women, Food and Diet in the Middle Ages: Balancing the Humours* (Amsterdam, 2020), 157–71. Vaughan found that medieval literature on female beauty did not make explicit reference to the size and shape of women's bodies. On medieval ideals for bust size see Kim M. Phillips, 'The Breasts of Virgins: Sexual Reputation and Young Women's Bodies in Medieval Culture and Society', *Cultural and Social History* 15 (2018), 1–19. On medieval aesthetic ideals for female and male bodies which do not encompass body size see Montserrat Cabré, 'Beautiful Bodies', in Linda Kalof (ed.), *A Cultural History of the Human Bodies in the Medieval Age* (London, 2014), 121–39. On medieval attitudes towards fatness see Georges Vigarello, *The Metamorphoses of Fat: A History of Obesity*, tr. Christopher Jon Delogu (New York, 2013), 3–30; Christopher Forth, *Fat: A Cultural History of the Stuff of Life* (London, 2019), 107–22.

Body size took on new significance in the German-speaking regions in the sixteenth century, and the material bodies of German men seem to have changed in conjunction with shifting bodily ideals. The sudden proliferation of images of burly German men most likely reflected an increase in fatness among Germans, while also reinforcing this physique as a fashionable ideal.[11] Yet this study offers a qualitative rather than quantitative account of body size by exploring the diverse cultural meanings assumed by fatness and thinness in connection with material experiences of the body. In so doing, it sheds new light on sixteenth-century German culture by revealing the enormous importance that early modern Germans attached to body size.

Historicizing Body Size

Despite the prominence of concerns about body size in early modernity, the cultural meanings of fatness and thinness in this period have only recently begun to receive sustained scholarly attention. An early exception was Elena Levy-Navarro's *The Culture of Obesity in Early and Late Modernity* (2008) in which she examined early modern literary characterizations of fatness to deconstruct twenty-first-century fat stigma.[12] Levy-Navarro's work aimed to challenge the view that bodily categories such as 'obesity' and 'overweight' are transhistorical and opposed the notion that fat bodies were celebrated to a greater extent in pre-industrial societies through a focus on early modern English literature.[13] The narrative of fat's development from something that was praised and idealized to that which was stigmatized and repudiated is one which numerous scholars have since sought to overturn. Ken Albala, for instance, argued that medical anxiety concerning obesity is not a recent phenomenon but may be dated to the seventeenth century.[14] Michael Stolberg went further in stating that 'virtually every major

[11] On the use of portraits as historical sources, see e.g. Peter Burke, *The Historical Anthropology of Early Modern Italy: Essays on Perception and Communication* (Cambridge, 2005), 150–67.

[12] Elena Levy-Navarro, *The Culture of Obesity in Early and Late Modernity: Body Image in Shakespeare, Jonson, Middleton and Skelton* (New York, 2008).

[13] On fat in premodern literature see also Christine Ott, 'Fette Körper in der Vormoderne. Überlegungen zu einer literarischen Geschichte des Dickseins', *Archiv für das Studium der neueren Sprachen und Literaturen* 256 (2019), 1–21; Christine Ott, 'Körperfülle als äesthetisches Problem in der Frühen Neuzeit', in Sofina Dembruk et al. (eds), *La Renaissance 'trop en corps'. Perspectives croisées sur le corps renaissant* (Heidelberg, 2023), 81–102; Christine Ott, 'Fat Carnival Princess in Renaissance Rome: Luigi Pulci's Political Misogyny', *Food and History* 21 (2023), 159–71; Christine Ott, 'Ein kleines dickes Mädchen. Körpernormen und -abnormitäten im 17. Jahrhundert', in Julia Saviello and Katharina Bedenbender (eds), *Dramaturgien von Bild und Raum* (Berlin, 2024), 139–49; David Lomersley, 'Why is Falstaff Fat?', *Review of English Studies: A Quarterly Journal of English Literature and the English Language* 47 (1996), 1–22; Patricia Parker, *Literary Fat Ladies: Rhetoric, Gender, Property* (London and New York, 1987).

[14] Ken Albala, 'Weight Loss in the Age of Reason', in Christopher E. Forth and Ana Carden-Coyne (eds), *Cultures of the Abdomen: Diet, Digestion and Fat in the Modern World* (Basingstoke, 2005), 169–83.

early modern medical author had something to say about obesity', while Sander Gilman has shown that obesity has been a cause for concern since Greek antiquity.[15] In French historian Georges Vigarello's influential study *The Metamorphoses of Fat*, he identified a 'definitive break' in attitudes towards fatness from the sixteenth century onwards, at which point people with wide waists began to be spoken of negatively and the medieval praise of large bodies disintegrated, resulting in a gradual 'privileging of lightness'.[16] Most recently Christopher Forth has emphasized that in premodern Europe fatness was viewed with ambivalence rather than appreciation. While mapping the shifting nature of this ambivalence, Forth traces the development of negative stereotypes about fat people over time.[17]

Existing studies have rightly drawn attention to the presence of negative attitudes towards fatness in past societies, yet in seeking to find explanations for present-day fat phobia, they frequently reinforce a narrative by which 'what was good...became bad'.[18] This trajectory is connected to larger, teleological theories of historical transformation, including Norbert Elias's 'civilising process' which has been deeply influential for historians of early modern Europe. Elias identified this period as one of shifting behavioural expectations, as standards regarding violence, sexuality, bodily functions, and table manners were gradually transformed through a strengthened sense of shame.[19] As natural human drives were increasingly suppressed, the unruly body became disciplined through new sets of behaviours and manners emerging in the sixteenth century, primarily among the aristocracy and then filtering down to the lower classes. Vigarello argues that the developing stigma around fatness reflected 'ever stricter rules and precise guidelines for physical appearance and the expression of self' in Western societies; he thus inserts the critique of fatness within Elias's understanding of increasing *civilité*.[20] Forth similarly suggests that by the end of the nineteenth century the attainment of a moderate physique was viewed as a marker of civility, and thus a close connection was made between the appreciation of fatness and non-Western

[15] Michael Stolberg, '"Abhorreas pinguedinem": Fat and Obesity in Early Modern Medicine (c.1500–1750)', *Studies in History and Philosophy of Science*, 43 (2012), 370–8, here 377; Sander L. Gilman, *Obesity: The Biography* (Oxford, 2010). See also Sander L. Gilman, *Diets and Dieting: A Cultural Encyclopaedia* (Abingdon, 2008) and Sander L. Gilman, *Fat Boys: A Slim Book* (Lincoln, NE, 2004). Sarah Toulalan has explored medical connections between fatness and infertility in early modern England. See Sarah Toulalan, '"To[o] Much Eating Stifles the Child": Fat Bodies and Reproduction in Early Modern England', *Historical Research* 87 (2014), 65–93. See also Alexander Pyrges, 'Fat Knowledge: The History of Corpulence', *Curare. Zeitschrift für Medizinethnologie*, 39 (2016), 126–35.

[16] Vigarello, *Metamorphoses of Fat*, p. x.

[17] Forth, *Fat*, 14–15.

[18] This quotation is taken from the title of Eknoyan's article, 'A History of Obesity, or How What was Good Became Ugly and Then Bad'. Alexander Pyrges has challenged such teleological narratives in relation to the visual representation of fatness in 'Frühneuzeitliche Verbildlichungen von Beleibtheit: Versuch einer körper- und kunsthistorischen Einordnung', in Michael Stolberg (ed.), *Körper-Bilder in der Frühen Neuzeit: Kunst-, medizin- und mediengeschichtliche Perspektiven* (Berlin, 2021), 103–25.

[19] Norbert Elias, *The Civilising Process: Sociogenetic and Psychogenetic Investigations*, ed. Eric Dunning, Johan Goudsblom, and Stephen Mennell (Oxford, 2000). First published in German in 1939.

[20] Vigarello, *Metamorphoses of Fat*, p. xi.

cultures.[21] Expanding on this association, Sabrina Strings argues that the stigmatization of fatness is fundamentally racist, originating with the Enlightenment view of fat as 'savage' and 'black'.[22]

Such narratives do not translate easily to sixteenth-century Germany.[23] Rather than scorned, large bodies were increasingly prized among German men, and this ideal followed one which was defined by slender elongation. Yet this too is not the only story to be told about body size in early modern Germany. As Mark Jenner has stated, the very term 'the history of the body' invites an approach to all bodies as though they were the same, when in reality early modern bodies were diverse.[24] Similarly, there was a diverse range of attitudes towards body size in early modern Europe. Body size represented various and complex meanings in German society, and it held significance beyond merely the availability of food or the refinement of contemporary manners. Ideals and experiences for women's and men's bodies varied across the lifecycle and within distinctive social and gender hierarchies. Body size was made to matter in early modern Germany in specific ways and in particular contexts, as part of cultural, embodied arguments about values and identities. Rather than examining historical fatness across vast time periods and regions, it is important, therefore, to study body size within a focused geographical, temporal, and cultural setting, to reveal the nuances in attitudes towards fatness and thinness in all their forms.

This book takes a new approach to the study of historical corporality by proposing a concept of 'doing body size'. This draws loosely on understandings of 'doing gender', a concept used in sociology and gender studies, by which gender is understood as something that people actively construct in their daily lives.[25] I suggest that meaning and identity in relation to body size, as for gender, can be constructed through socially guided actions. 'Doing body size' also incorporates anthropologist Annemarie Mol's method of 'praxiography' which reveals the multiplicity of the body in practice, as bodies are enacted differently depending on different actors, materials, bodily techniques, and contexts.[26] Body size can be

[21] Forth, *Fat,* 233–5. See also Christopher Forth, 'Fat, Desire and Disgust in the Colonial Imagination', *History Workshop Journal* 73 (2012), 211–39.

[22] Sabrina Strings, *Fearing the Black Body: The Racial Origins of Fat Phobia* (New York, 2019), here 210.

[23] Such narratives with regard to fatness are complicated in Roberta Colbertaldo and Christine Ott (eds), 'Fat Worlds: Feasters and Loafers in Medieval and Early Modern Europe', special issue of *Food and History* 21 (2023), see esp. 11–31.

[24] Mark S. R. Jenner, 'Body, Image, Text in Early Modern Europe', *Social History of Medicine* 12 (1999), 143–54, here 153–4.

[25] See Candace West and Don H. Zimmerman, 'Doing Gender', *Gender and Society* 1 (1987), 125–51. Judith Butler has written extensively about 'gender performativity' by which gender is communicated and constructed through the repetition of acts: Judith Butler, *Gender Trouble: Feminism and the Subversion of Identity* (New York and London, 1990) and *Bodies that Matter: On the Discursive Limits of Sex* (New York, 2011, first published, 1993).

[26] Annemarie Mol, *The Body Multiple: Ontology in Medical Practice* (Durham, NC, 2002). On the usefulness of Moll's theory for historians of the body see Iris Clever and Willemijn Ruberg, 'Beyond Cultural History? The Material Turn, Praxiography, and Body History', *Humanities* 3 (2014), 546–66.

lived and performed in various ways by different actors, drawing on cultural and contextual influences, and taking on meaning through interactions with others as well as in relation to the material reality of the body. 'Doing body size' can be both intentional and unintentional, and importantly the same body or bodily form may be enacted in different ways depending on the setting in which it is presented. The reformer Martin Luther's large body, for example, became a powerful symbol of his rejection of Catholicism in widely circulated printed portraits, yet among friends and followers Luther self-mockingly joked about the fatness of his body and his lack of discipline with food and drink.[27] Multiple enactments of Luther's body coexisted.

Body size was 'done' by early modern individuals who used clothing to mould their bodies into particular forms and make them behave in certain ways, or who followed dietary and health regimens to alter the natural shape of their figures. In this period, the physical body was thought to be generated through its interaction with external influences such as food and drink, and thus dietary practices aimed at actively creating the body as much as maintaining health.[28] Fatness and thinness were also enacted by letter-writers who referred to their changing bodies in correspondence with loved ones in hope of a response. Moreover, body size was used to stage male power among sixteenth-century German men, who performed masculine bulk in their portraits.[29] Crucially, the concept of 'doing body size' enables us to move beyond the recognition of a continued ambivalence towards fat across time which has dominated recent historiography. Rather than focusing on the positive or negative reception of fatness, we may instead think about the various ways in which fat or thin could be actively used and performed in different contexts, taking on culturally and historically specific meaning in dialogue with its material qualities. This book uncovers the various ways in which body size was lived and enacted in early modern Germany.

Beyond Fatness: Language and Body Size

Existing studies have focused their attention on fatness. The subject of body size instead enables a consideration of bodies of various forms. While fat bodies have frequently been subjected to particular discrimination and regulation, ideas

[27] Roper, 'Martin Luther's Body'.

[28] On the significance of food for constructing the body in this period see Rebecca Earle, *The Body of the Conquistador: Food, Race and the Colonial Experience in Spanish America, 1492–1700* (Cambridge, 2014); Rachel Winchcombe, 'Comfort Eating: Food, Drink and Emotional Health in Early Modern England', *English Historical Review* 138 (2023), 61–91. On early modern dietary practices see also David Gentilcore, *Food and Health in Early Modern Europe: Diet, Medicine and Society 1450–1800* (London, 2015) and Ken Albala, *Eating Right in the Renaissance* (Berkeley, CA, 2002).

[29] This approach is also inspired by Stefan Hanß's use of the concept 'face-work' to show how early modern people used the matter of hair, and especially beards, to make subjectivity a material reality. See Hanß, 'Face-Work', esp. 314–15.

about fatness are inevitably intertwined with those about thinness; attitudes towards one have repercussions for the other, and it is such complex, entangled relationships that must be examined and contextualized to get a fuller understanding of what either bodily form meant to early modern Germans.[30] Moreover, it was not merely extremes of body size that held meaning in sixteenth-century Germany—bodies between and within such categories also require consideration. It mattered which areas or parts of the body were fat or thin; the relationship between the form of separate body parts and that of the body as a whole was a key concern for early modern bodily ideals, since beauty was recognized to exist in the well-proportioned body.[31] The body's texture also held meaning; whether it was flabby or muscular, wobbly or firm, fleshy or bony. The umbrella term of 'body size' acknowledges these subtleties regarding the form and textural qualities of the body in ways that research on fat alone does not.

Recognizing the subtleties of body size requires sensitivity to the language early modern people used when describing bodies. In Early Modern High German, a range of terms were used for this purpose. Matthäus Schwarz used the words *dick* and *faist* which, along with *fett*, were the most common terms for describing fatness. *Dick* denoted thickness and breadth and could be used to describe the size of any object or being, rather than primarily the size or shape of a human body. Where it was used to describe the body, *dick* was understood in connection to terms such as to *fett* ('fat'), *fleischig* ('fleshy'), *kräftig* ('strong' or 'stout'), and *massig* ('bulky').[32] While often used to describe fat bodies, *dick* did not necessarily denote fattiness or fleshiness, but could also refer to bulk, density, and breadth. Similarly, terms such as *leibig* or *beleibt* suggested good nourishment, solidity, and stoutness without necessarily referring to fatness.[33]

Feist (also spelled *faist*, *feißt*, *feiszt*) specifically indicated corpulence and fleshiness in both humans and animals, and was also used to refer to heavy food and drink, or the fertility of landscapes.[34] *Feist* was often interchangeable with *fett*, a term which was derived from *feist* and made its way into High German via Martin Luther's vernacular translation of the Bible.[35] In some contexts, however, *feist* and *fett* could hold slightly different connotations; huntsmen were said to differentiate *feist* from *fett* in relation to animals who belonged to either the high

[30] Natalie Zemon Davis made a similar argument with regard to gender history. See Natalie Zemon Davis, '"Women's History" in Transition: The European Case', *Feminist Studies* 3 (1976), 83–103, esp. 90.

[31] This is a key argument in Albrecht Dürer's writings on beauty and proportion. See Chapter 3.

[32] 'Dik' *Frühneuhochdeutsches Wörterbuch* (FWB), digital edition: https://fwb-online.de/; 'dicke' *Mittelhochdeutsches Wörterbuch* (MHDWB), digital edition: https://www.mhdwb-online.de/ & 'dick' *Deutsches Wörterbuch von Jacob Grimm und Wilhelm Grimm* (DWB), digital edition: www.woerterbuchnetz.de/DWB/.

[33] 'Leibig', FWB.

[34] 'Feiszt', DWB.

[35] 'Feist', *Grammatisch-kritisches Wörterbuch der Hochdeutschen Mundart: Nach der Ausgabe letzter Hand, Leipzig 1793–1801* (*Adelung*) digital edition: www.woerterbuchnetz.de/Adelung/; 'fett', *Adelung*; 'fett', DWB.

or low hunt—a deer would be described as *feist* rather than *fett*, while a hare would be *fett* and not *feist*. This suggests that different categories of people, animals, and things could be described using a different language of fatness. Nevertheless, *feist* and *fett* were widely used to describe the fatness of humans, animals, food, landscapes, herbs and plants, and even the weather; one could refer to 'fat rain', suggesting volume or heaviness. Versions of both terms were also used as nouns to refer to the material substance of fat, primarily in relation to both animal and human bodies. Different terms could be used for fat found in different areas of the body. The Alsatian military surgeon Hans von Gersdorff, for example, differentiated between an external fatness of the skin which he termed *Feyßtigkeit* and an internal fatness of the stomach which he called *Schmär*.[36] This latter term was also used to refer to the internal fat of animals.[37] The language of fat thus repeatedly reveals how ideas about human fatness were closely connected to conceptions of animals, plants, and the wider environment in this period.[38]

The most common term for thinness was *mager* which indicated a lack of fat or flesh, and, once again, was used in relation to both humans and animals, as well as food and landscapes.[39] *Mager* was also connected to adjectives such as *schmächtig* and *schmal* both of which denoted slenderness or slimness, and could also be associated with weakness.[40] *Mager* was the opposite of *feist* and *fett*, while *dünn* was opposed to *dick*. The thinness referred to by *dünn* was thus conceived of in terms of size and width as opposed to fleshiness.[41] *Dürr* indicated leanness, or more specifically dryness, suggesting a more withered or scrawny thinness. The lack of moisture referred to by *dürr* could also be associated with infertility, primarily in relation to agriculture.[42] A further term, *gering*, connected small bodily girth to a sense of lightness, nimbleness, and agility.[43]

While early modern people did sometimes refer to the body as feeling heavy or light in relation to body size, weight was not as closely connected to ideas of fatness or thinness in this period as it is today. It was highly unusual to weigh people in early modern Europe.[44] Though weights, scales, and balances had been used for centuries to measure goods, it was not until the turn of the seventeenth century that such measures were applied to the human body and, even then, only

[36] Hans von Gersdorff, *Feldbuch der Wundartzney newlich getruckt vnd gebessert* (Strasbourg, 1528), fol. i^{v}.

[37] 'Schmer', DWB.

[38] This theme is explored in detail in Chapter 2.

[39] 'Mager', DWB.

[40] 'Mager', *Adelung* and 'mager' FWB.

[41] 'Dünn' DWB.

[42] 'Dürre' *Adelung*; 'dürr' DWB; 'dür' FWB.

[43] 'Geringe' *Adelung* and 'gering' DWB.

[44] In the early modern Indian Mughal Empire the Mughal would be weighed twice a year on his solar and lunar birthdays, a ritual which was commented upon in numerous European travel accounts in the seventeenth and eighteenth centuries. See Antje Flüchter, 'Weighing the Mughal: German Perception of Governmental Structures and the Staging of Power in the Early Modern Indian Mughal Empire', in Antje Flüchter and Susan Richter (eds), *Structures on the Move: Technologies of Governance in Transcultural Encounter* (Berlin and Heidelberg, 2012), 147–66.

in exceptional cases.[45] Occasionally the bodies of particularly large individuals were weighed as public spectacles. In Strasbourg in 1612, for example, a 36-year-old woman was found to weigh 480 pounds.[46] The limited use of weight as a measure of body size was likely due to the issue of accessing a scale large enough to weigh a person, as well as a different perspective on the significance of weight as a measure of health.[47] When the Paduan physician Sanctorius Sanctorius (1561–1636) devised one of the earliest known weighing chairs in the early seventeenth century, for example, it was not intended to measure how fat or thin the body was. Rather, Sanctorius sought to quantify the bodily evacuation that occurred through 'insensible perspiration' by noting the body's weight at various stages in relation to the consumption of food and drink and the excretion of urine and faeces.[48] While a connection between body size and weight was sometimes recognized, this was far from the primary framework through which early modern Germans understood or referred to body size, thus indicating a radically different conceptualization of fatness and thinness in this period.

Rather than gaining or losing weight, changes in the size of the body were typically described in terms of increasing or decreasing size, or fattening or slimming the body. For slimming, verbs such as, *ausmagern*, *ausmergeln*, and *auszeren* were associated with the removal of nourishment and the experience of hunger, as well as the emaciation, weakening, or wearing out of the body.[49] For fattening, the term *mästen* meaning to actively fatten, now typically used with reference to livestock, was also used in this period in relation to people's efforts to increase the size of their bodies, as well as for excessive consumption which was said to cause unnatural fatness. The verbs *zunehmen*, meaning to increase or gain, and *abnehmen*, meaning to decrease or reduce, were used to suggest change in body size without specific reference to fatness or thinness.[50] These terms were thus used by and for people who would not necessarily be understood to possess either a particularly fat or thin body, reinforcing the importance of examining body size as opposed to fatness alone.

[45] On the weighing of metal see Allison Stielau, 'The Weight of Plate in Early Modern Inventories and Secularization Lists', *Journal of Art Historiography* 11 (2014), 1–24.

[46] See Stolberg, 'Fat and Obesity', 372.

[47] There is also limited evidence for the weighing of livestock in sixteenth-century Europe. Bradford Bouley found that, while the owners of animals for sale in Rome would be taxed based on weight, the weight of the animals would be determined by visual inspection. Bradford Bouley, 'A Plague of Meat: Food, Politics, and Warfare in Early Modern Italy', *Isis* 114 (2023), 631–7, here 634.

[48] Sanctorius's weighing chair has received extensive scholarly attention. Recent publications include Teresa Hollerbach, 'The Weighing Chair of Sanctorius Sanctorius: A Replica', *NTM Zeitschrift für Geschichte der Wissenschaften, Technik und Medizin* 26 (2018), 121–49, and Jan Purnis, 'Sanctorius's Weighing Chair: Measurement, Metabolism, and Mind', in Simone Guidi and Joaquim Braga (eds), *The Quantification of Life and Health from the Sixteenth to the Nineteenth Century: Intersections of Medicine and Philosophy* (Cham, 2023), 111–32.

[49] 'Ausmagern', FWB, 'ausmergeln', FWB, 'auszeren', FWB.

[50] 'Zunehmen', DWB; 'abnemen', *Adelung*.

Materiality and Early Modern Bodies

As well as language, ideas about body size were shaped by the materiality of early modern bodies.[51] Body size is a physical, material, and embodied experience; the size and shape of a person's body determines the space they take up in a room, how they stand and move, and how they interact with other material things. In other words, body size informs our physical point of view on the world.[52] This book considers how body size felt, as much as what it signified, to early modern people, and it suggests that cultural meanings and corporeal experiences of body size were closely intertwined. Early modern bodies were characterized by the interconnectedness of mental and physical conditions and sensations. Corporeal experiences were thus shaped by the material conditions of life as well as a person's psychic world, both of which were dictated by a broad array of cultural, social, religious, and economic factors.[53] That thinness was frequently associated with sickness, infertility, and alienation from networks of care would have shaped the feeling of becoming slimmer in this period. Likewise, believing that a fat belly symbolized the sin of gluttony would have informed the material experience of a fleshy stomach.

The physical perception of body size depended upon early modern understandings of the body, including the medical view that bodies were composed of humours and fluids, the flows of which were subject to the emotions and determined physical health. Writing of such understandings, Ulinka Rublack has questioned whether early modern bodies were not only conceived of differently but actually behaved differently.[54] Bodies are not granted cultural meaning passively, but actively register, ground, and reformulate embodied experiences in relation to their cultural surroundings, processes which have physical consequences. Bodies need to be approached, therefore, as the 'existential ground of culture and self'.[55] The importance of selfhood for embodied perception, is especially noteworthy in relation to questions of body size, since every body consists of a unique

[51] On the materiality of the body see Lyndal Roper, *Oedipus and the Devil: Witchcraft, Sexuality and Religion in Early Modern Europe* (London, 1994), esp. 21 and Lyndal Roper, 'Beyond Discourse Theory', *Women's History Review* 19 (2010), 307–19.

[52] On the significance of the body in shaping external awareness see Maurice Merleau-Ponty, *The Primacy of Perception: And Other Essays on Phenomenological Psychology, the Philosophy of Art, History and Politics*, ed. James M. Edie (Evanston, IL, 1964), esp. 5. See also Maurice Merleau-Ponty, *The Phenomenology of Perception* (London, 1981).

[53] Laura Gowing, *Common Bodies: Women, Touch and Power in Seventeenth Century England* (New Haven, 2003), 4. See also Barbara Duden, *The Woman Beneath the Skin: A Doctor's Patients in Eighteenth-Century Germany*, tr. Thomas Dunlap (Cambridge, 1991).

[54] Ulinka Rublack, 'Fluxes: The Early Modern Body and the Emotions', *History Workshop Journal* 53 (2002), 1–16. On the physical consequences of emotions see also Ulinka Rublack, 'Pregnancy, Childbirth and the Female Body in Early Modern Germany', *Past and Present* 150 (1996), 84–110.

[55] Thomas Csordas, *Embodiment and Experience: The Existential Ground of Culture and Self* (Cambridge, 1994).

form which shapes that person's lived reality.[56] Experiences of body size remain diverse, therefore, in any period or culture. The diversity of experiences of body size in early modern Germany is clear from personal letters and diaries, known as 'self-narratives', which reveal how personal, material, and cultural perceptions of body size were intertwined in early modern people's descriptions of their bodies and bodily experiences.[57]

Weaving together the various factors which contributed to understandings of body size in early modern Germany, this book approaches body size from the perspective of the 'extended' early modern body. Stefan Hanß has worked with the concept of the 'extended body' to consider how the bodies of early modern women, as craftspeople and consumers, were extended through their interactions with material culture. He shows that artisanal training 'turned bodies into extended tools' as embodied practices of making and knowing remade the body and embodied behaviour.[58] Building on Hanß's use of this concept, I take a broader view which considers early modern bodies to be 'extended' through their engagement with a wide array of external forces, including material as well as social, cultural, and religious influences. Early modern bodies could be extended through the bodily care they shared and received within social networks, through embodied religious practices which drew on confessional beliefs, as well as through the body's engagement with its material environment. This understanding adds an embodied dimension to the arguments of cultural historians such as David Sabean and Thomas Robisheaux who have suggested that, in sixteenth-century Germany, personhood was essentially socially configured.[59] It also channels early modern theories of embodiment in which the flow of bodily fluids

[56] On the neglect of individual bodily experience and agency by discursive approaches to the body see Clever and Ruberg, 'Beyond Cultural History?', esp. 550.

[57] The extent to which we can access the embodied experiences of historical actors through such texts has been hotly debated. See Gudrun Piller, 'Private Body: What do Self-Narratives Bring to the History of the Body?', in Claudia Ulbrich, Kaspar von Greyerz, and Lorenz Heiligensetzer (eds), *Mapping the 'I': Research on Self-Narratives in Germany and Switzerland* (Leiden, 2015), 76–94, esp. 81–3. On the body in self-narratives see also Maren Lorenz, 'Tiefe Wunden: Gewalterfahrung in den Kriegen der Frühen Neuzeit', in Ulrich Bielefeld, Heinz Bude, and Bernd Greiner (eds), *Gesellschaft—Gewalt -Vertrauen: Jan Philipp Reemtsma zum 60. Geburtstag* (Hamburg, 2012), 332–54; Siglinde Clementi, *Körper, Selbst und Melancholie. Die Selbstzeugnisse des Landadeligen Osvaldo Ercole Trapp (1634–1710)* (Cologne, 2017). On early modern German self-narratives see Gabriele Jancke, *Autobiographie als soziale Praxis: Beziehungskonzepte in Selbstzeugnissen des 15. und 16. Jahrhunderts im deutschsprachigen Raum* (Cologne, 2002).

[58] Stefan Hanß, 'Gendering the Material Renaissance: Women Industriousness and the Female Body at the Court of Württemberg', *German History* 41 (2023), 367–99, here 380–2. On embodied practices of making and knowing see also Pamela Smith, *The Body of the Artisan: Art and Experience in the Scientific Revolution* (Chicago, 2004) and *From Lived Experience to the Written Word* (Chicago, 2022). On artisans' bodies see also Ulinka Rublack, 'Craft, Labour and Cabinets of Curiosities: Rethinking the Body of the Artisan', *German History* 41 (2023), 337–66.

[59] David Sabean, *Power in the Blood: Popular Culture and Village Discourse in Early Modern Germany* (Cambridge, 1984); Thomas Robisheaux, *The Last Witch of Langenburg: Murder in a German Village* (New York, 2009). Laura Kounine has qualified this view in *Imagining the Witch: Emotions, Gender, and Selfhood in Early Modern Germany* (Oxford, 2018).

ensured the body was not regarded as one whole but as 'something constantly changing, absorbing and excreting', as the boundaries between internal and external were porous, permeable, and unstable.[60] The early modern body was not understood to end at the skin, but rather the body's interior and exterior worlds were thought to be in constant material exchange.[61] Fatness itself was believed to result from an excess of blood in the body, and blood was one of the most important bodily fluids, the motion and consistency of which was constitutive of health and was subject to an array of external influences.[62] Early modern understandings of body size thus situated the body within its wider material environment, since fatness and thinness were conceived of in relational terms, as being determined by the body's fluid interaction with its surroundings. This focus on the extended early modern body enables a thorough contextualization and novel reconsideration of early modern conceptions of body size as situated material knowledge and experience.

German Bodies

The critical significance of body size for sixteenth-century Germans needs to be understood within the context of a growing discourse about German identity in this period. When seventeenth-century medical authors such as Friedrich Held, Franciscus Ignatius Hoassauer, and Karl Christian Leisner suggested that Germans had a predisposition towards fatness, they were following a longer tradition in which German people were thought to be naturally large of physique and prone to excessive consumption.[63] Len Scales has shown that a coherent image of Germanness had been gradually developing since as early as the thirteenth century which associated Germans with martial prowess, physical courage, and ruthless violence.[64] While French and Italian writers characterized Germans as 'bestial' due to their violent, wild, and uncultivated nature, German authors emphasized the physical virtues they possessed as a 'race of warriors'.[65] They 'spoke warmly of the immense stature and sturdy physique of [their] fellow-countrymen', and a contemporary origin myth even suggested that Germans were

[60] Rublack, 'Fluxes', 1–2.

[61] On the material interaction of the early modern body and its environment see Stefan Hanß, 'Eidechsenöl, Fledermaushirn, Bärenschmalz und Taubenkot: Haarpflege als Körper-, Medizin- und Materialwissen im 16. und 17. Jahrhundert', in Martin Mulsow (ed.), *Das Haar als Argument: Zur Wissensgeschichte von Bärten, Frisuren und Perücken* (Stuttgart, 2022), 55–80.

[62] On the significance of blood see Rublack, 'Fluxes', esp. 2.

[63] On these medical authors see Albala, 'Weight Loss', 177.

[64] Len Scales, 'German Militiae: War and German Identity in the Later Middle Ages', *Past and Present* 180 (2003), 41–82. See also Len Scales, *The Shaping of German Identity: Authority and Crisis, 1245–1414* (Cambridge, 2012).

[65] Scales, 'German Militiae', 71 and 47. The quotation referring to a 'race of warriors' is from Conrad von Megenberg, *Planctus Ecclesiae in Germaniam* in Richard Scholz (ed.), *Staatsschriften des späteren Mittelalters* (Stuttgart, 1977), vol. 2.1, 48.

descended from giants, emphasizing their natural robustness and vast size. At the same time, however, Germans were charged with 'troublesome barbarian failings—dull-wittedness, gluttony, drunkenness, *inurbanitas,* as well as a taste for blood' by their southern neighbours, which challenged German claims to serious military aptitude.[66]

The view of Germans as possessing barbarian impulses continued into the sixteenth century. Anti-German stereotyping was encountered by German humanists in classical literature and experienced directly by contemporary travellers. The Strasbourg humanist Jakob Wimpfeling (1450–1528) wrote with disdain about Italian fathers who would call little boys 'German pig' when they misbehaved.[67] With the rediscovery of Tacitus's *Germania* in the second half of the fifteenth century, German humanists began to consciously reconfigure this view of uncultured Germanness.[68] Drawing on the existing association between early Germans and plain warrior virtues, they interpreted Tacitus's text as evidence that Germans were a native race which was characterized by simplicity, resilience, strength, and violence. Once again, these traits were thought to have been materialized in the bodies of early Germans. Tacitus had written of the large stature of Germans, whose children '[fill] out amid nakedness and squalor into that girth of limb and frame which is to our people a marvel', thus '[reproducing] the vigour of their parents'.[69] Leading German humanist and poet laureate, Conrad Celtis, drew on Tacitus's text to argue that the German race had been created by a god called the Demogorgon, who had given them huge bodies, blonde hair, and pale eyes.[70] Celtis's writings and ideas had a huge impact on humanist culture, promoting a new proto-nationalist ideology that connected Germanness to male roughness, hardness, vigour, and physical heft from the beginning of the sixteenth century.

The modest, simple, yet robust and hardy bodies and appearances of original Germans were contrasted with the perceived softness and decadence of the *Welsch* (Romance-speaking foreigners).[71] Such perceptions of body size were part of a larger framework shaping German thought about the meaning of clothing and appearances in this period which sought to refute Italian claims of German

[66] Scales, 'German Militiae', 72.

[67] Ulinka Rublack, *Dressing Up: Cultural Identity in Renaissance Europe* (Oxford, 2010), 128.

[68] Ludwig Krapf, *Germanenmythus und Reichsideologie: Frühhumanistische Rezeptionsweisen der taciteischen 'Germania'* (Tübingen, 1979); Frank L. Borchardt, *German Antiquity in Renaissance Myth* (Baltimore, MD, 1971), 177–81 and 303–5. See also Rublack, *Dressing Up,* 127–32; Frederick G. Crofts, 'Visualizing Germanness through Costumes in the Sixteenth Century', *Historical Journal* 64 (2021), 1198–1229, esp. 1201, and Caspar Hirschi, *The Origins of Nationalism: An Alternative History from Ancient Rome to Early Modern Germany* (Cambridge, 2011), esp. 167–71.

[69] Publius Cornelius Tacitus, *Agricola. Germania. Dialogue on Oratory,* tr. M. Hutton and W. Peterson. Loeb Classical Library 35 (Cambridge and London, 1970, first published 1914), 293.

[70] Rublack, *Dressing Up,* 130. Celtis made this argument in his *Germania Generalis.* See Gernot Michael Müller, *Die 'Germania generalis' des Conrad Celtis: Studien mit Edition, Übersetzung und Kommentar* (Tübingen, 2001), 94–6.

[71] Herman Roodenburg has made a similar argument for the praise of 'Batavian plumpness' in contrast to the critique of luxurious 'courtoisie' in the Dutch Republic. See Hermann Roodenburg, *The Eloquence of the Body: Perspectives on Gesture in the Dutch Republic* (Zwolle, 2004), 44–6.

primitivism. A patriotic ideal of Germanness thus became connected with social ideals for bodily appearance and comportment.[72] Celtis warned students in Ingolstadt in 1492 that, under the influence of 'the south', Germans were becoming oppressed by an 'impulse of greed' and the 'acquirement of comfort and luxury'.[73] According to such humanist tropes, national rejuvenation required a return to past values. The anti-*welsch* sentiment which informed the celebration of strong and sturdy German bodies was exacerbated by the Lutheran Reformation and its rejection of the papacy. The successful presentation of Luther's stout body in his portraits from 1530 onwards thus owed much to the contemporary opposition constructed between southern pretension and German robustness.[74] The presentation of countless German men, notably among the elite and patrician classes, with similarly large and bulky bodies from the beginning of the sixteenth century must likewise be understood within this framework. Such bulk was not intended to appear soft or fleshy, rather their expansive bodies presented the robustness, solidity, and strength of German male authority.

In the second half of the sixteenth century, this relatively coherent presentation of German masculinity waned, as existing conceptions of Germanness came under pressure. The succession of Charles V to the imperial throne in 1519, who set his imperial sights well beyond the German lands, diminished the old motives for visualizing nationhood in terms of internal rejuvenation. Charles himself was said to be 'in very good shape', remaining moderate in his eating and drinking habits and thereby cultivating a strong and graceful body through which to fulfil his ambitious imperial agenda.[75] As the century progressed, confessional and dynastic motives for visualizing nationhood came to the fore, and a shift occurred in the loci of patriotism which turned from civic pride to territorial pride.[76] Patriotic visions of Germanness continued to be extolled which connected contemporary German values to early German morality and simplicity, yet the embodiment of such virtues in masculine bulk and solidity was never as prominent as in the first half of the century.[77] Nevertheless, body size had become established as a subject of cultural concern which maintained its significance throughout the period covered by this book. As German horizons expanded, fears of cultural instability grew, and this was imagined by some in terms of appearances and embodiment.[78]

[72] Rublack, *Dressing Up*, 131.

[73] Leonard Forster, *Selections from Conrad Celtis, 1459–1508*, edited with translation and commentary (Cambridge, 1948), 43–9.

[74] Roper, 'Martin Luther's Body', esp. 351–62.

[75] Geoffrey Parker, *Emperor: A New Life of Charles V* (New Haven, 2019), 66. On the relationship between the body of the ruler and the body politic see Ernst Kantorowicz, *The King's Two Bodies: A Study in Mediaeval Political Theology* (Princeton, 1957).

[76] On the shifting motivations of German patriotism in this period see Crofts, 'Visualizing Germanness', 1204–6.

[77] Alexander Schmidt, *Vaterlandsliebe und Religionskonflikt: Politische Diskurse im Alten Reich (1555–1648)* (Leiden, 2007), 174–89.

[78] Rublack, *Dressing Up*, 144–5.

In the first half of the seventeenth century, the satirist and statesman Johann Michael Moscherosch imagined an encounter between a court of old 'German Heroes' and a fictional German courtier. Laughing at the courtier's clothing and appearance, the Germans, who possessed 'great gravitas and strength (*grosse Gravität vnd Stärke*) of body', exclaimed 'Oh old manliness: Oh old German valour and integrity (*teutsche Dapfferkeit vnd Redlichkeit*), where have you gone? How can you be a German?'[79] They continued, 'What were you thinking you hulking (*vngeschlachte*) Germans, to weaken your strong German bodies with foreign medicine, foreign foods and spices, with foreign dress and foreign drink, and thus with foreign feminine softness (*Weichheit*)?'[80] Traditional Germanness was represented through bulky strength of body which had been weakened by cultural exchange. Moscherosch thus mourned for the imposing robustness which characterized the early German heroes and which had been embodied in the presentation of German masculinity from the early sixteenth century.[81]

This image of German strength, roughness, and solidity was distinctly male in character, just as the proto-nationalism with which it was associated was fundamentally patriarchal.[82] Although the original Germans in general, regardless of gender, were said to have possessed massive, powerful bodies, the expansive size which was cultivated by mature German men was not replicated among women. Yet contemporary discussions surrounding 'Germanness' still held implications for women's bodies. The ideal figure for German women remained relatively consistent across this period, centring on a compact slenderness of the upper body which was suggestive of controlled eating, drinking, and bodily comportment and was related to valorizations of self-discipline.[83] In German costume studies, the slim and modest figures of German women were contrasted with the voluptuous bodies and extravagant dress of Italians.[84] The robustness which was central to masculine German bulk, therefore, took a different form when it came to femininity, as the compact, neat, and firm bodies of German women continued to be opposed to the soft decadence of the *Welsch*.

As well as gender, differences in bodily ideals according to age qualify an image of German expanse. The youthful male body continued to be shown as tall, slim, and flexible with a narrow waist and shapely legs. Matthäus Schwarz, for example, appears to have lamented the expansion of his body as it began to depart from this graceful ideal, particularly since he remained unmarried at the time his nude portraits were produced. Typically, once men married and thereby gained

[79] Johann Michael Moscherosch, *Anderer Theil der Gesichte Philanders von Sittewalt* (Strasbourg, 1644), 63 and 101.

[80] Ibid. 105.

[81] On the comparison of ancient and early modern German bodies see Nancy Siraisi, *History, Medicine, and the Traditions of Renaissance Learning* (Michigan, 2007), 55–61.

[82] Rublack, *Dressing Up*, 130.

[83] Ibid. 126. [84] This point is expanded upon in Chapter 5.

authority as the head of a household, a shift which often occurred in tandem with the natural expansion of the body through age, they would be presented in portraiture as possessing a more imposing figure. Masculine German bulk was closely associated with notions of manliness and paternal authority, therefore, as marriage was understood to be a cornerstone of male maturity.[85] While the increasingly bulky presentation of mature German men was emblematic of a wider culture of body size which developed over the course of the sixteenth century, factors of age and gender contributed towards a more diverse range of bodily ideals and shaped the different embodied experiences of German women and men at various stages in their lives.

Sources and Methodology

To uncover widespread ideas and practices concerning body size within early modern German culture, and to explore the range of influences that informed these, the sources consulted in this book are deliberately wide-ranging. They include health regimens, herbals and recipe books, husbandry manuals, travel accounts, sermons and moralizing works, self-narratives such as letters and diaries, as well as images and material objects. Body size is not a topic with an obvious body of sources, yet it is mentioned in all manner of places, reinforcing the prominence of body size within this society. Uncovering such references is nevertheless a challenge and has depended upon the extensive digitization of early printed texts which has taken place over recent years, as well as the publication of manuscript sources in edited collections. Sources like the diaries of Hermann von Weinsberg or the letters of Magdalena and Balthasar Paumgartner will be familiar to scholars of early modern Germany, yet the analysis of such works through the lens of body size provides original insights into their contents. Moreover, the pursuit of references to body size in printed literature has brought to light forgotten texts which have rarely been analysed. These diverse sources are blended to reveal the complex mix of cultural, personal, and material influences for understandings and experiences of body size in this period.

Printed texts such as health manuals, moralizing works, husbandry guides, and travel accounts provide insights into cultural expectations and ideals for the body. They reveal, therefore, the cultural value that could be attached to body size. They also provide an indication of the language used to talk about body size, as well as insights into how the matter of fat or the flesh could be conceived of differently in medical or theological contexts. A limitation of these sources is the

[85] Scott Hendrix, 'Masculinity and Patriarchy in Reformation Germany', *Journal of the History of Ideas* 56 (1995), 177–93; Lyndal Roper, *The Holy Household: Women and Morals in Reformation Augsburg* (Oxford, 1989), 135–7. On Schwarz and marriage see Rublack, *Dressing Up*, 35.

difficulty of knowing how wide-reaching such understandings were, and for prescriptive literature, to what extent contemporaries actually followed such instructions. To counter this, lesser-known texts are deliberately mixed with more popular works which had a large readership, to ensure the exploration of influential and widely held views of body size alongside those with less obvious impact.

Self-narrative sources offer unparalleled insights into the personal experience of body size among early modern Germans. Texts in which authors described their own and others' bodies show how early modern people could conceive of their figures in relation to the cultural ideals of this period as well as narrate their own physical experiences. Such autobiographical texts reveal the great significance which early modern people attributed to body size, as they expressed care and concern about the size and form of their bodies and the bodies of their loved ones. I have taken care to include personal testimonies from both women and men, though they are inevitably individuals with the literary skills and leisure time to create such accounts.[86] Moreover, the personal nature of these texts means that the insights they provide are specific to the individuals who wrote them and, in some cases, such as the extraordinarily detailed diaries of Cologne townsman Hermann von Weinsberg, they are fairly exceptional. Exactly for this reason, self-narratives are remarkable entry points for uncovering and contextualizing early modern subjective experiences of body size as informed by the uniqueness of each body, thus providing nuance to broader cultural trends in attitudes towards fatness and thinness.

Images of dressed and naked bodies are key sources for considering how early modern people visualized body size. They also allow us the only possibility of 'seeing' the bodies of early modern people which no longer exist materially. Of course, images should not necessarily be taken as faithful replications of bodily appearances since all representations are mediated through the eyes and hands of their creators. They empower us, however, to consider how early modern people imagined bodies, and different bodily forms, as well as the associations they could hold. Visual sources provide insights, therefore, into bodily ideals for women and men, as cultural forces shaped the presentation of bodies. My approach to visual sources recognizes that the production and interpretation of images depends upon the contexts in which they are created and viewed.[87] Yet I also consider how personal embodied experiences would inform both the reception and production of images of the body.[88]

86 See Claudia Ulbrich, 'Schreibsucht? Zu den Leidenschaften eines gelehrten Bauern', in Alf Lüdtke and Reiner Prass (eds), *Gelehrtenleben: Wissenschaftspraxis in der Neuzeit* (Cologne, 2008), 101–12.

87 On this approach see Michael Baxandall's notion of the 'period eye' in Michael Baxandall, *The Limewood Sculptors of Renaissance Germany* (New Haven, 1980), 143–63.

88 On the significance of the artist's body for their material creations see Smith, *Body of the Artisan*; Smith, *From Lived Experience*; Hanß, 'Gendering the Material Renaissance'; Rublack, 'Rethinking the Body of the Artisan'.

Extant items of dress, which were worn by early modern bodies and show the forms such bodies could take, provide insights into material experiences of body size. As well as the measurements of the wearer, these garments reveal how clothing was used to mould early modern bodies through tailoring, padding, and boning, and can suggest the long-term material effects of such efforts on the physical body. Clothes literally extended the early modern body, creating idealized silhouettes and shaping everyday experiences of embodiment. They imposed particular ways of moving and dictated the wearer's posture.[89] They were also the primary means by which changes in body size would have been sensed and measured in this period. Extant garments thus play a key role in uncovering material perceptions of the body in relation to shifting fashionable ideals and revealing how early modern people could simultaneously experience and enact body size.

Structure

Attitudes towards body size are charted in relation to the main influences which shaped them during this period. Each of the first four chapters also highlights, therefore, a key contemporary development which contributed towards a growing culture of body size in sixteenth-century Germany. Chapter 2 explains how body size was understood from a health perspective, as fatness and thinness increasingly became subjects of medical enquiry. It explores early modern understandings of the relationship between body size and food consumption which it shows to be just one facet of a more holistic attitude towards size management. Drawing on the concept of extended early modern bodies, this chapter reveals how body size was implicated in wider understandings of the material interactions between bodies and their environments. This discussion then lays the foundations for the subsequent chapters which show how early modern bodies were 'extended' through complex matrices of social, cultural, aesthetic, religious, and personal influences, with profound consequences for understandings and experiences of body size.

Chapter 3 focuses on the growing significance of body size as a subject of artistic enquiry from the beginning of the sixteenth century. It centres on the figure of Albrecht Dürer, arguably the most influential German artist of this period, who produced the first theoretical text on bodily proportion in the German language. This chapter connects body size to embodied practices of making, as it reveals how Dürer's own embodied experiences shaped his creative and artistic exploration of bodies and their proportions. In so doing, the chapter highlights the interwoven nature of personal subjectivity and cultural construction with regard to body size and charts the impact of Dürer's study of proportion among a

89 Rublack, 'Renaissance Dress'.

subsequent generation of artists with lasting consequences for the representation of bodies in German art. Dürer's works were already widely collected in the sixteenth century, and as one of the first artists to capitalize on print as a new means to achieve broader circulation, his visual representations of bodies had wide-reaching impact.[90]

The religious significance of body size is the subject of Chapter 4, which reveals how bodily form was embedded within fundamental theological principles of the Lutheran Reformation. Reformation debates concerning the body elevated questions of body size and shape within German culture on a vast scale and across confessional divides, thereby contributing towards the developing culture of body size during this period. This chapter focuses on religious discussions regarding fatness and the belly, which took on metaphorical significance for Luther, and outlines a wider and more nuanced understanding of the emphasis which reformers placed on moderation, showing their teachings to permit the incorporation of various body types. Moreover, a distinction between 'natural' and 'unnatural' body size, which was similarly reflected in medical understandings of the body, is shown to have become increasingly important for the spiritual acceptability of fatness and thinness.

Chapter 5 examines body size in relation to clothing. It maps the development of dressed ideals for female and male bodies, relating these to proto-nationalist visions of Germanness which drew on gendered values of modesty, honour, and robustness. The material experience of body size is explored through extant garments, while tailor's practices are shown to have reinforced an awareness of body size in this period. Indeed, this was a crucial moment for the intimate relationship between body size and dress as the proliferation of tailored, figure-moulding clothing provided the primary means of perceiving changes in body size before it became common to weigh bodies in the following centuries. Dress is thus shown to be integral to conceptions of body size among early modern Germans, and the final section of the chapter considers the implications of this for German accounts of the bodies of enslaved and Indigenous people who were frequently described in terms of their nakedness.

The book's final chapter returns to personal experiences of body size by focusing on discussions of the body in self-narrative sources. It considers how individuals perceived of their bodies in relation to contemporary expectations and ideals for bodily form, showing body size to matter for these authors who used and performed their corporeality in various ways. While focusing on the personal, however, this chapter shows how embodied experiences of body size were nevertheless formed in connection with the broader networks of care and belonging

[90] On Dürer's significance see Ulinka Rublack, *Dürer's Lost Masterpiece: Art and Society at the Dawn of a Global World* (Oxford, 2023) and Edward H. Wouk and Jennifer Spinks (eds), *Albrecht Dürer's Material World*. exh. cat., Whitworth Art Gallery (Manchester, 2023).

within which a person was situated. Concern for body size forged and maintained relationships between spouses, family members, and friends, forming part of an emotional language of care in this period. Individuals made sense of their bodies in relation to the bodies of those around them, demonstrating the social dimension of the extended early modern body.

Body size in early modern Germany was a subject of social, personal, political, religious, artistic, and medical concern. Its growing significance across the sixteenth century shaped multiple dimensions of German culture in ways which have thus far been almost entirely overlooked. Studying body size, therefore, offers a new understanding of some of the most fundamental transformations of this period. This book provides a vital new chapter for the history of the body, and for historical corpulence in particular, offering a new framework through which to examine ideas about fatness and thinness in the past.

Body Size in Early Modern Germany. Holly Fletcher, Oxford University Press.
DOI: 10.1093/9780198972983.003.0001

2
Food, Health, and the Extended Body

In 1610 the Tyrolean physician and staunch Catholic Hippolytus Guarinonius (1571–1654) published the first volume of his 'Abomination of the Desolation of the Human Race' (*Die Grewel der Verwüstung menschlichen Geschlechts*), a wide-ranging work covering various phenomena which he understood to be destroying humanity. One such topic was the abomination of the 'fatness, thickness and bestial fattening (*Feyste, Dicke vnd bestialischen Außmästung*) of the body'.[1] While expansive size had become an ideal for German men in the sixteenth century, physicians nevertheless warned about the dangerous consequences of excessive fatness for the body. Guarinonius, whose views on fat were informed by his religious convictions as much as his medical training, called fatness a 'fleshly, onerous and harmful overloading' of the body. Writing at the end of the period considered by this book, his instructions for those who possessed such overloaded bodies focused on their food consumption. He stated that:

> The nourishment of the big-bodied (*groß leibigen*) can be divided into two points: First that they deprive themselves in the amount [of nourishment] at first by a quarter, then a third and then a half, and for that part suffer hunger. Then because they give their [internal] heat no other tinder, from which it might die away, they grasp at their excess and fatness (*Feyste*) and gradually consume it.[2]

This advice followed early modern medical understandings of the body as being like an oil lamp which needed to be maintained through a consistent supply of food which would in turn replenish the substance of the body which was consumed by this vital heat. According to this view, excessive consumption would oversupply the flame and ultimately extinguish it, preventing food from being properly concocted, the process by which food was broken down or 'cooked' in the stomach. Excess matter could then build up in the body, clogging the veins and causing swellings, ruptures, and illnesses.[3] Guarinonius suggested that, by

[1] Hippolytus Guarinonius, *Die Grewel der Verwüstung menschlichen Geschlechts* (Ingolstadt, 1610), 758.

[2] Ibid. 763.

[3] Ken Albala, *Eating Right in the Renaissance* (Berkeley, CA, 2002), 53–4.

gradually reducing the amount of food eaten by a fat person, their internal heat would be forced to instead 'consume' the sustenance that already existed in the body in the form of fatness and excess.

His second point concerned the substance of a person's diet, which he stated, should contain,

> namely those foods which have no power in them to make fat (*Feyste zu machen*), and instead [have the power] to emaciate and squeeze out (*abzuzehren vnd außzutrücken*), and because primarily it is meat which makes a fat paunch (*die feyste Wampen*), therefore above all other things eating meat should be wholly and completely, or for the most part, discontinued and instead fasting food should be used, especially salted fish, rice, millet, olives, and similar.[4]

To lose fat, Guarinonius thus recommended that people change their diet by first eating less food, the amount of which they should gradually reduce over time, and by eating foods which he considered to be less fattening, primarily those eaten during periods of fasting.

A relationship between what a person consumed and their body size was firmly established in the early modern period. In the Galenic-Hippocratic medical tradition, the category of food and drink was the foremost of the six non-naturals (the others being air, motion and rest, sleeping and waking, excretion, and the passions or emotions) understood to determine body size.[5] Medical advice on how to become fatter or thinner thus centred around changes in one's food habits, and health regimens and culinary texts from sixteenth- and early seventeenth-century Germany frequently referenced the effects of food and drink consumption on one's bodily form.[6] While Guarinonius's text focused just on the debilitating effects of fatness, other authors instructed on how to either increase or decrease the size of the body depending on their readers' personal requirements. These requirements would in turn be dictated by the 'natural' form of a person's body, as their humoral complexion, age, gender, and geographical location could encourage a tendency towards a particular body size.

The most prominent German medical author on the subject of fattening and slimming was the prolific popular science writer Walther Hermann Ryff

[4] Guarinonius, *Die Grewel der Verwüstung*, 763.

[5] On the importance of the non-naturals see Sandra Cavallo and Tessa Storey, *Healthy Living in Late Renaissance Italy* (Oxford, 2013) and Sandra Cavallo and Tessa Storey (eds), *Conserving Health in Early Modern Culture: Bodies and Environments in Italy and England* (Manchester, 2017).

[6] This challenges Ken Albala's view that early modern 'diet books' were not concerned with body size. Albala, *Eating Right*, 5. Albala has nevertheless shown that fatness was a concern among medical writers, though he suggests this was only the case from the seventeenth century onwards. See Ken Albala, 'Weight Loss in the Age of Reason', in Christopher E. Forth and Ana Carden-Coyne (eds), *Cultures of the Abdomen: Diet, Digestion and Fat in the Modern World* (Basingstoke, 2005), 169–83. On the relationship between digestion and body size in the eighteenth century see Kathryn Woods, 'Dismembering Appearances: The Cultural Meaning of the Body and its Parts in Eighteenth-Century Understanding' (PhD thesis, Warwick, 2014), n.p., ch. 'Digestion and Body Size'.

(*c.*1500-48).[7] Ryff's 'New Cookbook for the Sick' (*New Kochbuch für die Kranken*), first published in 1545, contained an extensive discussion of foods that should be eaten by those who were either too thin or too fat and is a key source for understanding medical attitudes towards body size in early modern Germany. Ryff's works were widely read. Between 1538 and 1548 he published more than forty books, which entered into almost 200 editions throughout the sixteenth and seventeenth centuries, chiefly concerned with medical subjects such as midwifery, pharmacopeia, anatomy, and surgery. During this period, he travelled around much of Germany and was active in Strasbourg, Metz, Frankfurt, Mainz, Nuremberg, and Würzburg, moves which were likely dictated by the publishing opportunities provided by these urban centres. Ryff addressed his works to the *gemeine* (common) man, and he repeatedly described his intended reader as the *Hausvater* or 'industrious householder'—his books were not the preserve of an educated elite but were widely owned.[8] During his lifetime, Ryff was recognized by his contemporaries as a blatant plagiarizer, since he took ideas from various sources which he rarely acknowledged.[9] It is likely, therefore, that the ideas he presented were also relatively widespread as he gathered his information from a variety of contemporary works, in turn giving these ideas a broader audience through his own popular and accessible style.

Guarinonius's text had less obvious impact. One of eight works published by the public health officer in Hall in Tyrol, the 'Abomination' was aimed specifically at German Catholics, as Guarinonius sought to establish a German Catholic medical tradition, drawing on the rhetorical and dramatic strategies of his Jesuit education.[10] There is limited evidence for its ownership or influence. By bringing together the writings of Ryff, Guarinonius, and their contemporaries, however, we gain a broad picture of medical attitudes towards fatness and thinness in sixteenth- and early seventeenth-century Germany.

[7] For Ryff's biographical information see Gundolf Keil, 'Ryff, Walther Hermann', *Neue Deutsche Biographie* 22 (2005), 310–11. See also Josef Benzing, *Walther H. Ryff und sein literarisches Werk: Eine Bibliographie* (Hamburg, 1959); William Eamon, *Science and the Secrets of Nature: Books of Secrets in Medieval and Early Modern Culture* (Princeton, 1996), 96–105; Katalin Rákóczi, 'Die Widerspiegelung der humanistisch-reformatorischen Tendenzen der Medizin im populärwissenschaftlichen Werk von Walter Hermann Ryff', *Orvostörténeti Közlemények* 28 (1982), 9–37; Katalin Rákóczi, 'Walter Hermann Ryffs charakteristische Stilmittel: Ein Vergleich mit H. Brunschwig, H. Gersdorf und O. Brunfels', *Orvostörténeti Közlemények* 30 (1984), 79–88.

[8] See Joachim Telle (ed.), *Pharmazie und der gemeine Mann: Hausarznei und Apotheke in der frühen Neuzeit* (Weinheim, 1988). The 1567 inventory of barber-surgeon Joachim Witthender included three books by Ryff. See Michael Hackenberg, 'Books in Artisan Homes in Sixteenth-Century Germany', *Journal of Library History* 21 (1986), 72–91.

[9] Alexander Marr, 'Walther Ryff, Plagiarism and Imitation in Sixteenth-Century Germany', *Print Quarterly* 31 (2014), 131–43; Eamon, *Science and the Secrets of Nature*, 98.

[10] For Guarinonius's biography see M. A. Katritzky, *Healing, Performance and Ceremony in the Writings of Three Early Modern Physicians: Hippolytus Guarinonius and the Brothers Felix and Thomas Platter* (Farnham, 2012), 29–44, and Jürgen Bücking, *Kultur und Gesellschaft in Tirol um 1600: Des Hippolytus Guarinonius' 'Grewel der Verwüstung Menschlichen Geschlechts' (1610) als kulturgeschichtliche Quelle des frühen 17. Jahrhunderts* (Lübeck and Hamburg, 1968), 1–10.

While food and drink were at the centre of such medical advice for slimming or fattening the body, numerous other factors were understood to contribute towards a person's size. These typically drew upon the other five non-natural things and included bathing, sleep, the emotions, and even the kinds of materials that came into contact with the body. Informed by the classical medical tradition, according to which 'diet' constituted a healthy lifestyle as opposed to just a food regimen, body size was conceived of as a holistic entity which was not purely the result of food consumption but was determined by the body's innate qualities as well as its interaction with a wide array of external forces.[11] Where food was concerned, early modern management of body size began well before diners encountered a dinner plate. The fatness of human bodies was understood to be closely related to the fatness of the foods, and specifically the animals, they consumed, as well as the fatness of the land where those animals were reared.[12] The interdependencies of food and body size were thus conceived of in complex material and multispecies terms, and animals played an active role in shaping contemporary ideas about fatness and thinness.[13] Within medical and dietary advice, therefore, body size is shown to be deeply implicated in early modern understandings of the body's extended nature.[14]

Food, Drink, and Body Size

Instructions on how to alter one's body size through the consumption of particular foodstuffs appear repeatedly in sources such as herbals, health regimens, and recipe books from early modern Germany. These had some late medieval precedents. The fifteenth-century surgeon Klaus von Matrei offered advice for 'one who will be thinner' in recipes which were later compiled by the Augsburg physician Jeremias Martius in 1572. Matrei advised the consumption of hare's-foot clover, for example, stating that those 'who wish to be thin (*mager*), should eat this herb like a salad, with salt and olive oil, twice or three times a week, before they go to sleep, and should do this for fifteen or sixteen weeks'.[15] Similarly in 1502

[11] On 'diet' see Cavallo and Storey, *Healthy Living*, 3.

[12] On the capacity of food to both alter and construct the body see Albala, *Eating Right*; Michael Walkden, '"You are What you Eat": Historical Changes in Ideas about Food and Identity', *Historical Research* 87 (2014), 377–92; Rebecca Earle, *The Body of the Conquistador* (Cambridge, 2014); Rachel Winchcombe, 'The Limits of Disgust: Eating the Inedible during Jamestown's "Starving Time"', *Global Food History* (2023), 1–23 (https://doi.org/10.1080/20549547.2023.2234252). On embodied effects of agricultural practices underpinning food practices see Sasha Handley, 'Lusty Sack Possets, Nuptial Affections and the Material Communities of Early Modern Weddings', *Environment and History* 28 (2022), 375–95.

[13] On the historical agency of animals see Erica Fudge, 'What was it Like to Be a Cow? History and Animal Studies', in Linda Kalof (ed.), *The Oxford Handbook of Animal Studies* (Oxford, 2014), 258–78.

[14] On the extended body see Introduction, 15.

[15] Klaus von Matrei and Jeremias Martius, *Artzneybuch Deß Hochberümbten und Weyterfahrnen Herrn Nicolai de Metri* (Augsburg, 1572), 158.

the physician and botanist Johannes Tallat von Vochenberg included a section 'for those who want to be thin' (*wer gern mager wer*) in his herbal remedy book, in which he recommended tartar mixed with mastic gum and diapenidion, a confection of barley water, sugar, and egg white. He stated that this remedy was used by the 'Saracens', a term used by Vochenberg to refer to Muslims, to counter fatness in the body.[16] Such early recipes focused on making the body thinner, likely reflecting the late medieval ideal of slender proportions. Tallat noted, however, that the seeds of the herb clary would 'make a person thin (*mager*) and dry out all moisture (*dörret all feüchtigkayt*)' from their body.[17] Since drying out the body entirely was very dangerous for a person's health, which depended upon maintaining a balance among the body's fluids, Tallat was not recommending the use of such seeds to reduce body size but rather warning against their consumption. Extreme thinness and dryness were always to be avoided.

Later in the sixteenth century, as advice on how to alter body size through food consumption proliferated, physicians increasingly noted specific foodstuffs that could make the body fatter. In his 'Little Book of Food' from 1583, for example, Bartholomäus Hubner, a physician in Erfurt, stated that butter 'nourishes well and makes fat (*machet feist*)'.[18] He continued by stating that 'a new, fresh, unsalted soft cheese gives good nourishment and makes fat (*macht fett*), is good for the stomach and for thin (*magern*) people'.[19] Hubner also stated that turnips which were boiled with 'good, fat meat' were 'good for a person's nourishment, make fat (*machen feist*), strengthen the manhood and the face wonderfully'.[20] With these comments Hubner presents a notably positive understanding of fatness which is associated with strengthened masculinity and good nourishment. His comments thus align with the presentation of masculine strength and power through physical heft in sixteenth-century Germany.

It was not only food that influenced body size. Georg Pictorius, a physician in Ensisheim noted that beer both fed and watered the body, and 'makes [one] fat (*machet feißt*)'.[21] Beer was a staple of early modern diets across northern Europe, and as Pictorius suggested, it was viewed as a foodstuff, which provided nourishment to the body, as much as a beverage.[22] Germans in particular were known for

[16] Johannes Tallat, *Artzney Büchlein der Kreutter, oder Margarita medicine* (Augsburg, 1502), fol. xxxiii^{v}.

[17] Ibid., fol. xx^{v}.

[18] Bartholomäus Hubner, *New Speisebüchlein: Darinnen kurtzer Unterricht von Essen und Trincken, auch von allerley Speisen und Getranck* (Erfurt, 1583), fol. G viii^{r}.

[19] Ibid., fol. G viii^{v}. [20] Ibid., fol. F iii^{r}.

[21] Georg Pictorius, *Leibs Artzney: Ein sehr Nutzliches Handtbüchlein vom grund und innhalt der gantzen Artzney* (Frankfurt am Main, 1566), fol. 58^{r}.

[22] On early modern beer and its nutritional importance see Susan Flavin et al., 'Understanding Early Modern Beer: An Interdisciplinary Case-Study', *Historical Journal* 66 (2023), 516–49; Craig Muldrew, *Food, Energy and the Creation of Industriousness: Work and Material Culture in Agrarian England, 1550–1780* (Cambridge, 2010), 65–83; David Gentilcore, *Food and Health in Early Modern Europe: Diet, Medicine and Society 1450–1800* (London, 2015), 157–80.

their indulgence in beer and alcohol more generally. In his condemnation of German drunkenness, the Lutheran pastor Matthäus Friderich claimed in 1552 that 'Germany in particular, above all other countries, has had the booze-devil (*Saufftеuffel*) again and again / who drives us Germans to booze day and night'.[23] In his famous book on the secrets of nature, first written in Latin in 1559 and translated into German in 1572, the Dutch physician Levinus Lemnius connected an indulgence in beer with body size as he suggested that Germanic people 'often become so fat (*fett*) from beer that their chins almost rest on their chests and they have good fleshy throats (*gute vnter kelen*)'.[24] Like Hubner, both Pictor and Lemnius presented the fatness of beer in a positive light, and since German masculinity was frequently expressed through communal drinking rituals, the bulkiness created through the consumption of alcohol likely contributed towards manly ideals for the body.[25]

As well as specifying particular food and drink for consumption, physicians offered more general recommendations for changing one's body size. Pictorius suggested that:

> those who are thin (*mager*) and use up their spirit quickly or do great [amounts of] work, they require food which will nourish them well, known as food of good quality, and those who are fat (*feist*), phlegmatic and idlers, they should have food which will satisfy the belly and not give much nourishment, called 'food of great quantity'.[26]

Simply put, the relationship between body size and food rested on the concept of nourishment. Those who wanted to increase the size of their body needed to consume food and drink which offered plenty of nourishment. Meanwhile those who were too fat should eat large quantities of food to satisfy their hunger, yet such food should be of a kind which would not be particularly nourishing.

The amount of nourishment one's food provided, and thus its effect on body size, was conceived of in such texts in terms of classical teachings concerning the four humours of the body (blood, phlegm, yellow bile, and black bile). Eichstätt

[23] Matthäus Friderich, *Wider den Saufftеuffel: Etliche wichtige Ursachen, warumb alle Menschen sich für dem Sauffen hüten sollen* (Leipzig, 1552), fol. A ii^{r}.

[24] Lemnius did not only refer to Germans as he stated this was particularly the case in Holland. Levinus Lemnius, *Von den wunderbarlichen Geheimnissen der Natur*, tr. Jakob Horst (Leipzig, 1572), fol. av^{r}. I have translated *gute vnter kelen* in terms of fleshiness due to the definition of 'Die Unterkêhle', in *Grammatisch-kritisches Wörterbuch der Hochdeutschen Mundart: Nach der Ausgabe letzter Hand, Leipzig 1793–1801* (Leipzig 1793–1801) (*Adelung*), digital edition www.woerterbuchnetz.de/Adelung/.

[25] On German drinking rituals and masculinity see Lyndal Roper, *Oedipus and the Devil: Witchcraft, Sexuality and Religion in Early Modern Europe* (London, 1994), 110–13. B. Ann Tlusty, *Bacchus and Civic Order: The Culture of Drink in Early Modern Germany* (Charlottesville, VA, and London, 2001), esp. 115–46. See also Beat Kümin, *Drinking Matters: Public Houses and Social Exchange in Early Modern Central Europe* (New York, 2007).

[26] Pictorius, *Leibs Artzney*, fol. 8^{r}.

physician Jakob Oetheus, for instance, wrote that those who wanted to relieve their body of excess should practise fasting, as by ceasing to eat and drink altogether (presumably for a fixed duration of time), and thus cutting off all nourishment to the body, 'fattened and fat (*mastigen vnd faisten*) people' would reduce 'the great phlegmatic mucous they have'.[27] Despite the bulky ideal for German men in the sixteenth century, German physicians generally agreed on the unhealthiness of excessive fatness, or obesity, which they understood to be caused by an excess of the interconnected humours of blood and phlegm, which derived primarily from food and drink.[28] Galen had written of obesity as being caused by a surplus of blood which was then transformed into fat, and sixteenth-century medical authors drew on this understanding in their own theories on the origins of fatness.[29] Thomas Erastus in Heidelberg, for instance, provided an early synthesis of the physiology of fat in the human body in 1580, as he explained that fat resulted from the airy parts of the blood, produced in the liver and derived from food and drink.[30] The physician and pharmacist Christoph Wirsung made a similar argument, stating that fat 'is a spreading out of nourishment in the skin which in such parts becomes tightly packed together and impervious'. He stated that fat (*Feistin*) 'has its origins in the fattest part of the blood, which flows through the most tender veins of the skin' and it would accumulate on the body 'when it met with a cold or bloodless place and like oil it would become hard'.[31] As fat was, by nature, 'of the utmost moistness', fat bodies were typically understood to possess a phlegmatic temperament, characterized as cold and wet. Conversely bodies that were hot and dry, possessing a choleric temperament, were often excessively thin.

Such understandings shaped advice concerning the foods which should be eaten to alter body size. Since fat itself was 'nothing other than cooked blood', as Wirsung suggested, some writers advised that those who were already too fat should avoid consuming food and drink which were rich in blood since this would only increase their humoral imbalance. Guarinonius, for instance, recounted the case of a man who had suffocated under the weight of his own fat at the age of 35, yet who could have lived to 90 if he had taken medical advice and allowed 'his veins to be opened because he was of a blood-rich nature, and drank vain blood-rich wine, and ate blood-rich foods'.[32] In his 'New Cookbook for the Sick', Ryff

[27] Jakob Oetheus, *Gründtlicher Bericht, Lehr unnd Instruction, von rechtem und nutzlichem brauch der Artzney* (Dillingen, 1574), fol. 147^{r-v}.

[28] On the relationship between fat, blood, and phlegm see Georges Vigarello, *The Metamorphoses of Fat: A History of Obesity*, tr. Christopher Jon Delogu (New York, 2013), 10–12.

[29] See Niki S. Papavramidou, Spiros T. Papavramidis, and Helen Christopoulou-Aletra, 'Galen on Obesity: Etiology, Effects and Treatment', *World Journal of Surgery* 28 (2004), 631–5. See also Michael Stolberg, '"Abhorreas pinguedinem": Fat and Obesity in Early Modern Medicine (c.1500–1750)', *Studies in History and Philosophy of Science* 43 (2012), 370–8, here 373.

[30] Stolberg, 'Fat and Obesity', 372.

[31] Christoph Wirsung, *Artzney Buch* (Heidelberg, 1568), 538.

[32] Guarinonius, *Die Grewel der Verwüstung*, 764.

advised specifically against the consumption of any foodstuff produced with blood, such as black pudding, by those who wanted to become thinner as he suggested, 'like human blood, it transforms easily and quickly into nourishment and sustenance', indicating that this excess nourishment would then increase the person's fatness.[33] The significance of nourishment for body size was thus embedded in humoral theory, as blood-rich foods were understood to be especially nourishing for the body.

Ryff's text, which entered into at least five editions between 1545 and 1608, contains the most extensive discussion of methods for altering the form of the body in sixteenth-century Germany.[34] His account of the relationship between food and body size reveals the complexities involved in dietary guidance on fatness and thinness, and given his lengthy exploration of this topic and his popular appeal, it is worth unpicking his instructions in detail. Ryff began with a discussion of how to fatten the body as he offered instructions on how to 'care and attend to a person who has become completely thin and emaciated (*gantz vnnd gar mager worden vnd abgefallen*) so that they may return to their body (*wider zum leib kommen*) and increase [in size] (*zunemmen*)'.[35] His suggestions in this case were based on humoral understandings of opposition. As thin bodies were thought to be dried out, he stated that 'all food and drink should tend towards moisture'.[36] He also structured his care recommendations around the seasons of the year. Ryff stated that in winter, autumn, and spring it was not necessary that a thin person should eat a lot of food, because the internal heat was reduced during these seasons, but what one did eat should provide very rich nourishment. It would be enough, Ryff claimed, for one to merely eat once a day in such periods. This was especially the case in winter when the internal heat would struggle to concoct much food at all and so one should not eat much at any meal. In the summer, however, it was necessary to eat much more often, even four times a day, in the manner, Ryff stated, of artisans.[37] He also suggested eating particular foodstuffs depending on the season, for instance, during summer goat's milk was the best drink for a thin person, yet during the winter they would benefit most from sheep's milk or cow's milk.[38] He did not give a reason for this distinction, yet as the Swiss naturalist Conrad Gessner stated that goat's milk, after human milk, provided the greatest nourishment and strength to the body, it likely stemmed from Ryff's understanding that a person required greater nourishment in the summer months.[39]

[33] Walther Hermann Ryff, *New Kochbuch für die Kranken* (Frankfurt am Main, 1545), fol. 143v.
[34] See editions of this work in 'Verzeichnis der im deutschen Sprachbereich erschienenen Drucke des 16. und 17. Jahrhunderts' (VD 16 and 17) which includes editions from 1545, 1555, 1564, 1580, and 1608.
[35] Ryff, *New Kochbuch*, fol. 138v. [36] Ibid. [37] Ibid., fol. 139r. [38] Ibid., fol. 140r.
[39] Conrad Gessner, *Thierbuch, das ist ein kurtze beschreybung aller vierfüssigen Thieren* (Zurich, 1563), fol. lixv.

Drawing on the significance of nourishment for body size, Ryff recommended that thin people should eat foods which were easily digestible and gave 'excessive nourishment'. This included the meat of young hens, capons, and cockerels, and soft eggs. He stated that 'all noble birds which live in mountains and forests are also of use and good for this condition', indicating how an animal's environment could determine the nourishment it provided. Ryff also drew on teachings by which the humoral and temperamental qualities of particular foodstuffs would influence the balance of humours within the body. He stated for instance that it was most appropriate for sauces to be made 'from wine rather than vinegar, for in this case vinegar is very harmful'.[40] Vinegar was repeatedly stated by medical authorities to cause thinness due to its dry nature. Citing the great Persian physician Rhazes as his source, Hubner for instance stated that vinegar would 'reduce the natural seed and make the body thin (*mager*)', connecting such thinness to infertility.[41] The botanist and physician Hieronymus Bock similarly wrote of vinegar as 'weakening the whole body and making [one] thin (*mager*)'.[42] The dryness of vinegar would exacerbate the existing dryness of the thin body, making it a dangerous foodstuff for those who were already emaciated. While following such humoral teachings, however, Ryff recommended that thin people should avoid overloading their bodies with 'slimy, phlegmatic, moist food'. He seemed concerned that efforts to fatten the body, by opposing the heat and dryness of the thin figure, might accidentally lead to an 'increase in phlegmatic or melancholic moisture from which their veins become blocked'.[43] Humoral balance rather than an excess of moisture was the goal.

To increase the fatness of the body, Ryff emphasized the importance of sweetness. Honey, for instance, was 'extremely useful and good'.[44] The best cheese for thin people was sweetened with sugar, and many foods could be improved for a thin person's constitution through 'sweet almond oil'.[45] Finally red wine, which was not watery but thin, subtle, with a good smell and sweet flavour, was the best drink for those who were emaciated.[46] Sweet foods were understood to provide the most wholesome nourishment to the body, since they were rich in moisture.[47] Yet the importance of sweetness for the treatment of thin people also went beyond humoral understandings. It was part of a wider perspective which associated comfort, pleasure, and happiness with fatness, and connected thinness with discomfort, displeasure, and unhappiness. In order to become fatter or thinner, one needed to pay attention to the comfort in which one lived, and this included the pleasure that one received from food. In this period, sweetness was associated

[40] Ryff, *New Kochbuch.*, fol. 139v. [41] Hubner, *New Speisebüchlein,* fol. Nviir.

[42] Hieronymus Bock, *Kreutterbuch* (Strasbourg, 1580), fol. 439v.

[43] Ryff, *New Kochbuch*, fol. 139r.

[44] Ibid., fol. 139v. [45] Ibid., fols 140r–v. [46] Ibid., fol. 140v.

[47] Hannah Newton, *Misery to Mirth: Recovery from Illness in Early Modern England* (Oxford, 2018), 108.

with comforting passions of joy and mirth, as well as sensual pleasure, and the love of God.[48] The process of becoming fatter was thus one of sweetness and comfort, while efforts to slim the body frequently involved opposing sensations and emotions.

Ryff understood 'immoderate fatness (*vnmessige Feyste*)' to be 'a great impediment and burden to the body in all things' and he instructed those who suffered from this burden to observe 'particular rules' regarding food and drink.[49] First, to become thinner he stated that 'one should maintain moderation, and arise from every meal with good want and hunger'.[50] To achieve this, Ryff suggested that at the beginning of a meal one should eat filling appetizers to subdue the longing for food. He recommended eating fat or greasy morsels such as small pieces of bread with lots of butter, or which had been dunked in olive oil, which should then be eaten as quickly as possible. This advice seems somewhat counter-intuitive, yet Ryff warned that this should only be practised by those who 'have no particular preference for fatty foods'.[51] He thus indicated an understanding by which those with fat bodies were not necessarily thought to be gluttonous or to possess a desire for fattening foods which they were unable to control. Such fatty appetizers, Ryff stated, would ensure that one began the meal with little appetite and so would not overindulge in the main dishes.

In terms of food preparation, Ryff stated that boiling was better than frying because fried meat would provide the body with greater nourishment. He also claimed that the nourishment of fried meat was more 'enduring' (*bestendiger*) than that of boiled meat, which was 'more fluid and more likely to melt'.[52] In order to become thinner, therefore, one required not merely less nourishment but also less durable nourishment, as this was easier to concoct and less likely to build up in the body. Ryff thus recommended that all meat should be 'boiled until it was tender and close to deterioration'.[53] Methods of preparing food could fundamentally alter the material qualities of food substances, and this in turn could affect their capacity to transform the bodies which consumed them. This understanding was linked to a contemporary interest in food preservation, methods of

[48] Rachel Winchcombe, 'Comfort Eating: Food, Drink and Emotional Health in Early Modern England', *English Historical Review* 138 (2023), 61–91, esp. 84 and 89–90; Hannah Newton, 'Inside the Sick Chamber in Early Modern England: The Experience of Illness through Six Objects', *English Historical Review* 136 (2021), 530–67, esp. 539; Elizabeth Swann, *Taste and Knowledge in Early Modern England* (Cambridge, 2020), 201. On sugar in the early modern world see Urmi Engineer, 'Sugar Revisited: Sweetness and the Environment in the Early Modern World', in Anne Gerritsen and Giorgio Riello (eds), *The Global Lives of Things: The Material Culture of Connections in the Early Modern World* (London, 2015), 198–220; Wendy Wall, 'Just a Spoonful of Sugar: Syrup and Domesticity in Early Modern England', *Modern Philology* 104 (2006), 149–72; Jason Moore, 'Sugar and the Expansion of the Early Modern World-Economy: Commodity Frontiers, Ecological Transformation, and Industrialization', *Review: A Journal of the Fernand Braudel Center* 23 (2000), 409–33.

[49] Ryff, *New Kochbuch*, fol. 142^{r}. [50] Ibid., fol. 142^{r-v}. [51] Ibid., fol. 142^{v}.

[52] Ibid., fol. 143^{r}. [53] Ibid., fol. 143^{v}.

which were at the forefront of material experimentation in this period and generated new knowledge about how materials behaved and transformed over time.[54] Ryff suggested that it was not only methods of cooking that would shape food's effect on the body, but earlier stages of preparation too. He wrote, for instance, that wheat and spelt bread should be avoided because of their rich nourishment, whereas bread made from barley, for which the bran was less refined, would be more suitable for those seeking to become thinner.[55]

While tender meat was preferable, in general meat should only rarely be consumed. To reduce their nourishment, Ryff instructed those with fat bodies to favour fish, a view which Guarinonius echoed with his recommendation of fasting foods. Different varieties of fish were more fattening than others. Ryff stated that one should avoid 'fat fish' (*feiste Fisch*) such as salmon, eel, tench, and especially crab; the fatness of the body would thus be influenced by the fatness of the creatures it consumed.[56] The temperature and seasoning of a dish was also important. Suitably thin fish should be eaten cold, and salted fish was better than unsalted fish. Ryff also suggested that fish should be accompanied by good sauces, seasoning, vinegar and onion.[57] This reflected his initial statement that, as a general rule, fatness should be treated with foods which had a 'subtle or dry power, which are sour and bitter', since these produced the least nourishment.[58] Similarly those wanting to become thinner should not drink freshly made red wine, which was sweet and thus particularly nourishing, but should content themselves with 'common, white, sour wine'.[59] Such instructions for slimming the body through diet thus directly inverted those for fattening the figure, including Ryff's references to specific ingredients such as vinegar, as well as the general consumption of sour and bitter, as opposed to sweet, food and drink.

The advice of Ryff and his contemporaries reveals a close connection between food and body size, as fatness and thinness could be countered or encouraged by consuming specific types of food or drink, or changing the amount which one ate. Yet the size of a person's body was not just the result of their food practices, as medical experts believed individuals could possess a natural tendency towards fatness or thinness regardless of their dietary regimen. Various factors contributed towards the 'natural' form of the body, including age, gender, and geography, each of which held consequences for those seeking to alter their body size through food consumption.

[54] Lucy J. Havard, '"Preserve or Perish": Food Preservation Practices in the Early Modern Kitchen', *Royal Society Journal of the History of Science* 74 (2020), 5–33.

[55] Ryff, *New Kochbuch*, fol. 143^{r}.

[56] This point is expanded on later in this chapter, see pp. 50–5.

[57] Ryff, *New Kochbuch*, fols 143^{v}–144^{r}.

[58] Ibid., fol. 143^{r}.

[59] Ibid., fol. 144^{v}.

'Natural' Body Size

The Swiss physician Theophrastus von Hohenheim, known as Paracelsus, wrote around 1530 that 'every creature is twofold: the one comes from the *sperma*, [and] the other from the nourishment'.[60] Nourishment was what provided the body with its form as 'fat and other such tissues increase with nourishment'.[61] Yet the *sperma*, or seed, constituted the nature of a person, and this could have bodily consequences which were not the result of nourishment but were innate. As an example, Paracelsus wrote of *Specifica pinguedo*, a fatness in which 'someone gets fat (*feist*) and the fault does not lie in the food' and *Specifica Macredo*, in which 'one is thin (*mager*) and no amount of eating helps'.[62] Paracelsus thus suggested that while food was typically the main factor in dictating whether one was fat or thin, this was not always the case. Indeed, it 'often' happened that food held little influence over these extremes of body size. Paracelsus also used 'semen', connected to the *sperma* which he understood to construct the natural body size of a person, to conceptualize material creation more generally. He believed semen to be present in all materials, which when animated would result in material transformation and the creation of new matter. His interest in the sources of fatness and thinness, therefore, was embedded within his broader, and hugely influential, conceptualization of material transformation and the body.[63]

Following his discussion of innate body size, Paracelsus wrote that 'physicians have recorded nothing about this in their *scientia specifica*, instead cozying up to the ignorant *astronomi*, [who say]: "it is *melancholia*, etc. [or] *Saturnus*," [which means:] in the nature of the ascendant', yet one is 'made by the hand of God, not by ascendants, planets, constellations, or anything else of the kind—as if these were to force anyone to be thin or fat (*dür oder feist*)'.[64] Paracelsus insisted that a person's body size was created by God and was not dictated by the planets, as some medical authors suggested. Such astronomical explanations for body size may indeed be discerned in several texts from early modern Germany. In his updated 'Field Book of Surgery' from 1528, for instance, Hans von Gersdorff wrote that those born under Saturn who had a phlegmatic complexion were 'fat

[60] Theophrastus von Hohenheim (Paracelsus), 'Opus Paramirum', in Andrew Weeks (ed. and tr.), *Paracelsus (Theophrastus Bombastus von Hohenheim 1493–1541): Essential Theoretical Writings* (Leiden, 2008), 297–501, here 388, translation 389. Quotations from this text use Weeks's translation unless otherwise stated.

[61] Ibid. 386, translation 387.

[62] Ibid. 492, translation 493. I have adapted Weeks's translation since he interprets the phrase *einer mager ist* as 'people waste away'.

[63] See Hiro Hirai, *Le concept de semence dans les théories de la matière à la Renaissance: De Marsile Ficin à Pierre Gassendi* (Turnhout, 2005), 179–216; Amy Eisen Cislo, 'Paracelsus's Conception of Seeds: Rethinking Paracelsus's Ideas of Body and Matter', *Ambix* 55 (2008), 274–82; and Katharina Dück, *Materia prima: Zur Semantik des Begriffs in naturkundlichen Sachschriften des 16. Jahrhunderts* (Wiesbaden, 2019). On Paracelsus and fat see Christopher Forth, *Fat: A Cultural History of the Stuff of Life* (London, 2019), 132–3.

[64] Paracelsus, 'Opus Paramirum', 492, translation 493.

and sluggish', while those of a phlegmatic complexion who were born under Jupiter would be 'not too fat' and instead were of 'moderate' size.[65] Similarly the lawyer and astrologer Martin Pegius repeatedly mentioned the importance of the planets for determining body size and shape in his 'Book of the Hour of Birth' from 1570. He stated for instance that if, at a person's hour of birth, Venus overlapped and was well-placed against the sun, they would be born with a 'middling and beautiful length of body' and 'would be fat'.[66]

Paracelsus and his followers dismissed the view that astronomy could influence body size, and rejected several of the fundamental tenets of traditional Galenic medicine more generally; notably Paracelsus worked with a concept of similitude rather than the logic of opposition, meaning illnesses would be treated with substances resembling the nature of the illness itself.[67] Paracelsus would likely have rejected Ryff's recommendations to treat moist, fatty bodies with dry substances like vinegar and pepper, therefore. The increasing popularity of Paracelsus across the German-speaking lands complicated early modern understandings of body size, and such ambiguities fostered lively debate on the causes and treatment of fatness and thinness. Despite their differences, however, the notion of a natural form of the body which did not result from food consumption was shared by both Paracelsian and humoral medical understanding and was most frequently expressed in relation to fatness.

Following Hippocrates, for instance, Christoph Wirsung wrote that those who were naturally fat had narrow veins and therefore a more limited flow of blood in comparison to those who were naturally thin. As they grew old, the natural heat of those who were born fat would weaken and die out much sooner than those who were born thin and who thus had a greater supply of blood. Wirsung continued by stating that,

> those who are middling (*mittelmässiger*) from nature, but become fat (*feyst*) from delicious foods and many sweet and fat dishes, constantly eating meat and frequently drinking, and in sum living in lust and pleasure, and thereby applying themselves, they retain their larger veins despite increasing the flesh and fatness (*fleisch vnd Feystin*) they have; therefore there is less danger that they will extinguish their natural heat.[68]

[65] Hans von Gersdorff, *Feldbuch der Wundartzney newlich getruckt vnd gebessert* (Strasbourg, 1528), n.p.

[66] Martin Pegius, *Geburtsstundenbuch darinen eines jetlichen Menschens Natur und Eigenschafft sampt allerley Zufählen auß den gewissen Leuffen deren Gestirn nach rechter warhafftiger und grundtlicher Ahrt der Gestirnkunst mit geringer Müh außgereitet und derselb vor zufelligem Unfahl gewarnet* (Basel, 1570), fol. Ji ii^r.

[67] Paracelsus's insistence on similitude nevertheless drew on sympathetic medicine which was Galenic in origin. See Frederick W. Gibbs, *Poison, Medicine and Disease in Later Medieval and Early Modern Europe* (Abingdon, 2019), 201.

[68] Wirsung, *Artzney Buch*, 538.

According to Wirsung, an unnaturally fat person would ultimately be healthier than a naturally fat person as they would retain some of the advantages of their middling body despite increasing their size through excessive consumption. Nevertheless, Wirsung suggested that the unnaturally fat deserved greater moral condemnation than those who were fat by nature, since they had caused their own fatness by 'living in lust and pleasure'.

Guarinonius was even more scathing in his condemnation of those who made their naturally slim bodies fat. He wrote,

> When one doubles the size and heaviness (*Grösse vnd Schwere*) of the unchaste flesh, with such skill what can one be other than a double brute and purely conceited unnecessary excrement and earthly burden? This adds to the difference [between such fat] and that fatness and thickness of the body which is innate (*angebornen Feyste vnd Leibs Dicke*), which however, despite being innate, can also be increased through gluttony.[69]

For Guarinonius therefore, an increase in 'unnatural' fatness appears as the greatest sin in relation to the fat body, as through gluttony one increases the 'unchaste flesh', causing oneself to be more thoroughly grounded in base desires. This position drew strongly on Guarinonius's religious convictions and his rejection of the flesh as sinful and unchaste was not universal, as fatness took on different meaning with the Lutheran Reformation.[70] Nevertheless, Guarinonius's position provides a particularly interesting example of how this distinction between natural and unnatural body size could be conceptualized in terms of morality and sinfulness. He even suggested reintroducing the ancient Spartan custom by which 'all grown young people' would be measured every ten days and 'if in any part of their body (not to mention in the whole body) they had become a bit thicker or fatter (*dicker oder feyster*)...then one would chase and beat the fat ones (*die Feyste*) and then arrest them'.[71] Guarinonius was extreme in his hatred of fat but strikingly he stated that such young people should be fully grown before this practice started, and thus what was measured would be any deviation from their natural, adult form.[72] The condemnation of fat among authors such as Guarinonius and Wirsung in the late sixteenth and early seventeenth centuries may have resulted from the increase in fatness, particularly among German men, from the beginning of the previous century as indicated by contemporary portraiture. Despite such warnings about the burdens of fat, however, the ideal of masculine bulk continued throughout this period, indicating that cultural practice often diverged from medical prescription.

69 Guarinonius, *Die Grewel der Verwüstung*, 758.

70 See Chapter 4.

71 Guarinonius, *Die Grewel der Verwüstung*, 760.

72 The Ragusan statesman Nicolo Vito di Gozzi also sought to revive this custom. See Forth, *Fat*, 157.

Bodies were understood, therefore, to possess a natural form which was innate, yet which could change with the influence of external factors. The advice of authors such as Ryff could thus be aimed at both those who were trying to change their natural form and those whose bodies had increased or decreased in size unnaturally and who wished to return to their original proportions. Most authors agreed that alterations to the natural body were the most difficult to achieve. Paracelsus stated, for instance, that 'what is inborn cannot be eradicated', while Guarinonius wrote that 'for those who bring this curse [of fatness] with them from their mother's bodies, it is not easy to change'.[73] Moreover, since the natural body was understood to be given to one by God, efforts to alter this natural form could be morally questionable.[74]

Of course, the very concept of an unnatural form of the body suggested that the natural body could be altered, and this was typically through practices of food and drink. Yet, the relationship between eating and body size was far from simple; factors of age, gender, and geography were understood to inform a person's humoral complexion and thus dictate what foodstuffs a person should eat to maintain or change their body. Age was a particularly important factor for determining body size and ordering health. Guarinonius for instance, wrote that the 'nourishment of grown young people [between 17 and 34], should tend towards the cool and moist, since they are increasing in their heat and dryness', and by avoiding hot and dry foods they would therefore avoid humoral imbalance.[75] Due to their natural heat and dryness, young people would therefore take great pleasure in bathing and swimming, drinking cool wine and eating fresh salads and fruits. With their hot and dry natures, young people were generally understood to be thinner than middle-aged people, for whom the natural heat had begun to decline (typically around the age of 30), meaning that they could no longer digest the same amount of food, and excess would begin to accumulate in their bodies if they did not take pains to reduce their food intake. Though this was a general rule, Guarinonius acknowledged that some people may reach adulthood with a body that is already fat. This fatness was not so unhealthy during youth, he suggested, since the strength of their internal heat would counteract fat's negative effects. Yet as the internal heat declined with age the wetness and coldness of their fat bodies could cause worrying illnesses such as dropsy. Similarly, if a person entered adulthood with a thin body, they needed to take care that the declining heat of the body did not cause it to become too cold in nature and lead to illnesses of the spleen. With old age, the body was understood to dry out while the internal heat continued to decline, thereby reducing the body's capacity to digest and

[73] Paracelsus, 'Opus Paramirum', 486, translation 487; Guarinonius, *Die Grewel der Verwüstung*, 761.

[74] See e.g. Hans Jacob Wecker's dedication in Girolamo Ruscelli, *Weiber Zierung*, tr. Hans Jacob Wecker (Basel, 1575), fol. ii^{v}.

[75] Guarinonius, *Die Grewel der Verwüstung*, 543.

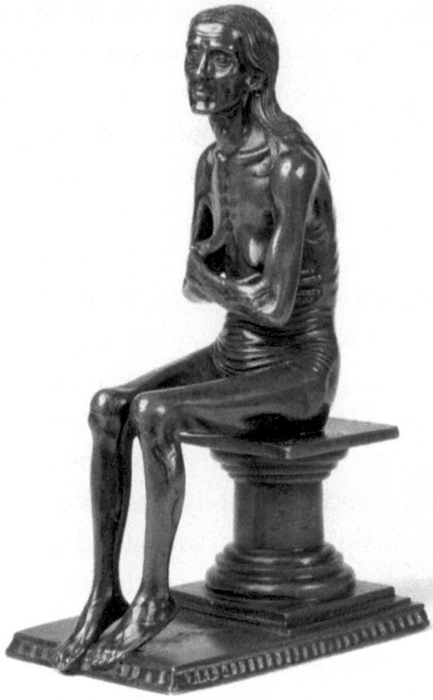

Figure 2.1 Artist unknown, Old Woman Seated, c.1520s. Bronze, 15.7 × 9.3 cm. Fitzwilliam Museum, University of Cambridge. © Fitzwilliam Museum/Bridgeman Images. The presentation of this elderly woman as emaciated drew on humoral understandings of old age in which the body became colder and drier, and thereby thinner. For old women in particular such dryness was associated with the end of menstruation.

encouraging the consumption of less and less food.[76] The body would thus become thinner, as it grew both colder and drier, and for women such dryness was also associated with the end of menstruation (Figure 2.1).[77]

In general, women were understood to be colder and moister than men, meaning their bodies were also thought to be naturally fatter.[78] As part of his explanation for how fat formed on the body, by which he stated that fat within the blood would solidify when reaching a cold area of the body, Wirsung stated that those with cold bodies 'such as women and certain animals who hide themselves in the winter are often immoderately fat (*vber die maß feyst*), whereas the hot-bodied

[76] Albala, *Eating Right,* 53 and 154–6. See also Kaspar von Greyerz, *Passagen und Stationen: Lebensstufen zwischen Mittelalter und Moderne* (Göttingen, 2010), 200.

[77] Holly Fletcher, 'Age, Gender and the Body in the Bronze and Pearwood Statuettes of 1520s' Germany', *Gender and History* 32 (2020), 341–72.

[78] On the temperamental differences between women and men see Katherine Crawford, *European Sexualities, 1400–1800* (Cambridge, 2007), 102–5.

remain thin and slender (*Magern vnd rhan*).'[79] This recognized tendency towards fatness among women, particularly as they entered adulthood, may have contributed to a practice to which Guarinonius vehemently objected. He wrote that 'several misguided and tyrannical parents, especially mothers, have a custom that they starve their daughters while they are growing children, and particularly make them struggle for thirst, so that they retain their thin and slender bodies (*dünn vnd ran*) and do not become too large and powerful (*groß vnd kräfftig*).'[80] The ideal for German women's bodies was consistently defined by slenderness from the late fifteenth to the early seventeenth centuries, despite vast changes in the cultural ideal for male bodies. While Guarinonius's moralizing condemnation is characteristically hyperbolic, his statement suggests how intersecting ideas about gender and age in relation to food could, at the very least, be imagined to result in acts of deprivation that aimed to physically mould the female silhouette to match this cultural ideal. Though thinness was frequently connected with modesty and self-control, Guarinonius warned that such young women were only suitable for 'love affairs' (*Bulschafft*) because they would be too weak and feeble to make good housewives or to bear children.

Slimming practices among young women were particularly worrying for medical authors since extreme thinness was recognized as a central cause of infertility and miscarriage. Both fatness and thinness could result in difficulties regarding conception, and in general, it was believed to be easier for thin women to conceive than those who were fat.[81] However, extreme thinness was thought to result in a lack of nourishment being provided to an unborn child, ultimately resulting in miscarriage. The most famous German authority on childbirth and midwifery, Eucharius Rösslin, wrote that for women

> who are pregnant and emaciated (*verzert*), the food that they consume is needed for their own sustenance and the replacement or extension (*ersetzung oder erstreckung*) of their own bodies, and for that reason, not very much food is left over for the nourishment of the child and therefore the child becomes weak in its mother's body and will not want to stay and will, from necessity, leave the body.[82]

[79] Wirsung, *Artzney Buch*, 538.

[80] Guarinonius, *Die Grewel der Verwüstung*, 547.

[81] On the relationship between body size and fertility see Sarah Toulalan, '"If slendernesse be the Cause of Unfruitfulnesse; you Must Nourish and Fatten the Body": Thin Bodies and Infertility in Early Modern England', in Gayle Davis and Tracey Loughran (eds), *A Handbook of Infertility in History: Approaches, Contexts and Perspectives* (London, 2017), 171–97, and Toulalan, '"To[o] Much Eating Stifles the Child": Fat Bodies and Reproduction in Early Modern England', *Historical Research* 87 (2014), 65–93. In the German translation of Albert the Great's 'Secrets of Women' from 1581, it was explicitly stated that 'all fat women are maladapted for conception to a greater extent than thin women'. Albertus Magnus, *Dauraus man alle heimligkeit dess Weiblichen geschlechts erkennen kan* (Frankfurt am Main, 1581), fol. Aii^r.

[82] Eucharius Rösslin, *Der schwangeren Frawen vnd Hebammen Rosengarten* (Augsburg, 1528), fol. Gi^r.

Interestingly, when Wirsung made a similar argument in his discussion of thinness, he stated that it was women who were thin 'in the extreme and by unnatural means (*zu gar vnd gleich vnnatürlicher weis mager*)' who were particularly likely to miscarry.[83] He implied, therefore, that those with naturally thin bodies, which did not result from deprivation, would not necessarily face the same difficulties.

As well as age and gender, geography could influence the form of the 'natural' body. Early modern 'geohumoral' understandings of the body suggested that climate created temperamental differences among humans. In general, those living in northern climates were understood to be cold and moist, while southerners were hot and dry.[84] Since cold and moist bodies were also understood to be fatter than hot and dry bodies, northern Europeans were typically thought to be fatter than their southern counterparts. Such views were particularly prominent later in the seventeenth century as Germans gained a reputation for being particularly fat and large in connection with the cold and northerly climate of the German lands.[85] This reputation likely stemmed from the physical expansion of German men in the previous century.

Writing at the beginning of the seventeenth century, Guarinonius also recognized such national, geographical differences. He wrote, for example, that 'we Germans like to drink wine because we are, from nature, much colder than the Italians or Spanish.'[86] Germans were drawn to the warm nature of wine because of their own cold bodies, just as Italians, like young, thin people, who had hot and dry temperaments, liked to eat salad and fruits which were cold and moist. Moreover, Guarinonius stated, 'a German will eat more than two *Welschen* [romance-speaking people]' accounting for both age and season. While he suggested that such German coldness was 'from nature', however, he complicated this view by commenting that, a *welsch* person in Germany 'would eat not only the same amount as the Germans but would overstep them by a lot.'[87] With this statement Guarinonius indicated that the greater consumption of Germans was due to situational or climatic factors, rather than a natural difference, yet in commenting that southern Europeans would eat more than Germans if they lived in a German climate, he nevertheless suggested that there were some innate differences between *welsch* and German bodies and appetites. The distinction between the natural and unnatural body could be blurry, and throughout early modern medical texts the supposedly natural temperament and complexion of the body were rarely shown to be insurmountable.[88] The significance of geography for body size, therefore, was as much about the material surroundings of the body as national temperaments.

[83] Wirsung, *Artzney Buch*, 446.
[84] Mary Floyd-Wilson, *English Ethnicity and Race in Early Modern Drama* (New York, 2003), 3.
[85] Stolberg, 'Fat and Obesity', 373–4. See also Albala, 'Weight Loss', 177.
[86] Guarinonius, *Die Grewel der Verwüstung*, 546. [87] Ibid. 548.
[88] See Sara Miglietti, 'Mastering the Climate: Theories of Environmental Influence in the Long Seventeenth Century' (PhD thesis, Warwick, 2016), 18 and 107. See also Earle, *Body of the Conquistador*.

External Influences

Though food took precedence in medical advice on how to alter body size, it was also believed that changes to the body's external environment could influence its form. This understanding drew on the contemporary conception of the body as existing in a constant state of material exchange with its surroundings, and thus external influences had the capacity to dictate both physical and emotional health.[89] Included within Ryff's advice for those who were too thin or fat, therefore, was a discussion of 'all external things' (*eusserlichen dingen*) which could determine body size.[90] The interaction of the body with its exterior world was commonly understood in terms of the non-naturals of Galenic-Hippocratic tradition—the six spheres of life which required careful regulation for the preservation of health. Following this teaching, Ryff structured his discussion of 'external things' around the other five non-naturals besides food and drink: air, movement, sleep, evacuations, and emotions. These categories also subsumed concerns such as bathing and sex, which were sometimes considered as exercise, but more often as evacuations.[91]

Ryff considered the management of external influences to be especially important for those seeking to become fatter. In this case, he stated that dry and windy air should be avoided, and particularly cold air. To prevent dryness, a person's chamber could be sprinkled with fresh water from a fountain mixed with a little wine and vinegar. One should also make sure that the chamber had a pleasant smell, which could be achieved with

> noble, good-smelling things, herbs, and spices such as amber, aloe vera or paradise wood, the good-smelling storax [similar to vanilla], and from these substances make small balls by grinding them to a fine powder and mixing them with gum dragon [tragacanth] and then placing these balls on glowing coals so that they smoke the chamber.[92]

This emphasis on scent was connected to the importance of healthy air, as aromatic substances were used to balance the humoral composition of ambient air in this period.[93] Indeed, Ryff's focus on air quality in relation to body size reflects a broader shift in concerns about air circulation in sixteenth-century health regimes, as extremes of air temperature and humidity began to be viewed as more serious

[89] Ulinka Rublack, 'Fluxes: The Early Modern Body and the Emotions', *History Workshop Journal* 53 (2002), 1–16.

[90] Ryff, *New Kochbuch*, fol. 140^{v}.

[91] Sandra Cavallo, 'Introduction—Conserving Health: The Non-Naturals in Early Modern Culture and Society', in Cavallo and Storey, *Conserving Health*, 1–20, here 3.

[92] Ryff, *New Kochbuch*, fol. 141^{r}.

[93] Sandra Cavallo, 'Health, Air and Material Culture in the Early Modern Italian Domestic Environment', *Social History of Medicine* 29 (2016), 695–716, here 711.

health concerns than disease-infected air.[94] Ryff's recommendations align with the increasing attention paid towards the humoral characteristics of air, which he understood to hold consequences for body size. His suggestions for preventing dry air once again follow humoral teachings of opposition, as thin and emaciated bodies were already dry and thus required moisture to become fatter.

In terms of exercise, Ryff recommended moderate movement, but warned against over-exertion. To become fat, one should ensure they never became tired. If they found pleasure from exercise however, Ryff recommended they should practise 'gentle walking', particularly 'while food is in movement (*speiß im gang ist*), so that the juices (*gesäfften*) should be drawn on [to the body]. That is commonly six or seven hours after one has taken in the food'.[95] Exercise during the period of digestion was thus said to encourage the accumulation of body mass. In place of exercise one could also rub various parts of the body, such as the thighs, the shoulders and arms, and lastly the chest, since these 'body parts will then be strengthened and empowered (*gestercket vnnd bekrefftigt*) and the nourishment will be applied to the same parts more forcefully'. A warm towel should be used to rub these regions until they received 'a warm feeling and the body parts begin to be visibly red'. Head massage could also help to fatten the body. Ryff stated that the scalp 'should be combed softly with an ivory comb, from which the brain will receive great help, as the steam and damp from which the natural heat is suppressed, will steam away'.[96] Here, Ryff connects thinness to the suppression of the natural heat which meant that less food could be digested and therefore less nourishment would be applied to the body. Ryff seems to suggest that a comb made specifically of ivory would provide the correct pressure or sensation to prevent the dampening of the natural heat. Gessner wrote that ivory could strengthen the heart and encourage conception and fertility, and such associations likely encouraged Ryff's recommendation of this material to strengthen and replenish the thin body.[97]

Concluding his discussion of exercise, Ryff stated that, for thin bodies, 'rest is altogether more useful and suitable, and the above exercise of the body should occur for no other reason than to encourage delight'.[98] Ryff thus connected the two non-naturals of movement and the emotions, emphasizing the importance of positive feelings for those wanting to become fatter. He specifically stated that it is 'useful and good in this case, that one ensures the patient remains happy'.[99] Such advice chimed with his guidelines on consuming sweet foods, which were associated with pleasure and enjoyment. Indeed, all of the non-naturals were understood to be interconnected and reciprocal, reinforcing the holistic quality of early modern health advice.[100]

[94] On the growing importance of air see Cavallo and Storey, *Healthy Living*, esp. 70–112, and Cavallo, 'Health, Air and Material Culture'.

[95] Ryff, *New Kochbuch*, fol. 141r.

[96] Ibid., fol. 141v.

[97] Gessner, *Thierbuch*, fol. lxxviiiv.

[98] Ryff, *New Kochbuch*, fol. 141v.

[99] Ibid., fol. 142r.

[100] Cavallo, 'Conserving Health', 10.

Healthy sleep too was frequently connected to happiness in the early modern period, and Ryff prescribed plenty of sleep for those wanting to become fatter.[101] He stated that 'a lot of sleep is much better than a lot of waking, because sleep moistens (*befeuchtigt*) the body, whereas waking presses the body and dries one out (*erdrücknet vnd verdörret*).'[102] It was commonly observed that sleeping a lot could make the body fatter, as it was during sleep that digested food would be distributed throughout the body.[103] To increase one's fatness, therefore, Ryff stated that a person should sleep for eight or nine hours at least and if they were unable to sleep for that time 'one should at least lie in bed and rest, and this should be in a soft and tender bed, and this not-sleeping will count as a half sleep.'[104] In connection to sleep, therefore, Ryff emphasized the importance of material comfort for increasing body size.

Ryff's final point concerning the external care of thin bodies was particularly emphatic. He stated that 'unchastity' was highly forbidden and extremely harmful, and so 'one should completely avoid it, as one would a harmful and deadly enemy.'[105] While pleasure could encourage fatness this did not include sexual pleasure. This advice likely centred on ideas about temperature and moisture and the importance of balancing the humoral composition of the body. Since sexual activity was understood to both dry out and heat the body, Ryff suggested it could have dangerous consequences for the thin body which was already hot and dry.[106]

Once again, Ryff's advice for those with fat bodies inverted his suggestions for thin bodies. Beginning with air quality he wrote,

> choose warm air, or quite cool [air], because temperate air is unsuitable in this case, this will then stifle the attracting power (*ansichziehendt krafft*), so that the nourishment is pulled on [to the body] to a lesser extent, which is a central cause of thinness (*magerkeit*). Indeed, it is better in this case that one should often change the air, beginning with hot and then changing to cold.[107]

101 Sasha Handley, 'Sleep-Piety and Healthy Sleep in Early Modern English Households', in Cavallo and Storey, *Conserving Health*, 185–209, here 189.

102 Ryff, *New Kochbuch*, fol. 141v.

103 Albala, *Eating Right*, 136, and Sasha Handley, *Sleep in Early Modern England* (New Haven, 2016), 22–9.

104 Ryff, *New Kochbuch*, fol. 141v–142r.

105 Ibid., fol. 142r.

106 On the humoral consequences of sex see Jon Arrizabalaga, 'Medical Responses to the "French Disease" in Europe at the Turn of the Sixteenth Century', in Kevin Siena (ed.), *Sins of the Flesh: Responding to Sexual Disease in Early Modern Europe* (Toronto, 2005), 33–55, here 46. Stefan Hanß has shown that the body's increased heat from sexual activity could be thought to result in hair loss. Stefan Hanß, 'Eidechsenöl, Fledermaushirn, Bärenschmalz und Taubenkot. Haarpflege als Körper-, Medizin- und Materialwissen im 16. und 17. Jahrhundert', in Martin Mulsow (ed.), *Das Haar als Argument: Zur Wissensgeschichte von Bärten, Frisuren und Perücken* (Stuttgart, 2022), 65.

107 Ryff, *New Kochbuch*, fol. 145r.

Frequently changing the ambient air between extremes of hot and cold would was said to alter body size by preventing nourishment from being retained in the body. This view likely also connected to notions of comfort as temperate air, which was neither too hot nor too cold, was typically understood to be the most comfortable and healthy.[108]

To become thinner, Ryff noted that exercise was particularly important; 'the body should be worked hard, especially when one is hungry'.[109] Rest should be taken just before eating, however, and so it was most suitable for one to sleep immediately before a meal. Connecting bathing to exercise, Ryff noted that 'sweat-baths' or steam baths would work the body and were particularly useful for this 'affliction'. The expulsion of sweat in a steam bath was thought to dry out the body, thus correcting the fat body's excess of moisture. This may account for why contemporary artists like the brothers Sebald and Barthel Beham repeatedly used particularly fleshy figures in bathhouse scenes, since these bodies were understood to benefit the most from such bathing practices (Figure 2.2).[110] As well as releasing sweat, Ryff advised letting blood twice a year, following the view that fatness could be caused by an excess of this humour.

A key point for Ryff was that those who were too fat should not sleep too much because, he wrote, 'everyone knows how greatly the natural power is strengthened' through sleep.[111] To reduce the amount of sleep a person had, and thereby decrease their size, Ryff advised doing increased exercise in the evening and diverting oneself with pastimes or other business. It was also necessary to stay awake for at least four hours after a meal so that food could settle in the stomach prior to rest. Ryff added that to prevent sleep the underside of the thighs should be 'well rubbed' so that moisture was drawn down them, since such moisture was 'a particular cause of longer sleep'. Finally, 'one should sleep in a hard bed' to ensure they were less comfortable and their sleep would be hindered.[112]

To counter fatness, Ryff again emphasized the importance of the mind and emotions. He stated that movement of the mind was 'good and useful', therefore one should 'load oneself with worries and great business and be somewhat angry', though he warned, 'everything in moderation'. Just as happiness could cause fatness, Ryff indicated that anger and worry would encourage thinness, reflecting the contemporary understanding that emotions had bodily consequences.[113] How one thought and felt impacted on body size, and becoming thinner was shown to involve those emotions, thoughts, and sensations which were relatively unenjoyable. Reducing the size of the body was not just a case of managing external influences on the body, therefore, but also making life more uncomfortable and unpleasant.

[108] See Hannah Newton, '"She Sleeps Well and Eats an Egg": Convalescent Care in Early Modern England', in Cavallo and Storey, *Conserving Health*, 104–32, here 120.

[109] Ryff, *New Kochbuch*, fol. 145r.

[110] See Chapter 3, 80–2 and Chapter 5, 195.

[111] Ryff, *New Kochbuch*, fol. 145r.

[112] Ibid., fol. 145v.

[113] Rublack, 'Fluxes'.

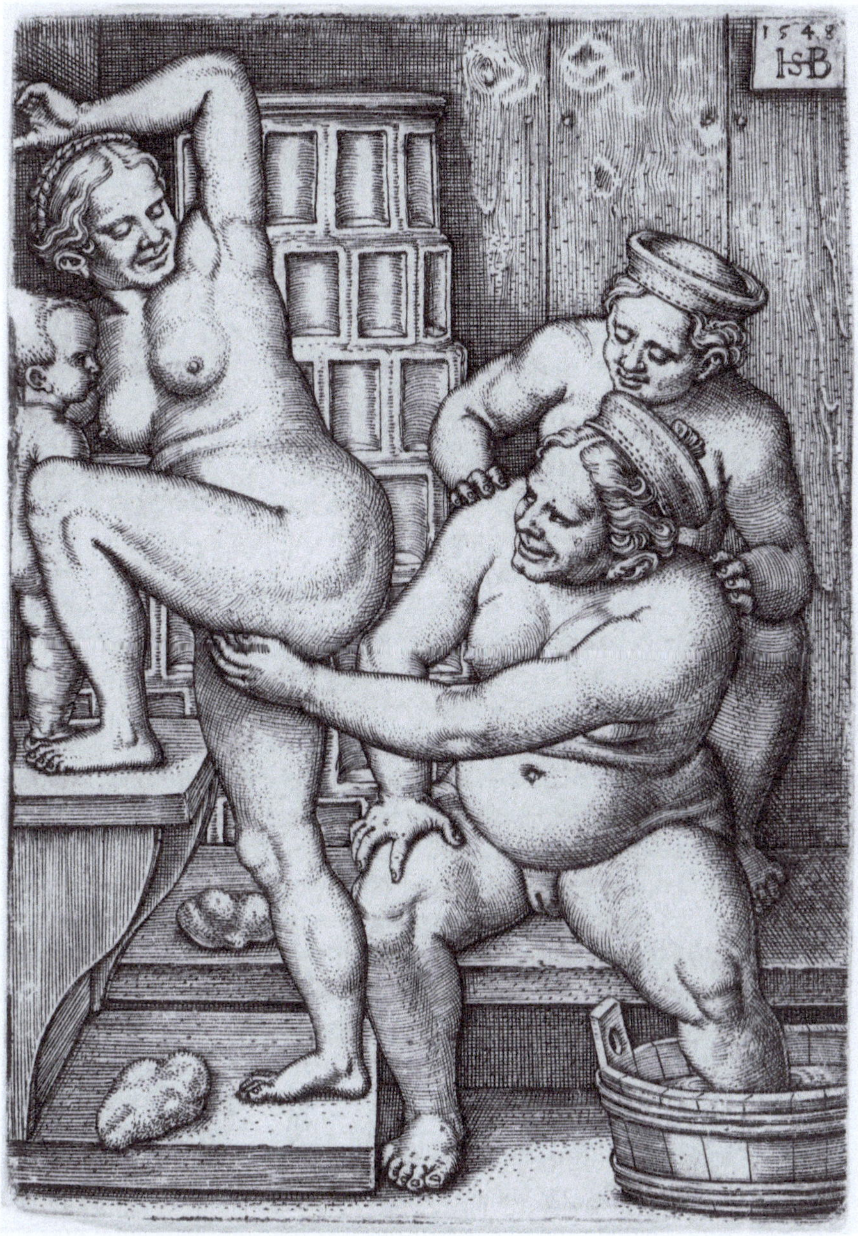

Figure 2.2 Sebald Beham, Three Women Bathing, 1548. Engraving 8.3 × 5.7 cm. National Gallery of Art, Washington, DC, public domain. Sebald Beham and his brother Barthel repeatedly depicted bathhouse scenes containing women with notably fleshy bodies. This may have related to a medical association between bathing and the reduction of body size. The fatness of the women in Beham's print is central to its eroticism, evoking the carnal and sensual elements of their interaction.

This understanding of slimming appeared in a satirical 'recipe', reportedly from 1626, intended for those who were 'so fat and wide (*feist vnd dick*) that they can't walk'. It stated:

> First, take at breakfast one pound of worry boiled in unboiled love; for lunch eat two pounds of melancholy; for a snack take on a lot of debt with no money to pay it back; then for the evening meal take a sack full of badly funded trials, then lay in a bed which is overflowing with lice, fleas, bedbugs, and similar creatures, then you will certainly become thin (*mager*).[114]

This 'advice' satirized the guidance of authors such as Ryff and exaggerated their suggestions for slimming the body. Appearing in the first quarter of the seventeenth century, it appears to mock the proliferation of printed advice for the management of body size from the previous century, taking aim at the cycle of cause and effect such printed regimens initiated by strengthening concerns about fatness and thinness and thus increasing the demand for such instructions. Playing with the form of a dietary regimen, the text conflates advice regarding food consumption with that concerning the discomfort, anxiety, and sleep loss involved in becoming thinner. In so doing it not only suggests the unpleasantness connected to slimming, but also the ridiculousness of those who followed such guidance, since becoming thin was only difficult for those with comfortable, worry-free lives.

Though Ryff's text contained the most extensive discussion of interconnected material, sensory, and emotional practices for the alteration of body size, the importance of 'external' care in relation to fattening and slimming was reiterated throughout printed health regimens. Bathing practices in particular were frequently connected to the management of bodily form. Concerns included the timing of baths in relation to mealtimes and evacuations. The German physician Johannes Wittich, for instance, wrote that 'fat (*fetten*) people who want to be thin (*mager*)' should make sure that they passed a stool, thus ensuring that the body was not weighed down with excess moisture, prior to entering the bath. They should also not eat or drink before or in the bath, and they should take warmer baths than thin people.[115] As well as its temperature, the content of the bath was significant. Pictorius stated that milk baths were very beneficial for those who were thin, and possessed hot complexions, as the cooling qualities of milk would help to cool their bodies. Drawing on Avicenna, he stated that one should use milk from which butter could be drawn but was not sour, indicating how the nature of the milk itself would dictate its effects upon the body.[116] In relation to

[114] S. Maurer, *Inventorium Universale* (1626), quoted in Anton Birlinger (ed.), *Alemannia: Zeitschrift für Sprache, Litteratur und Volkskunde des Elsaszes, Oberrheins und Schwabens* 16 (1888), 58. I have been unable to find the original text.

[115] Johannes Wittich, *Praeservator Sanitatis* (Leipzig, 1590), 182.

[116] Georg Pictorius, *Baderbüchlein* (Mülhausen, 1560), fol. 5^{v}.

the benefits of steam baths for the fat body, Wittich specified that a broth in which herbs had been steeped should be poured on hot stones and coals to encourage the body to sweat out its excess moisture. Such herbs could also have the same effect when cooked and laid upon the body. He wrote that helpful herbs for this purpose would be calamint, oregano, hay flower, camomile, pennyroyal, wild thyme, and lavender.[117] The aromatic nature of these herbs suggests how the senses were deeply involved in methods for reducing body size.

Even when a bath merely contained water, the properties of that water could determine its effect on body size. The botanist and physician Jacobus Theodorus's 'New Water Treasure' from 1581 discussed the different kinds of water in which one could bathe or drink, and their usefulness for altering the form of the body. These included sour water, or acidulous spring water, salt water, sea water, nitre (potassium nitrate) water, and alum water. Theodorus stated that all of these waters will 'make fat people thin', yet they acted in different ways depending on their qualities.[118] Salt water, for instance, was helpful for reducing swelling, and Theodorus suggested it could also be used to treat growths on the thighs, feet, and penis.[119] Nitre water would dry out the body, removing the excessive moisture of fatness.[120] Yet, Theodorus stated, alum water, would promote fever in a thin or otherwise hot-bodied person and was therefore dangerous for them to bathe in, suggesting that it was this increase in natural heat that helped slim down fatter bodies.[121] The minerals contained in different kinds of bath water thus altered the body in slightly different ways, and Theodorus connected the effects of such bath water to specific locations. Listing the healing properties of spa waters in various towns and villages throughout the Holy Roman Empire, he indicated a connection between the water's effect on the body and the local environment from which it originated.[122] Similarly, in his book on bathing from 1602, Johann Bauhin particularly recommended the thermal water from Balaruc in Languedoc for 'fat and corpulent (*feisten vnd leibigen*)' people, who should 'drink, bathe in and wash themselves with [the water]', 'smear themselves with its waste' and even 'distil the water and use what remains instead of salt in their food and drink'.[123] It seems likely that the natural heat of such thermal waters made them especially useful for combatting cold and moist fat bodies.

[117] Wittich, *Praeservator Sanitatis*, 182–3.

[118] Jacobus Theodorus, *New Wasserschatz* (Frankfurt, 1581), 483, 495, 503, 517, 546.

[119] Ibid. 495. [120] Ibid. 502. [121] Ibid. 547.

[122] On bathing in early modern Germany see Birgit Studt, 'Die Badenfahrt: Ein neues Muster der Badepraxis und Badegeselligkeit im deutschen Spätmittelalter', in Michael Matheus (ed.), *Badeorte und Bäderreisen in Antike, Mittelalter und Neuzeit* (Stuttgart, 2001), 33–52; Frank Fürbeth, 'Zur Bedeutung des Bäderwesens im Mittelalter und der frühen Neuzeit', in Heinz Dopsch and Peter F. Kramml (eds), *Paracelsus und Salzburg* (Salzburg, 1994), 463–88; Matthias Bitz, *Badewesen in Südwestdeutschland 1550 bis 1840: Zum Wandel von Gesellschaft und Architektur* (Idstein, 1989); Ute Lotz-Heumann, *The German Spa in the Long Eighteenth Century: A Cultural History* (Abingdon, 2022), 25–57; Hannah Murphy, 'Der Körper im Bad: Baden und Gesundheit im frühneuzeitlichen Deutschland', in *Stay Healthy*, exh. cat., Draiflessen Collection, Mettingen (Mettingen, 2021), 19–34.

[123] Johann Bauhin, *Ein New Badbuch* (Stuttgart, 1602), 8.

The view that external, material conditions could influence body size is most fascinatingly demonstrated by Pictorius, who suggested that to ensure health and manage body size even 'the nature of clothing should be considered'. He stated that materials like linen, silk, and cotton would cool the body, while fur acted on the body following the nature of the animal from which it came. According to Pictorius, 'fox and marten fur are warm and dry and suit those who have weak and moist nerves, such as those with gout in the feet and limbs, or those who are fat and want to be thin (*feißten die da begerend mager züwerden*)'. Moreover, 'sheep's wool is warm and moist, therefore it builds up those who are melancholy or are thin (*mageren leuthen*), as it disperses moisture throughout the body'.[124] The properties of the materials that came into contact with the body were recognized to influence the nature of the body itself, altering its complexion and ultimately determining body size. In this case, Pictorius built on existing, though rare, medical advice concerning the bodily effects of different fabrics. A medical manuscript from late fifteenth-century Germany indicates that fabrics like linen and silk would, by their nature, cool the body, while wool would confer heat to the body's limbs.[125] Reflecting the increased awareness of fatness and thinness in his time, Pictorius applied such understandings to the manipulation of body size. That Pictorius connected the properties of such fabrics to the complexions of the animals from which they originated shows how body size could be conceptualized within a broader system of understanding in which human bodies were known to be entangled with those of non-human agents and their material environments. Like humans, the complexions of animals depended not merely on their natural tendencies but also on their living conditions and the food they ate, and as animal complexions were known to affect the bodies of the humans who consumed them and used their products, the relationships between humans, animals, and environments formed a complex network of interactions within which ideas about fatness and thinness were interwoven.[126]

Body Size, Animals, and Environments

Early modern people's lives were deeply enmeshed with those of the animals with whom they lived and worked, whom they trained and bred, and whose products they consumed and used for a multitude of purposes including craft, medicine, and construction. People relied on animals just as animals frequently relied on them for their food, shelter, and bodily maintenance. This close interaction with

[124] Pictorius, *Leibs Artzney*, fol. 6^{v}.

[125] *Deutsches salernitanisches Arzneibuch*, John Rylands Library, University of Manchester. Late fifteenth century. German. MS 24. fol. 27 r. I am grateful to Stefan Hanß for bringing this manuscript to my attention.

[126] On such interactions see Hanß, 'Haarpflege'.

animals fundamentally shaped ideas about body size, particularly with regards to practices of fattening the body.[127] The very concept of what fat was, as a material substance, would have been informed by the widespread use of animal fats in everyday life. Animal fats were frequently used in medical recipes; Hieronymus Bock, for instance, claimed that pig fat smeared over wounds would heal them wonderfully, while Gessner stated that dog's fat was good for gout and would remove blotches from the face.[128] They were also used for cooking, with *Schmalz* (lard) being a commonplace ingredient. Artisans would likewise rely on animal fats in their making processes; cow's fat, Bock stated, was especially good for clockmakers.[129] In early modern Germany, human fat was used much like any other form of animal fat. It was prescribed by, and could be bought from, executioners for use in medical recipes, particularly to treat fractured bones, sprains, and arthritis.[130] A common proverb stated, 'melted human fat (*Menschenfett*) is good for lame limbs, if one rubs them with it, they become right again.'[131] Such human fat, procured from executed criminals, was understood to have potent healing powers which differentiated it from the fat of other animals. Yet its commonplace use as an unguent meant that the materiality of human fat was conceptualized in very similar ways to that of animals. Everyday interactions with animal lard and grease would have shaped how early modern people thought about the matter of fat which was present in their own bodies.

It is not surprising therefore that ideas about how to alter the size and shape of the body were closely connected to ideas about fattening animals. Understanding the means by which an animal's body size could be altered, and particularly fattened, was a concern for all those who owned or interacted with livestock in this period. Husbandry manuals and agricultural literature frequently discussed various methods for fattening animals as part of their care and maintenance. Johannes Coler's 'Oeconomia', an early, genre-shaping example of 'housefather literature' (*Hausväterliteratur*) included instructions for fattening cows and oxen, pigs, sheep, geese, and doves.[132] As for human bodies, this advice included specifying particular foods, and the amount of such foodstuffs, that should be eaten to fatten animal bodies. Coler stated that oxen, for example, should be fattened with chaff, hay, and groats. He also specified that they could be fattened with turnips which

[127] On the importance of material fats for shaping responses to fat bodies see Forth, *Fat*, esp. 17–56. See also Christopher Forth, 'The Qualities of Fat: Bodies, History and Materiality', *Journal of Material Culture* 18 (2013), 135–54, and 'On Fat and Fattening: Agency, Materiality and Animality in the History of Corpulence', *Body Politics: Zeitschrift für Körpergeschichte* 3 (2015), 51–74.

[128] Bock, *Kreutterbuch*, fol. 435r and Gessner, *Thierbuch*, fol. lxxxviiiv.

[129] Bock, *Kreutterbuch*, fol. 435r.

[130] Kathy Stuart, *Defiled Trades and Social Outcasts: Honor and Ritual Pollution in Early Modern Germany* (Cambridge, 2009), 157.

[131] 'Fett', in Hans Bächtold-Stäubli (ed.), *Handwörterbuch des deutschen Aberglaubens*, vol. 2 (Berlin, 1929/1930), 1383–5. Quoted in Stuart, *Defiled Trades*, 157.

[132] On Coler see Philip Hahn, *Das Haus im Buch: Konzeption, Publikationsgeschichte und Leserschaft der 'Oeconomia' Johann Colers* (Epfendorf, 2013).

had been 'finely chopped', suggesting that the preparation of food was significant. Such fattening was structured around the time of day, as Coler suggested that oxen be fed mashed cabbage leaves in the morning, and in the afternoon receive good, ripe acorns which were yellow and sweet, again indicating the significance of sweetness for fatness.[133] Seasonal shifts were also of great importance, as cattle would be brought in from the fields in the winter to avoid the cold weather and would then need to regain their strength on their return and be prepared for fattening. Thus, Coler wrote, every morning after they returned to the field they should receive fodder of oat-straw or hay 'so that they can revive and strengthen themselves'.[134]

The fattening of animals typically focused on food consumption yet, as with human bodies, other non-natural influences, sensory experiences, and material environments were also understood to impact on an animal's body size. Gessner noted that bears would become so fat during long periods of sleep in the winter that they would hardly be able to move, and he attributed their fatness to this extended sleep since they consumed nothing until their re-emergence in spring.[135] He also wrote of the practice of playing pipe music to sheep in 'Arabia' by which, he stated, they became fatter than from food alone.[136] Further appealing to the senses, Gessner suggested that the eyes of geese should be poked out in order to fatten them, since this would reduce their visual stimulation.[137] Similarly, he remarked upon a practice of fattening doves, in which their owners would break their legs so that they could not move, indicating the perceived importance of an animal's movement (or lack of movement) in relation to fatness. On this point, however, the German translator of Gessner's text intervened, commenting beneath: 'this breaking of the legs does not make [the bird] fat (*feißt*) but thin (*mager*), because they suffer in pain for a long time'.[138] The translator suggested that, for animals too, pain or discomfort was believed to cause thinness. Comfort was also shown to be important for fattening geese as Gessner wrote that 'the place where one wants to fatten them must be clean and pure, as they like to be in a clean place'.[139] Coler likewise noted that geese 'like community' and therefore it was easier to fatten two or three geese together than one on its own.[140]

Gessner's 'Book of Birds' demonstrates that animals, like humans, were understood to possess a 'natural' body size. Writing of falcons for instance, he stated that one should 'pay attention to its condition, whether it is thin or fat (*mager oder feißt*), and whichever state you find it in, you should maintain it, for some are better for field sports when they are fat, and others when they are thin, while

[133] Johannes Coler, *Oeconomia oder Haußbuch* (Wittenberg, 1599), vol. 4, fol. T^{v}.
[134] Ibid., fol. Z 4^{v}. [135] Gessner, *Thierbuch*, fol. xvi^{r}. [136] Ibid., fol. cxxxix^{r}.
[137] Gessner, *Vogelbuch Darin[n] die art, natur und eigenschafft aller vöglen, sampt jrer waren Contrafactur, angezeigt wirt* (Zurich, 1557), fol. lviii^{r}.
[138] Ibid., fol. ccxlii^{v}. [139] Ibid., fol. lviii^{r}. [140] Coler, *Oeconomia*, fol. Ddd^{v}.

others and the best ones, when they are middling'.[141] Similarly, Coler gave advice on how to tell if a horse was naturally fat or had been fattened temporarily for a higher sale price at market. His instruction included gripping the horse at the neck where one would find two layers of skin—if the under-layer was thin, the horse did not have a natural tendency towards fatness.[142] As for humans, the fatness or thinness of an animal would be determined by their individual nature, as well as factors of age and sex. Coler stated, for instance, that it was easier to fatten geese when they were young as opposed to when they were old.[143] He also claimed that an uncastrated male pig would not become fat, no matter how much one fed it, and thus it was not worth the effort to try.[144] Gessner meanwhile stated that 'particularly the male' bear would become fat during its winter sleep, while young pigs had moister bodies than those which were old.[145]

This comparison of animal fatness with ideas about human body size is not intended to suggest that animal and human bodies were understood in exactly the same way. Yet there are clear similarities between processes of altering the bodies of both animals and humans, including the awareness of 'natural' and 'unnatural' body size, the significance of the senses, variation depending on factors of age and sex, as well as material environments. The connection between fattening animals and fattening people is also suggested by the contemporary use of the verb *mästen*, which in modern usage typically denotes the fattening of animals but was also used during this period to refer to human bodies. The verb could be used in a derogatory way (suggesting that fat people were bestial), such as when Guarinonius explicitly complained about the abomination of 'bestial fattening (*Außmästung*) of the body'.[146] Yet it was also used by individuals to describe their own bodies, such as the Nuremberg merchant Balthasar Paumgartner who, having become thinner on a trip to the baths at Lucca, promised his wife that he would take time to 'fatten' (*mesten*) himself again.[147] Like animals, human bodies could be deliberately fattened through processes of feeding and the management of non-natural influences. Later in the seventeenth century this connection was expressed explicitly by Gottfried Christian Winckler: 'we see that hens and geese are better fattened (*gemästet*) when they are shut in, than when they can run around. We also see it often that people who sit locked away and are well fed, become immoderately fat (*über die massen fett werden*).'[148] Since the importance of fattening animals predated the culture of body size that emerged in sixteenth-century Germany, it seems highly likely that methods of altering human bodies

[141] Gessner, *Vogelbuch*, fol. cxlviii^{v}. [142] Coler, *Oeconomia*, fol. B 2^{r}.
[143] Ibid., fol. Ccc 4^{v}. [144] Ibid., fol. Qq^{r}. [145] Gessner, *Thierbuch*, fols xvi^{r} and cxlv^{v}.
[146] Guarinonius, *Die Grewel der Verwüstung*, 758.
[147] Georg Steinhausen (ed.), *Briefwechsel Balthasar Paumgartners des Jüngeren mit seiner Gattin Magdalena, geb. Behaim (1582–1598)* (Stuttgart, 1895), 44. See the discussion of Balthasar's letters in Chapter 6, 212–13.
[148] Gottfried Christian Winckler, *Wunder der Natur/Nach der Menschen Unterschiedlichen Beschaffenheit* (Frankfurt and Leipzig, 1690), 85.

were influenced by those for animal bodies rather than vice versa, as Winckler also implied.

This relationship between animal and human bodies took on further importance in relation to consumption of meat and animal products and their effects on body size. Ryff stated, with reference to cattle for instance, that 'fat meat (*feyßt fleisch*) gives better, stronger and much more nourishment, than from a thin (*magern*) cow, especially one which had been fat (*feyßt*) but has wasted away (*abgefallen*).'[149] Similarly Gessner suggested that fat geese provided the best nourishment, while the flesh of hens, which was fat and easy to digest, gave excellent moisture to the body. 'The stomachs of all birds give good nourishment', Gessner stated, 'especially if they are fat (*feißt*).'[150] As we have seen, nourishment was recognized to be particularly important for influencing body size, and therefore the greater provision of nourishment from such fatty flesh would have been understood to promote fatness in human bodies. This understanding took effect in instructions directed to those seeking to alter their body size, as when Ryff advised that those wanting to become thinner should not eat 'fat fish' and should avoid the meat of pigs and calves and instead favour beef, which was not as fatty.[151]

To alter or maintain one's body size, therefore, a person needed to pay attention to the rearing of the animals which they consumed, as this would dictate the condition of the animals' bodies and in turn affect the consumer's body. This included an awareness of the environments which such animals inhabited. Gessner for instance stated that the best hens were those which grazed freely in green meadows.[152] He further stated that, in an 'overflowing' pasture, sheep would become 'so fat (*feißt*) from it and produce so much meat that it would be unbelievable.'[153] Hubner similarly suggested that sparrows could provide good nourishment if they were young, fat, and lived in beautiful, pure forests, suggesting that such fattened flesh, created through moist land, provided better nourishment to human bodies.[154] Ryff similarly stated that the health and fatness of cattle depended 'not a little on the pasture' as 'the meat of cattle who are put out to pasture mostly with good grass and herbs has less excessiveness (*Uberflüssigkeit*) than those which graze in deep, polluted, boggy and watery meadows.'[155] Meanwhile the German translation of Lemnius's 'Secrets of Nature' stated that oxen who grazed in moist pastures became fat and thus their meat could be more easily absorbed into a person's body, increasing their own fatness in turn.[156]

Such discussions of environment also applied to animal products, particularly dairy.[157] Georg Pictorius, for example wrote that cheese made in places with 'healthy, subtle and fat (*feißte*) pastures' would 'without doubt' be better, and

149 Walther Hermann Ryff, *Spiegel der Gesundheit* (Frankfurt am Main, 1555), fol. 62^{v}.
150 Gessner, *Vogelbuch*, fol. lviii^{v}.
151 Ryff, *New Kochbuch*, fols 143^{v}–144^{r}.
152 Gessner, *Vogelbuch*, fol. lxxxi^{r}.
153 Gessner, *Thierbuch*, fol. cxxxviii^{v}.
154 Hubner, *New Speisebüchlein*, fol. J vii^{v}.
155 Ryff, *Spiegel der Gesundheit*, fol. 62^{v}.
156 Lemnius, *Von den wunderbarlichen Geheimnissen der Natur*, fol. av^{r}.
157 Handley, 'Lusty Sack Possets'.

provide better nourishment, than that produced in regions with 'course, smoky or thin (*mageren*) herbs and grass'.[158] Similarly Coler wrote that cows who lived in pastures with red or white clover, three-fingered cinquefoil (plants of the potentilla genus), as well as those in fat, green and lovely fields with many yellow flowers would produce the best milk.[159] Meanwhile Gessner claimed, 'that such cows which become fat (*feyßt*) from clover produce much milk is commonly known among farmers', indicating a widespread awareness of how particular pastures were known to impact on the fatness of an animal and have a knock-on effect on their products.[160]

In the works of these sixteenth-century German authors, there appears a clear chain of influence between the human body, the animals and animal products it consumed, and the environments in which such animals lived and grazed.[161] Methods of fattening animals, including both their fodder and their material and sensory experiences, were understood to materially impact on the form of the bodies which consumed them, since such bodies were porous and unstable, thus requiring constant engagement and attention.

Webs of Meaning

As part of the growing medical discourse concerning body size in sixteenth-century Germany, Hieronymus Bock's 1546 'Book of Herbs' included a recipe to make the fat body thin. Bock wrote, 'several people teach that if one crushes ash leaves for a short while and drinks the resulting juice with wine, that will make fat people thin (*die feißten Leut mager machen*) in little time'. This recipe likely drew on an understanding of the warming nature of wine, and the hotness and dryness of ash leaves, which would counter the cold moisture of the fat body. Bock then admitted however, 'I have not tried this, and I also don't need to, rather I might need the opposite'.[162] As Bock's comments indicate, the consumption of particular food and drink was understood to affect one's body size in this period, and similar instructions regularly appeared in contemporary dietary and medical manuals. Such advice was not merely directed towards those who were considered too fat but was also aimed at those who were perceived to need fattening up, or to 'return to their body' as Ryff termed it. Practices of altering the body's form thus depended on a person's innate tendency towards a particular size, just as Bock suggested that his figure, which tended towards thinness, might require fattening rather than slimming.

158 Pictorius, *Leibs Artzney*, fol. 19^{r}.
159 Coler, *Oeconomia*, fol. Aa 4^{v}.
160 Gessner, *Thierbuch*, fol. cxviii^{r}.
161 See Forth, *Fat*, 135–6.
162 Bock, *Kreutterbuch*, fol. 395^{r}. Bock does not mention the nature of the leaves but they were generally understood to be of a hot and dry nature in early modern herbals. See e.g. Nicholas Culpepper, *Pharmacopœia Londinensis* (London, 1653) 18.

Instructions for altering body size went beyond food and drink, encompassing all the non-naturals of Galenic medicine. Body size could be shaped by a person's emotional state, what they wore, what substances they bathed in, the temperature of their homes, and even how comfortable their bed was. The advice offered by Ryff, Pictorius, and others shows that the early modern body was understood to exist in dialogue with its material surroundings and that ideas about body size were embedded within these interactions. This is particularly evident in the significance of animals and animal products for understanding body size. The nature of an animal's meat, the very foodstuff which Guarinonius stated to have the greatest impact on human fatness, was known to depend on the material environment which the animal inhabited. Fresh, green, and fertile environments were thought to produce the most nourishing meat and animal products, and these in turn would increase the fatness of the human bodies that consumed them. Ideas about body size were thus entangled within complex webs of meaning, as animals, environments, materials, humours, and health converged within dietetic instructions on body size.

Significantly, though none condemned fatness as damningly as Guarinonius, the majority of the authors considered here viewed the fat body as a 'burden' in need of reduction through practices of diet and non-natural influences. How can these perspectives be reconciled with the increasing popularity of a large, bulky, and even fat silhouette among sixteenth-century German men? On one level this was a question of extremes, as physicians such as Ryff differentiated between a plump and healthy fat body, nurtured through sweet foods and positive emotions, and excessive fatness which hindered mobility and encouraged illness. On another level, however, the divergence of medical guidance from gendered ideals for the body presents the coexistence of differing attitudes towards fatness and thinness within this period. These physicians were German men themselves and their medical counsel could depart from the reality of their own bodies. Paracelsus, who suggested that overeating created a body that was too fat, 'like a field that has become too rich, and is thereby ruined', was shown in his portraits to have a fleshy figure and prominent double chin.[163] His monumental form aligned with the bulky German ideal, seeming to embody his formidable reputation and robust medical learning.[164]

Body size was understood, and enacted, in various ways in different contexts. Medical and culinary texts repeatedly described processes of growing fat in association with sensory pleasure, comfort, and luxury. Through the presentation of their bulky masculine bodies, these were often the very things that German men were rejecting, instead presenting the hardy robustness that connected them to

[163] Paracelsus, 'Opus Paramirum', 466, translation 467.

[164] Forth, *Fat*, 132–3. For Paracelsus's portrait see, after Quentin Metsys, *Presumed Portrait of the Physician Paracelsus* (1493–1541), Louvre, Paris (RF1730).

their forebears. It seems unlikely, therefore, that they would have viewed their bodies as 'fat' in the terms which such authors described. Nevertheless, the association between the fatness of human beings, their livestock, and environments, meant that fat Germans could present the fertility and prosperity of the German lands and the creatures which inhabited them. This would no doubt have appealed to many contemporary Germans, particularly in view of a growing proto-nationalist ideology in this period which inspired individuals, like cartographer Sebastian Münster, to praise Germany's natural landscapes, abundant wildlife, and rich mineral deposits.[165]

Attitudes towards fatness and thinness were complex and multivalent, and the presence of debates about body size is testament to its growing prominence within this society. With their advice for fat and thin bodies, physicians were both responding to and encouraging an increasing bodily vigilance among early modern Germans for whom body size mattered like never before.

DOI: 10.1093/9780198972983.003.0002

[165] Jasper van Putten, *Networked Nation: Mapping German Cities in Sebastian Münster's Cosmographia* (Leiden, 2018), 40.

3
Visualizing Body Size

> Albrecht Dürer told me of Maximilian that the thickness of his arms (*dick an den armen*) was the same size as the thickness of his own thigh. And yet Albrecht was of middling stature. And Maximilian, when he was in Augsburg at a tournament, although by then already an old man, was competing with his nobles. They were setting up stakes and contending with lances to see who might hit the most targets. Then Maximilian pierced two stakes with one throw, which none of the nobles was able to match. Maximilian was then 59 years of age. Nowadays men's bodies are no longer so robust, they are growing weaker.[1]

This anecdote, reportedly from the reformer Philipp Melanchthon, was recorded in the lecture notes of Erich Vendenhaimer of Nuremberg in 1557. The observation, which probably originated from the Imperial Diet in Augsburg in 1518, seems unlikely to be true since Emperor Maximilian I died from a fatal illness just months later, yet it offers fascinating insights into contemporary conceptions of body size.[2] That Vendenhaimer chose to record it at all is suggestive of the significance he accorded this account of Maximilian's robust size in connection to his sporting prowess. Moreover, in his retelling of the event, Melanchthon used body size not only to praise the power and strength of the former emperor, but also to lament what he perceived to be the increasing enfeeblement of men's bodies. His comments reflected the idealization of robust masculinity in sixteenth-century Germany. Yet Melanchthon also used body size to make an eschatological argument. His view that men's bodies were becoming weaker echoed a narrative of earthly deterioration prior to the impending end of the world which was particularly prominent among Lutherans, and which increased in urgency over the second half of the sixteenth century. The sun was said to have sunk in the sky and the heavens had grown tired and decrepit.[3] The earth itself was ageing, while its creatures were becoming weaker, and its natural materials were softening. Reflecting the interconnectedness of early modern bodies with their material surroundings,

[1] Hans Rupprich, *Dürer: Schriftlicher Nachlass* (Berlin, 1956), vol. 1, 325. Translation from Jeffrey Ashcroft, *Albrecht Dürer: Documentary Biography* (New Haven, 2017), vol. 2, 1025. Translations are taken from Ashcroft unless otherwise stated.

[2] This dating is suggested by Hans Rupprich in *Dürer*, 325.

[3] See Robin B. Barnes, *Astrology and Reformation* (Oxford, 2015), 267.

Melanchthon extended this belief in the weakening and ageing of the earth to the bodies, and body size, of its inhabitants.[4]

This was Melanchthon's interpretation of the tale, yet its supposed originator, the Nuremberg artist Albrecht Dürer (1471–1528), likely viewed the disparity between his and Maximilian's limbs in different terms. By the time of this alleged encounter, Dürer had been concerned with the representation of the body for over two decades. He had devoted countless hours to studying the body's appearance and proportions, both by observing bodies from life and by using geometry to construct idealized figures. Indeed, Dürer had already started drafting his 'Four Books on Human Proportion' which, after its posthumous publication in 1528, became the first theoretical text on bodily proportion in the German language. This artistic training meant that Dürer was particularly conscious of, and fascinated by, the diversity of human figures. Dürer's observation of the size of Maximilian's arms in comparison to the thickness of his own thigh was almost certainly indebted, therefore, to his intense personal study of bodily difference in terms of size, mass, and proportion.

Dürer's investigation of human proportion was both a product of and a contributing factor in the growing cultural significance of body size within German society. Growing up in the late fifteenth century, Dürer lived through a period which saw a fundamental shift in the popular ideal for the male body in the German-speaking lands.[5] Slender gothic figures, which dominated his early work, began to morph into the oversized bodies of male elites. At the same time, body size was assuming new meanings as it became a subject of critical concern for early modern Germans. Though his study of proportion has traditionally been viewed as resulting from his engagement with classical antiquity, informed by his travels in Italy and his familiarity with the Vitruvian canon of proportions, Dürer's interest in the body was also shaped by influences which were closer to home.[6] In sixteenth-century Germany, fatness could be associated with happiness, nourishment, comfort, and prosperity, yet it could also be associated with gluttony, immorality, and excess. Equally, thinness could signify control, elegance, and athleticism, as well as sickness, infertility, and death. In his depiction of the human body, Dürer drew on these ambivalent contemporary understandings of body size, moulding them according to his own requirements for a particular

[4] The significance of body size for apocalyptic belief is explored in greater detail in Chapter 4.

[5] On Dürer and the German patriotism associated with this trend see Larry Silver, 'Germanic Patriotism in the Age of Dürer', in Dagmar Eichberger and Charles Zika (eds), *Dürer and his Culture* (Cambridge, 1998), 38–68.

[6] See Erwin Panofsky, *The Life and Art of Albrecht Dürer* (Princeton, 2005, first publ. 1943), esp. 80–131; Kenneth Clark, *The Nude: A Study in Ideal Form* (Princeton, 1990, first publ. 1956), 321–9; Andrew Morall, 'Dürer in Venice', in Larry Silver and Jeffrey Chipps Smith (eds), *The Essential Dürer* (Philadelphia, 2010), 99–114. On the combination of Italian and German models in Dürer's representation of the body see Anne-Marie Bonnet, *'Akt' bei Dürer* (Cologne, 2001), esp. 84–7, and Anne-Marie Bonnet, *Albrecht Dürer: Die Erfindung des Aktes* (Munich, 2014), 8–10.

image. Dürer thus used body size to create meaning in his artworks and he experimented with constructing bodies of various forms which could embody different meanings and emotions.[7]

As well as his cultural context, Dürer's own corporeality shaped the ways in which he investigated bodily form. Dürer possessed a human body which consisted of a particular size, and which underwent changes with age and sickness. Moreover, as an artist, Dürer had a particular awareness of his body, its movements, and capabilities due to the physical training, labour, and skill involved in producing his works.[8] The early modern period involved an intense engagement with materials and processes of making, as 'almost all members of society engaged in transforming matter in some way'.[9] Understanding early modern conceptions of the body thus requires a consideration of bodies as the vehicles through which objects and images were created and materials transformed.[10] This chapter examines Dürer's representation of bodies and their proportions as being fundamentally informed by his own embodied experience in combination with cultural conceptions of body size.[11] Dürer thus serves as a case study through which to examine the interwoven nature of personal subjectivity and cultural construction with regard to body size, yet his works also held immense significance for the representation of bodies throughout the visual culture of early modern Germany.[12]

[7] On cultural influences which informed Dürer's work see Dagmar Eichberger and Charles Zika, 'Dürer and his Culture: An Introduction', in Dagmar Eichberger and Charles Zika (eds), *Dürer and his Culture* (Cambridge, 1998), 1–10.

[8] On the significance of the artist's body see Pamela H. Smith, *From Lived Experience to the Written Word: Reconstructing Practical Knowledge in the Early Modern World* (Chicago, 2022), 125–6; Pamela H. Smith, *The Body of the Artisan: Art and Experience in the Scientific Revolution* (Chicago, 2004); Stefan Hanß, 'Gendering the Material Renaissance: Women Industriousness and the Female Body at the Court of Württemberg', *German History* 41 (2023), 367–99; Ulinka Rublack, 'Craft, Labour and Cabinets of Curiosities: Rethinking the Body of the Artisan', *German History,* 41 (2023), 337–66.

[9] Ulinka Rublack, 'Matter in the Material Renaissance', *Past and Present* 219 (2013), 41–85, here 45. See also Ulinka Rublack, 'Renaissance Dress, Cultures of Making, and the Period Eye', *West 86th: A Journal of Decorative Arts, Design History and Material Culture* 23 (2016), 6–34.

[10] On the influence of Dürer's physical training on his artistic production see Otto Benesch, *The Art of the Northern Renaissance: Its Relation to the Contemporary Spiritual and Intellectual Movements* (London, 1965, first publ. 1945), 8.

[11] This approach is indebted to pioneering studies which centre Dürer's own psychological landscape and experiences as informing his artworks. See Joseph Leo Koerner, *The Moment of Self-Portraiture in German Renaissance Art* (Chicago, 1993); Mitchell B. Merback, *Perfection's Therapy: An Essay on Albrecht Dürer's Melencolia I* (New York, 2017), esp. 177–211; Ulinka Rublack, *Dürer's Lost Masterpiece: Art and Society at the Dawn of a Global World* (Oxford, 2023). Art historical scholarship focusing on the significance of the artist's body more generally has tended to examine artists' use of their bodies as both subjects and objects for their work, but this approach understands the artist's body as the vehicle through which all artworks are produced. See Tracey Warr and Amelia Jones (eds), *The Artist's Body* (London, 2000).

[12] Dürer is the ideal case study in this regard as he left an unparalleled collection of written sources concerning his life and work which enable an investigation of his embodied subjectivity to an extent which would simply not be possible for other contemporary artists. These are compiled in Ashcroft, *Documentary Biography*, vols 1 and 2.

Dürer's study and theorization of the proportions of the human body profoundly shaped the ways in which bodies were represented in German art throughout the sixteenth and seventeenth centuries and beyond. Dürer was the most influential German artist of the early modern period; during his lifetime he was venerated as a 'new Apelles', and later a 'German Apelles', referencing the fourth-century Greek painter considered to be the most exceptional artist to have ever lived.[13] While his books on proportion did not result in the widespread application of his theories by young painters in the way he had hoped, they were highly influential in terms of the conceptualization of differences in body size, form, and movement, as well as the aesthetic judgement of bodies. Moreover, since Dürer's artworks were already widely collected by his contemporaries, and as one of the first artists to distribute his artworks in large numbers through the innovations of print culture, Dürer arguably had the most significant impact on the visual representation and perception of bodies of any contemporary artist.[14] Dürer's works, and especially his proportion studies, are thus essential sources for understanding how early modern Germans viewed, experienced, and evaluated body size.

The Artist's Body

The body was critical to an early modern artist's work. A painter's workshop was the site of intense bodily labour. Many hours would be spent smoothing a panel in preparation for the application of pigment which had to be finely ground over long periods of time and with great effort to create the best possible shade.[15] Popular medical author Walther Herman Ryff's suggestion that thin people wanting to increase the size of their body should 'eat much more often, such as four times a day, as is common practice among artisans', gives a sense of the energy that such craftspeople were known to expend in the workshop.[16] Ryff singled out artisans as needing to regularly replenish their bodies through food in order to support the work they performed. Writing from experience, Dürer likewise recognized the importance of the body for a painter's creations. In a draft of his 'Manual for Painting' from 1508 he described the bodily requirements of a young apprentice painter. While artisans needed a greater amount of food than others, they should nevertheless avoid excess, and Dürer insisted the apprentice painter

[13] Conrad Celtis was the first to refer to Dürer as a new Apelles. See his 'Four Epigrams on Albrecht Dürer', in Ashcroft, *Documentary Biography*, vol. 1, 77. See also Andrea Bubenik, *Reframing Albrecht Dürer: The Appropriation of Art, 1528–1700* (Farnham, 2013), 14.

[14] On the significance of Dürer's prints see Edward H. Wouk and Jennifer Spinks (eds), *Albrecht Dürer's Material World*, exh. cat., Whitworth Art Gallery (Manchester, 2023). For Dürer's impact on representations of the body see also Bonnet, *'Akt' bei Dürer* and *Die Erfindung des Aktes*.

[15] Smith, *Body of the Artisan*, 110–11.

[16] Walther Hermann Ryff, *New Kochbuch für die Kranken* (Frankfurt am Main, 1545), fol. 139^{r}. See Chapter 2, 32.

should 'be kept moderate in his eating and drinking, likewise in his sleeping'. Moreover, they should be 'kept away from the female sex, not allowed to live in the same house with them, not see or touch any naked woman, and be protected from uncleanness. Nothing debases the mind more than impurity.'[17] Dürer's comment that sexual contact would debase the mind suggests an understanding that such 'impurity' might impact on an apprentice's artistic ability, as it was through both mind and body that artworks were produced. Such requirements for apprentices were not unusual, and authors of Renaissance treatises repeatedly advised artists not to have excessive sex, which would cause their hands to 'shiver and tremble [more] than a leaf in the wind'.[18]

Yet Dürer's own mind and body were not as free from impurity as the ideal he described. While he suggested that apprentices should not see or touch naked women, Dürer is believed to have based his early nude studies on live female bodies observed at the public bathhouse, including his first nude image which was produced before his marriage in 1494.[19] Dürer may have considered these requirements to be more important for the malleable minds and bodies of young apprentices, and his text also needs to be understood within the common register of moral writing in this period. Nevertheless, even for established artists, the female nude could be an ambivalent subject, being associated with both indecency and impurity, as well as intrigue, pleasure, and artistic skill. Melanchthon's one-time student Johannes Manlius, for example, included this passage among his collection of the reformer's stories and anecdotes from 1565:

> When Apelles was painting Venus, he took the trouble to have thirty of the most beautiful maidens selected for him to inspect. Dürer—that respectable painter of Nuremberg—did similarly, and various highly respectable matrons and maidens put themselves at his disposal. Alluding to this, the painter Lukas Cranach's father, an excellent and most respectable old man, used to jest that maidens stripped themselves bare in the ladies' quarters for painters in ancient times, who found out the proportions of their bodies—by feeling their way (*contrectando*).[20]

[17] Rupprich, *Dürer*, vol. 2, 92. Ashcroft, *Documentary Biography*, vol. 1, 246. The original manuscript draft is held in the British Library, BL 5230, fol. 5^{r-v}.

[18] Apprentices in early modern London, for instance, pledged themselves not to commit fornication or marry. See Steven R. Smith, 'The London Apprentices as Seventeenth-Century Adolescents', *Past and Present* 61 (1973), 149–61, here 150. See also Stefan Hanß, 'Face-Work: Making Hair Matter in Sixteenth-Century Europe', *Gender and History* 33 (2021), 314–45, here 329. Quotation in Ulrich Pfisterer (ed.), *Die Kunstliteratur der italienischen Renaissance: Eine Geschichte in Quellen* (Stuttgart, 2002), 61.

[19] See Walter L. Strauss, *The Complete Drawings of Albrecht Dürer*, 6 vols (New York, 1974), vol. 1, 140–1, no. 1493/3 and Jeffrey Chipps Smith, *Dürer* (London, 2012), 69–70.

[20] Ashcroft, *Documentary Biography*, vol. 2, 1029. For Melanchthon's original Latin text see Rupprich, *Dürer*, vol. 1, 327.

Despite repeated references to respectability, there is a sense of titillation to this passage, alluded to by the comment that these women 'put themselves at [Dürer's] disposal'. The tale of Cranach the Elder, who himself produced numerous paintings of female nudes, portrays Dürer in a slightly scurrilous manner, linking his painting of the female body to ancients who would 'feel' their models' proportions.[21] Given Dürer's own extensive study of bodily proportion, it seems that the reader is meant to connect Dürer himself to this practice, and the use of the verb *contrecto* appears as a double entendre, implying not only to feel or touch, but to 'sexually harass' or even 'violate'.[22]

Also included in Manlius's book was a description of Charles V's entry into Antwerp in 1520, where it was reported that 'there were some very attractive and beautiful girls who were almost naked, except for the flimsiest of veils'. According to Manlius, Dürer reported to Melanchthon that the emperor himself 'did not even cast a glance' at them, though Dürer was delighted to 'properly view the perfection of these most lovely girls. He said, "I, being a painter, had a good look at every little thing, quite shamelessly!"'[23] Despite warning against the debasement of the mind, therefore, Dürer himself took pleasure in viewing the naked bodies of beautiful women, justifying his voyeurism through his artistic interests. These examples suggest how the artist's body could be a site of conflict, where the ideal of a pure and chaste mind and body was set against the requirement to observe the human figure from life, as well as one's personal desires.

Dürer's instructions concerning moderate eating, drinking, and sleeping, as well as the avoidance of sex, would also have had consequences for the size of an artist's body. Given contemporary understandings concerning the relationship of the non-naturals with body size, such moderation would have been thought to prevent either an unnatural fattening or slimming of the body which could result from the excess or restriction of these non-natural factors.[24] Through practices of moderation the apprentice would maintain the natural size of his body which he had been granted by God, aligning with Dürer's emphasis on purity. Dürer's draft hints that there could even be an ideal body size and shape for a painter, as in creating a provisional list of topics to be discussed in the book he included a heading concerning the measurement of the apprentice's 'form and limbs (*geschtalt vnd glidmos*)'.[25] As the text was never completed, however, we do not know what these ideal proportions were, and it may have been that Dürer himself could not decide upon them. Regardless, it is clear that Dürer recognized the significance of an artist's body, including its size, for their creations.

[21] On Cranach see pp. 100–4 of this chapter.

[22] Ashcroft, *Documentary Biography*, vol. 2, 1029 n. 3.

[23] Ibid., vol. 2, 1028. In his account of his travels in the Netherlands, Dürer himself wrote of 'beautiful girls...the like of which I have scarcely ever seen'. Ibid., vol. 1, 563.

[24] On the relationship between the non-naturals and body size see Chapter 2, esp. 43–50.

[25] Rupprich, *Dürer*, vol. 2, 92. Ashcroft, *Documentary Biography*, vol. 1, 246.

The connection between an artist's body and the work they created was expressed explicitly by the humanist scholar Joachim Camerarius when he described Dürer's figure in a foreword to the Latin edition of the 'Four Books on Human Proportion' (1532). Camerarius wrote:

> Nature granted him a physique remarkable in its proportions and stature, and a match for the brilliant intellect which it was to house...As she has clothed the ridiculously minded ape with a ridiculous body, so she is accustomed to envelop outstanding minds with corresponding bodies. He has a *caput argutum* [graceful head], a keen glance, a noble nose, the kind that the Greeks call *tetragonon* [four-square, symmetrical], quite a long neck, a broad chest, a taut belly, muscular thighs, sturdy legs.[26]

Camerarius connected Dürer's 'outstanding mind', the creative genius which enabled him to create his artworks, with the form of his body, matching its greatness by describing a figure he considered to be particularly beautiful. Unsurprisingly for a humanist scholar, Camerarius derived his descriptions of bodily beauty from classical authors, with the phrase *caput argutum* originating in Virgil's description of a thoroughbred horse.[27] Through his comments on Dürer's broad chest and taut belly, Camerarius shows body size to be implicated in this understanding of an ideal artistic figure. It is no coincidence that this description appears in the preface to Dürer's works on proportion. Camerarius suggests that the 'remarkable...proportions and stature' of Dürer's body is mirrored in the figures which the reader may learn to create, which were themselves the result of his 'brilliant intellect'.

In considering the ideal proportions for an apprentice, Dürer must surely have reflected on his own body. Did he, like Camerarius, believe that he possessed the ideal artist's body? And how did this body relate to the ideal body in art? Though there is no extensive surviving statement from Dürer regarding his appearance, he is known to have taken great pride in his looks, selecting distinctive outfits for his self-portraits and carefully grooming his curled hair and unusual beard.[28] His friend, the humanist Lorenz Behaim (1458–1521) commented to their mutual close friend Willibald Pirckheimer in 1507: 'Let me know if he's still trimming and crimping his beard', suggesting the effort that went into creating Dürer's image.[29] A couple of months later, Behaim wrote to Pirckheimer stating that he had cast a horoscope for Dürer, claiming 'he has Leo as ascendant house, which is

[26] Ashcroft, *Documentary Biography*, vol. 2, 952. This text was not reproduced by Rupprich.

[27] Ashcroft states that Virgil coined the phrase in *Georgics* 3.80 and it remained an unusual expression, indicating the Camerarius is consciously quoting Virgil. Ibid. 958 n. 3.

[28] See Ulinka Rublack, *Dressing Up* (Oxford, 2010), 33–4.

[29] Rupprich, *Dürer*, vol. 1, 253. Ashcroft, *Documentary Biography*, vol. 1, 186. On the relationship between Dürer, Pirckheimer, and Behaim see Rublack, *Dürer's Lost Masterpiece*, 55–73.

why he is lean'.[30] While Behaim suggested Dürer's lean body was determined by astrology, it seems likely that Dürer would have taken steps to cultivate and maintain the kind of body he desired, just as he crimped and managed his hair.[31] Though slim by nature, Dürer may have implemented practices involving food, sleep, exercise and the other non-naturals to ensure his figure remained lean and muscular over time.

Returning to our opening anecdote, though Melanchthon used the comparison of Dürer's thigh and Maximilian's arm to present the superior strength of the Emperor, it seems possible that Dürer was reflecting on the slimness of his own body. In 1493, Dürer produced a study of two legs, bent at the knee and at different angles, which are generally thought to be his own (Figure 3.1).[32] In this drawing Dürer's legs are notably thin, and he depicts the shadowy contours of his elongated thigh muscles through the lines of his pen. It is quite easy to imagine an arm being of similar size and proportion to Dürer's thigh in this drawing. The image was produced at a time when the gothic fashion for thin bodies with slender legs was repeatedly reflected in Dürer's work. In his image of a 'Young Couple Walking' from 1492 (Figure 3.2), for instance, the viewer's attention is drawn to the narrow but shapely leg of the young man. His trim waist is emphasized through the fastening of his clothing, while his pointed shoes elongate his limbs. The drawing echoes those produced by the Master of the Housebook, whose impact on Dürer's early drawings has long been noted.[33] Dürer's observation of slender bodies and thin limbs in contemporary artworks would have influenced both how he presented bodies in his works and how he viewed and experienced his own figure. In depicting his thin legs in 1493, Dürer must have observed the correspondence of his body with the ideals of contemporary art, including the images which he himself created. Dürer's study of his slender body and his depiction of idealised elongated bodies were thus mutually reinforcing activities.

Dürer's view of his body was closely connected to his impression of his own talents and achievements. On a material level, the physical labour and discipline of mind and body that went into producing his artworks would have shaped Dürer's figure, contributing towards his lean but muscular form. In 1500, Dürer created an image of the classical hero Hercules which bears a striking resemblance to Dürer himself (Figure 3.3). Through the figure's extremely muscular yet elongated limbs, Dürer shows his body to bear the traits of this exemplary hero,

30 Ashcroft, *Documentary Biography*, vol. 1, 187. See Rupprich, *Dürer,* vol. 1, 254, for Behaim's original Latin text with a German translation in the footnotes.

31 On the significance of astrology for body size see Chapter 2, 36–7.

32 Panofsky, *Life and Art of Dürer*; Johann Eckart von Borries, *Albrecht Dürer: Christus als Schmerzensmann* (Karlsruhe, 1972), 30. Panofsky stated that the drawing shows Dürer's own left leg in two views, sketched from a reclining position. Johann Eckart von Borries commented that the legs are indeed Dürer's own but viewed from a sitting position.

33 The influence of the Housebook Master on Dürer was first noted in print in Carl Hachmeister, *Der Meister des Amsterdamer Kabinetts und sein Verhältnis zu Albrecht Dürer* (Heidelberg, 1897).

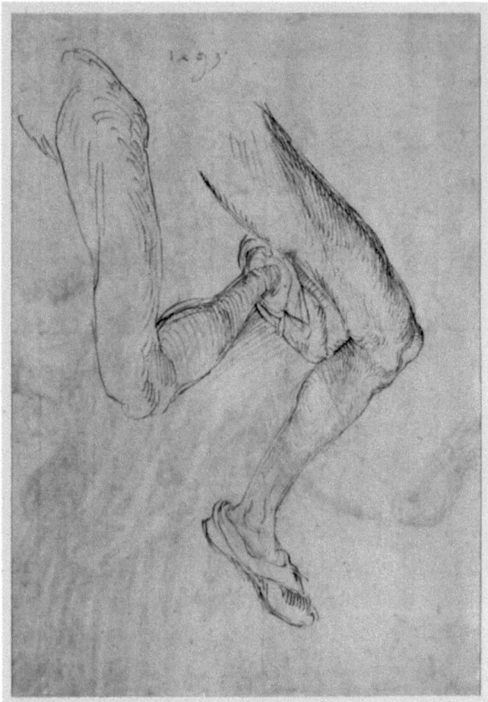

Figure 3.1 Albrecht Dürer, Study of a Left Leg from Two Viewpoints, 1493. Pen and ink, 29.1 × 20.2 cm. The Courtauld, London (Samuel Courtauld Trust). Photo © The Courtauld. Dürer depicted his own left leg from two different angles, likely from a seated position. Through his pen lines, Dürer emphasized the contours of his lean muscles which aligned with late fifteenth-century ideals.

while the drawn bow may reflect his taut intellect and virtue as an artist.[34] Yet Dürer also reflected on his bodily appearance at moments when he felt particularly vulnerable professionally and physically. Though Dürer was generally confident in his abilities as an artist, he was distinctly aware of his lack of education and was plagued by financial anxieties.[35] In 1506 Dürer wrote to his close friend Pirckheimer: 'nothing annoys me more than when they say you are growing handsome whereas I'm getting ugly. It's enough to drive me mad. I've just spotted a grey hair. What's made it grow is sheer poverty and the way I exert myself. I believe

[34] Ulrich Pfisterer, '"Here's Looking at You": Ambiguities of Personalizing the Nude', in Jill Burke, Thomas Kren, and Stephen J. Campbell (eds), *The Renaissance Nude*, exh. cat., J. Paul Getty Museum (Los Angeles, 2018), 307–23, here 309–10. See also Irving Lavin, *Past-Present: Essays on Historicism in Art from Donatello to Picasso* (Berkeley, CA, 1993), 34–5.

[35] Evidence of Dürer's confidence with regard to his work appear in his surviving letters to Willibald Pirckheimer and Jakob Heller. Ashcroft, *Documentary Biography*, vol. 1, 163 and 212. On Dürer's insecurities see Ashcroft, *Documentary Biography*, vol. 2, 710.

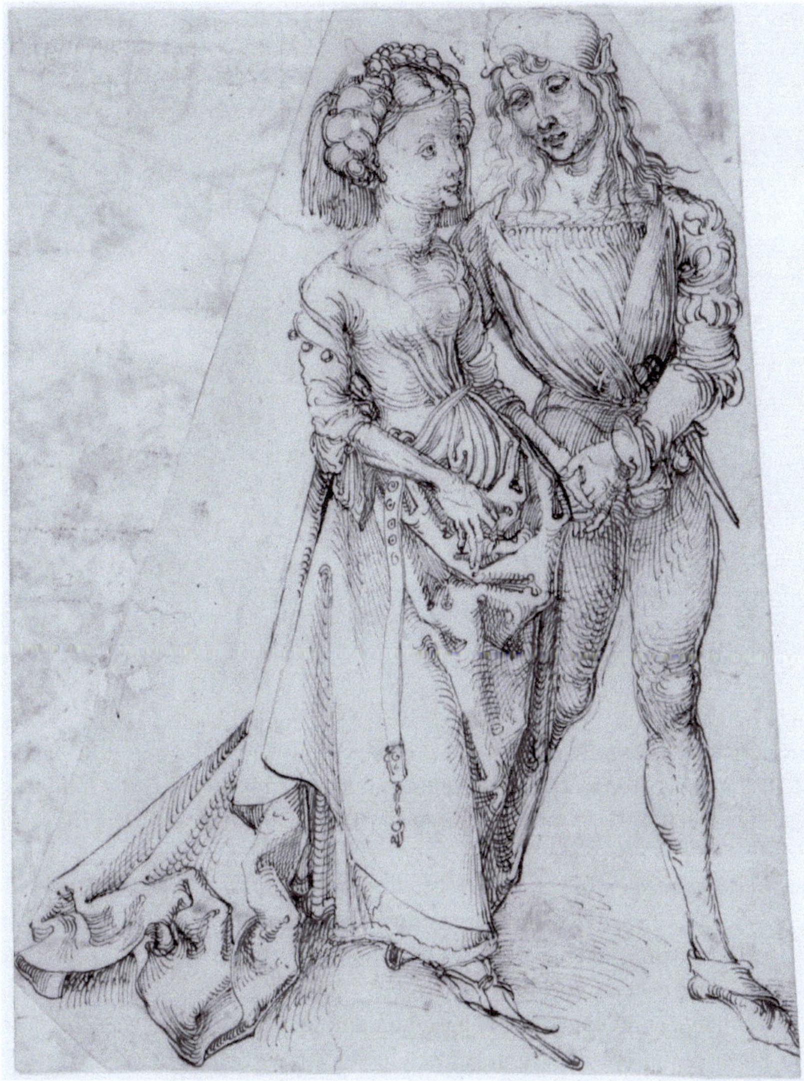

Figure 3.2 Albrecht Dürer, Young Couple Walking, c.1492. Pen and ink, 25.8 × 19.1 cm. Kunsthalle, Hamburg. © bpk/Hamburger Kunsthalle/Christoph Irrgang. In accordance with contemporary ideals for the body, slender male figures populate Dürer's early works. Here Dürer draws attention to the narrow waist and shapely leg of the young man.

it was in the stars that I get a raw deal in life.'[36] While joking with his friend, Dürer expressed a serious and long-standing belief that his life was especially difficult, despite his talent and success. By 1506, Dürer was not yet at the peak of his career but he was already a highly esteemed artist. Only a few years later he would

[36] Ibid., vol. 1, 163.

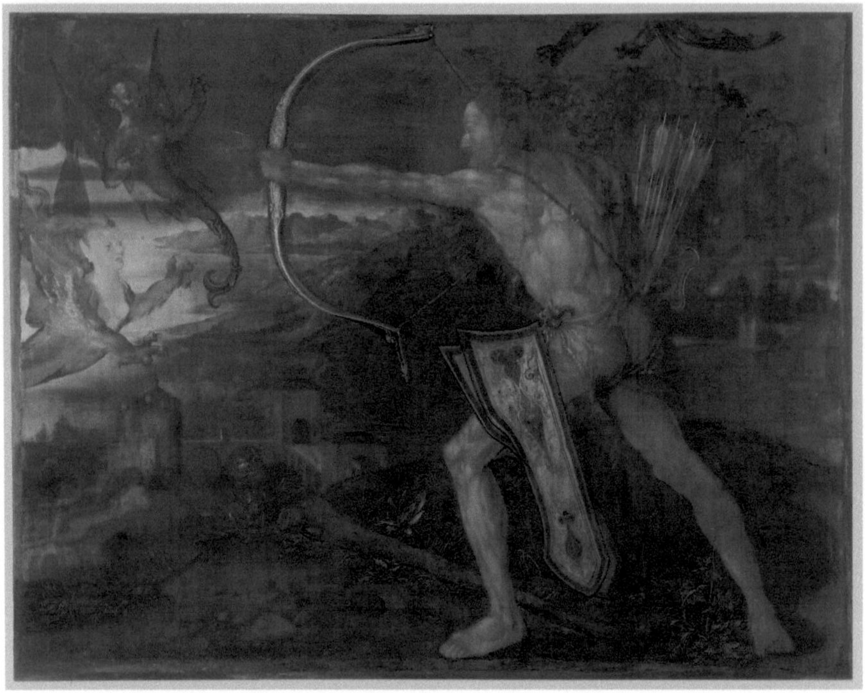

Figure 3.3 Albrecht Dürer, Hercules Killing the Stymphalian Birds, 1500. Tempera on canvas, 87 × 110 cm. © Germanisches Nationalmuseum, Nuremberg. Leihgabe BStGS. Photo: M. Runge. Hercules bears a striking resemblance to Dürer himself, suggesting that the artist's own body bears the traits of the classical hero.

be appointed to the Great Council of Nuremberg and buy his large house near the city's castle.[37] Underlying this humorous exchange was thus an insecurity which Dürer connected explicitly with his body and appearance, as he referenced his ageing and even ugliness.

Dürer had a conflicted view of his talent and success, and this was intertwined with his sense of his own appearance. In his 'Nude Self-Portrait' (Figure 3.4), Dürer carefully depicted his muscular body, highlighting his toned torso through the use of the chiaroscuro technique. Yet there is a lumpiness to his form as his knees turn inwards and the right side of his body wrinkles and sags, an impression which is enhanced through Dürer's use of cross-hatched lines at varying angles. Dürer likely produced this image while he was engrossed in the study of the human body, perfecting his methods of proportion, and depicting the ideal male figure in his famous engraving of 'Adam and Eve' from 1504 (Figure 3.5). The form of Dürer's torso, his muscular arms and lean chest, do not appear so far from Adam's ideal body. Yet, in depicting his imperfections, Dürer also noted his

[37] See Jane Campbell Hutchison, *Albrecht Dürer: A Biography* (Princeton, 1990), 119–20. See also Rublack, *Dürer's Lost Masterpiece*, 83–4.

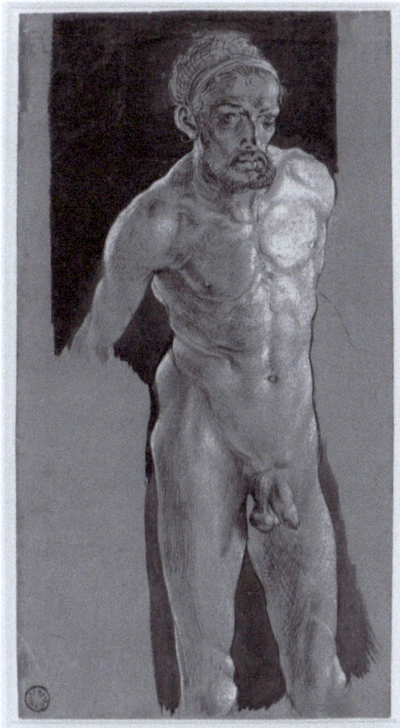

Figure 3.4 Albrecht Dürer, Nude Self-Portrait, c.1499–1509. Pen and brush, 29 × 15 cm. Schloss Weimar. © bpk/Klassik Stiftung Weimar/Olaf Mokansky. Dürer created this nude self-portrait at a time when he was engrossed in the study of ideal human proportions. This pursuit likely informed the way in which he perceived his own body, in terms of how it aligned with, and diverged from, such ideals.

weakness and fallibility, a view encouraged by the dating of this image to 1503, shortly after Dürer suffered a period of illness.[38] In his first representation of his naked form, we thus see Dürer's conflicted impulses in relation to his own body, as he recognized his bodily beauty and skill whilst also being highly aware of his mortality and human frailty.[39]

[38] The dating of this image has been heavily contested. Erwin Panofsky first suggested the year 1503, considering Dürer to have created the image in the same year as his *Head of the Dead Christ* which, according to the inscription, was sketched 'in my sickness'. See Panofsky, *Life and Art of Dürer*, 90, and Chipps Smith, *Dürer*, 154–6. Joseph Leo Koerner agreed with Panofsky's view in *Moment of Self-Portraiture*, 241–2. Christine Demele suggested that it was in fact created later, around 1509, based on the dark background of the image, see *Dürers Nacktheit: Das Weimarer Selbstbildnis* (Münster, 2012). Both Bonnet and Erwin Pokorny argue this is not persuasive and the latter dates it to 1499. See Anne-Marie Bonnet, *Albrecht Dürer: Die Erfindung des Aktes* (Munich, 2014), 38, and Erwin Pokorny, 'Dürers Selbstakt', in Christof Metzger (ed.), *Albrecht Dürer*, exh. cat., Albertina, Vienna (Munich, 2019), 70–3, here 72.

[39] See Koerner, *Moment of Self-Portraiture*, 242; Pfisterer, 'Personalizing the Nude', 311–12; Panofsky, *Life and Art of Dürer*, 90.

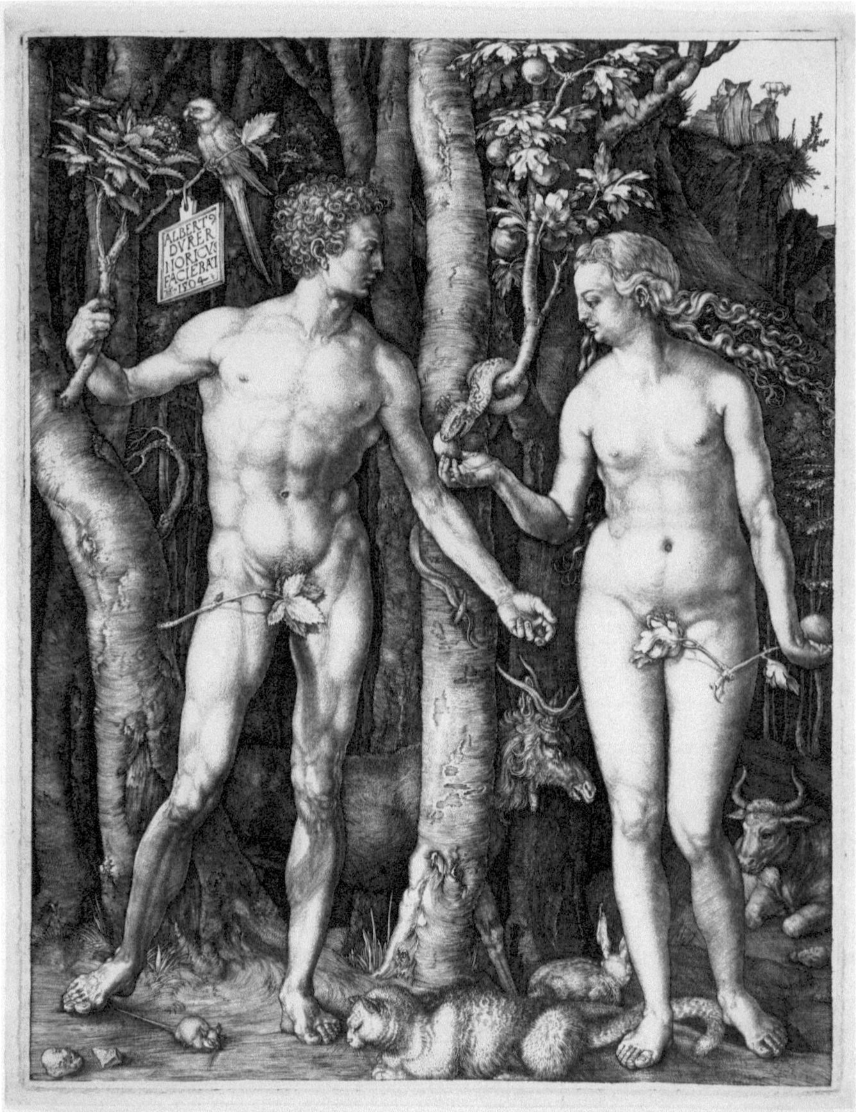

Figure 3.5 Albrecht Dürer, Adam and Eve, 1504. Engraving, 25.1 × 20 cm. Metropolitan Museum of Art, New York, public domain. Dürer's famous engraving presents the first couple immediately before the Fall—the final instant at which they represented ultimate humanity. Dürer sought to convey this perfection through the ideal proportions of their bodies.

Interestingly, almost every surviving image of Dürer's naked body was reportedly made in a time of illness. A second figure from around 1509 shows Dürer pointing to a 'yellow spot' on his side, locating the area of his pain or sickness.[40] Similarly, in a final image from 1522, Dürer presented himself in the image of 'Christ as the Man of Sorrows' (Figure 3.6) and again his body is shown as lean, with slightly withered but muscular arms and a fleshy stomach.[41] In 1521, Dürer had recorded that he was 'struck down by high fever and drastic weakness, nausea and headache', further writing that he 'suffered a mysterious illness that no one had ever heard of, and this sickness has never left me'.[42] Whilst his weakness is

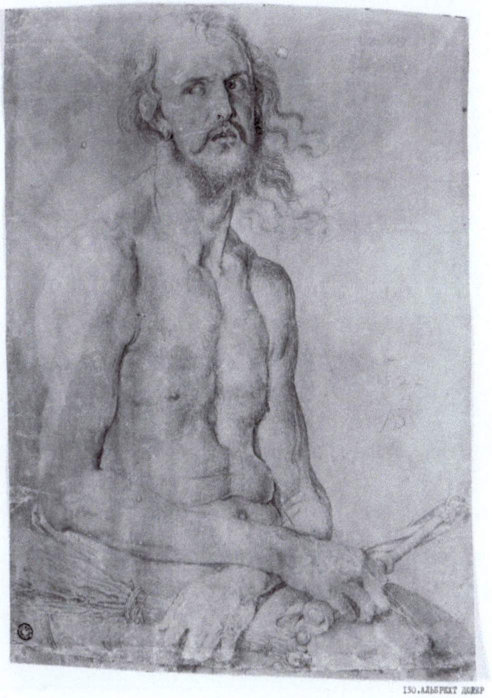

Figure 3.6 Albrecht Dürer, Self-Portrait as Man of Sorrows, 1522. Metal point and white highlights on green prepared paper, 40.8 × 29 cm. © Kunsthalle Bremen—Der Kunstverein in Bremen, Kupferstichkabinett, inv. 1851/7 Z (war loss). Dürer presented himself in the image of Christ as the Man of Sorrows, an iconic devotional image depicting Christ's suffering during the Passion. Dürer recorded his own suffering during this period in which he was afflicted with a 'mysterious illness'.

[40] See Koerner, *Moment of Self-Portraiture,* 177; Merback, *Perfections Therapy,* 190–3.

[41] Mitchell Merback views this image as exemplifying the autotherapeutic aspect of Dürer's project of self-portraiture. Merback, *Perfection's Therapy*, 198–9.

[42] Rupprich, *Dürer*, vol. 1, 169. Ashcroft, *Documentary Biography,* vol. 1, 579. Dürer has been retrospectively diagnosed with numerous ailments, with suggestions including malaria, tuberculosis,

conveyed through his limp, sagging form, that he chose to present himself as Christ, whose figure Dürer himself considered 'the most beautiful in all the world', suggests he retained a certain admiration for his body.[43]

Dürer's representation of himself as particularly lean, even emaciated, during periods of illness reinforces the vulnerability he experienced during such times. This is emphasized by the contrasting figure he presents in his dressed self-portraits which are included in panel paintings such the 'Feast of the Rose Garlands' (1506) (Figure 3.7), 'The Martyrdom of the Ten-Thousand' (1508), and the 'Landauer Altar' (1511).[44] In these works, Dürer presents himself with an imposing body,

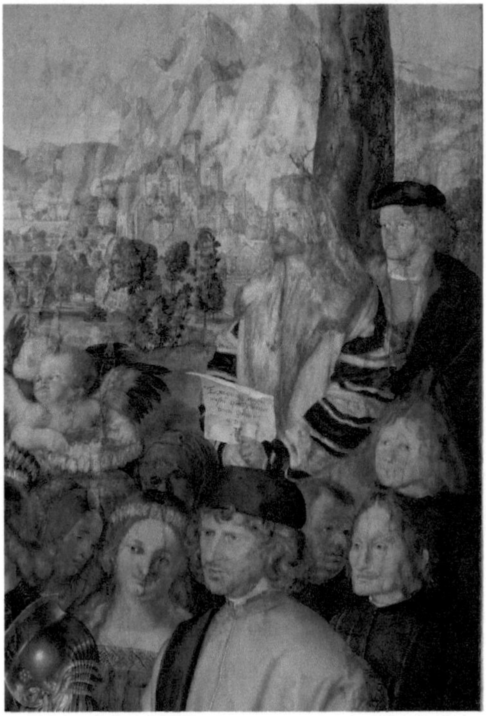

Figure 3.7 Detail from Albrecht Dürer, Feast of the Rosary, 1506. Oil on panel, 161.5 × 192 cm [full image]. National Gallery, Prague. Photo © National Gallery Prague 2025. Dürer included this self-portrait within a commissioned panel painting as a proclamation of his authorship and artistic mastery. His dressed figure in his gown appears imposing.

and syphilis. See R. F Timken-Zinkann, 'Medical Aspects of the Art and Life of Albrecht Dürer (1471–1528)', *Proceedings of the XXIII International Congress of the History of Medicine, London, 2–9 September 1972* (London, 1974), 870–5.

[43] Rupprich, *Dürer*, vol. 2, 104. Ashcroft, *Documentary Biography*, vol. 1, 339.

[44] Albrecht Dürer, 'Feast of the Rose Garlands', National Gallery, Prague, Inv. No. O 1552; Albrecht Dürer, 'Martyrdom of the Ten-Thousand', Kunsthistorisches Museum, Vienna, Inv. Nr. Gemäldegalerie, 835; Albrecht Dürer, 'Landauer Altar', Kunsthistorisches Museum, Vienna, Inv. Nr. Gemäldegalerie, 838.

appearing tall and dressed in clothing which bulks out his frame. These self-portraits proclaim his authorship of great commissions, thus presenting not only his artistic talent, but also his increasing prosperity and elevated social position. The disjuncture between these and his nude self-portraits heightens our sense of the conflict Dürer experienced in relation to his success. Though he acknowledged his wealth and prestige through such dressed portraits which were included in paintings commissioned by wealthy clients, in times of illness, when Dürer was reminded of his own mortality and vulnerability, he depicted this in private drawings of his naked body, presenting his fallibility through his weakened bodily form.

For Dürer the body could be a site of personal conflict, and the form of the body could play a critical role in the representation of such anxieties. Intertwined with this tension was an awareness that the body was central to artistic creation, and Dürer recognized this both in terms of his own figure as well as in his instructions concerning young apprentices. This latter point was something with which he had considerable lived experience; while the exact number of pupils and journeymen active in Dürer's workshop is unknown, it is estimated that almost every major painter and printmaker active in Nuremberg between 1500 and 1528 either trained with Dürer or worked in his atelier.[45] Dürer played a critical role as teacher to a generation of German artists. In so doing he shared knowledge concerning the construction of bodily proportions which had been hard won; Jacopo de' Barbari had been reluctant to share his own theories of proportion with Dürer, who wrote that 'I could not get out of him his method'. With help from the writings of classical author Vitruvius, Dürer thus, 'found my own way forward'.[46] Dürer recognized that the very practice of art and the acquisition of knowledge could be marked by conflict and struggle, and this was especially the case for his study of bodily form.

With regard to his own body, though he acknowledged an ideal for the artist's figure, Dürer knew that he did not always align with such ideals. Similarly, though he took pains to fashion and mould his appearance, he was aware that this was not without limits, noting the effects of age and sickness on his embodied form. This conflict in Dürer's bodily perception reflected his broader engagement and fascination with the elements of himself and his life which he could not control.[47] He was particularly interested in his dreams, for example, writing in 1512, 'Ah, how often I see great arts and fine works in my sleep, the like of which do not

[45] Jeffrey Chipps Smith, *Nuremberg, a Renaissance City, 1500–1618* (Austin, TX, 2021), 46.

[46] Rupprich, *Dürer*, vol. 1, 103. Ashcroft, *Documentary Biography*, vol. 2, 712. See Chipps Smith, *Dürer*, 130–3.

[47] Shira Brisman, 'Sternkraut: "The Word that Unlocks" Dürer's Self-Portrait of 1493', in Daniel Hess and Thomas Eser (eds), *The Early Dürer*, exh. cat., Germanisches Nationalmuseum (Nuremberg, 2012), 194–207. On Dürer's engagement with chance through the figure of Fortuna, see Merback, *Perfection's Therapy*, 204–11.

occur to me in waking hours'.[48] In 1525 he made great efforts to remember a dream he had in which 'great masses of water fell from the sky', recording his vision in watercolour. Beneath the image he wrote: 'when the first torrent to reach the earth was about to strike, it was falling at such speed, with wind and roaring, that in my terror, when I awoke, my whole body was trembling'.[49] Dürer recorded this experience as being grounded in his body, provoking an embodied response. Through the very act of recording he attempted to impose some level of control over this unconscious experience, working through what he saw and felt while being aware that it was inexplicable.

These complexities in Dürer's psyche suggest that the relationship between ideal and natural, between what can be constructed and what is simply observed, involved deep layers of meaning for Dürer. Considering such complexities in relation to his representation and investigation of the body, in which he combined natural observation with artistic construction, a wider-reaching story emerges in which the subtleties of Dürer's own lived, embodied experience were embedded.

Meanings in the Flesh

Dürer was particularly interested in conveying meaning in his artworks through engagement with the matter of the fleshy body. This is evident from his earliest studies of his appearance, confirming the extent to which Dürer's conception of the body was related to an awareness of his own corporeality. Already in Dürer's first surviving drawing, a self-portrait at the age of 13, Dürer took pains to depict the contours of his face and features. On his cheeks, Dürer used curved lines to emphasize the softness of his youthful face in contrast to his straight nose, which he defined with a dark, thick outline. In this image the young Dürer experimented with form and texture, depicting firmness and plasticity through shading alone.[50] In 1491, Dürer again studied his face, this time showing himself supporting his head with his hand.[51] He observed the effect of this posture on his fleshy cheek, which was pushed up to meet the skin of his bottom eyelid. On the recto of this image, Dürer had drawn the Holy Family and in the self-portrait the folds of skin beneath Dürer's eye are represented with the same cross-hatching as the virgin's cloak on the sheet's reverse.[52] In this drawing of his face, therefore, Dürer appears interested in the way that flesh and skin may be folded and manipulated in a

[48] Rupprich, *Dürer*, vol. 2, 115. Ashcroft, *Documentary Biography*, vol. 1, 380 n. 11.

[49] Rupprich, *Dürer*, vol. 1, 215. Ashcroft, *Documentary Biography*, vol. 2, 767.

[50] See Chipps Smith, *Dürer*, 24–6.

[51] 'Selbstbildnis des etwa zwanzigjährigen Dürer' (Self-Portrait of Dürer around the Age of Twenty), 1491/2, in Friedrich-Alexander-Universität Erlangen-Nürnberg, Graphische Sammlung, UER-Zeichnungen B 155.

[52] See Christopher Heuer, 'Dürer's Folds', *Anthropology and Aesthetics* 59–60 (2011), 249–65, here 253.

similar manner to clothing and fabric. The image represents a starting point for what would become an important element in Dürer's depiction of the body, as he began to use bodily form and the flesh in much the same way as he used drapery; to convey emotional significance.

Writing of this image, David Freedberg has stated that Dürer's pose, with hand supporting head, 'establishes the mood of anxiety, melancholy and compassion'. Freedberg draws on German art historian Aby Warburg's notion of the *Pathosformel*, a term Warburg first used to describe the expression of pathos through bodily movement in Dürer's drawing of the 'Death of Orpheus' from 1494.[53] Building on this concept, Freedberg suggests that the superior artist 'consciously or unconsciously knows how best to convey the emotions he or she wishes to convey through the movements of the body' and argues that this 'consists of arousing in the viewer the activation of the same neural circuits that underlie movement'. According to Freedberg, the viewer, when faced with an image of bodily gesture, undergoes an inward simulation of the same movement, optimally resulting in 'the arousal of the correct emotions' in the viewer themselves.[54] Viewers, as well as artists, encounter images as embodied beings, which determines how they experience and understand such images. Yet Freedberg's specific argument does not stand up to considerations of body size, seeming to rely on all viewers possessing the same figure. The inward simulation of particular movements and postures would surely be influenced by the form of the viewer's body and their perception of how this form related to the bodies they were observing. Taking the example of the 'Death of Orpheus', a fatter person would experience the central figure's posture differently to a thinner person, and this would not require their bodies to actually replicate the movement. The experience of living in a large body, where one's flesh would be more likely to roll or bunch up around the waist and joints would influence even the imagined sensation of this position. The affective resonances of such an image would therefore be shaped by the viewer's own bodily form.

Dürer recognized, consciously or unconsciously, that it was not merely the posture and movement of the body which constructed emotional meaning, but also the body's shape and fleshiness. In his 1491 self-portrait the image of melancholy, anxiety, and concentration is created by his pose and by his depiction of the flesh and the imposition of this posture upon it.[55] By showing flesh which was taut and flat, or rolling, wrinkling, folding, and sagging, Dürer utilized the affective

[53] David Freedberg, 'Dürer's Limbs', in Stephanie Buck and Stephanie Porras (eds), *The Young Dürer: Drawing the Figure* (London, 2013), 37–56, here, 45. For Warburg's writings on the *Pathosformel* see for instance: Aby Warburg, *The Renewal of Pagan Antiquity: Contributions to the Cultural History of the European Renaissance*, introduction by Kurt W. Forster, tr. David Britt (Los Angeles, 1999), 553–8. This image is in the Hamburger Kunsthalle, Kupferstichkabinett Inv. Nr. 23006.

[54] Freedberg, 'Dürer's Limbs', 47–8.

[55] This use of folding flesh is of particularly significance given that the representation of emotion through folded drapery was a central component of Warburg's *Pathosformel*. Ibid. 53.

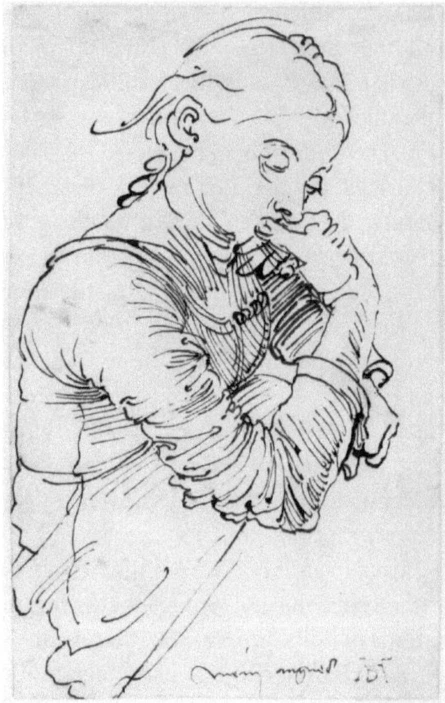

Figure 3.8 Albrecht Dürer, Agnes Dürer, 1494. Pen and ink, 15.7 × 9.8 cm. Albertina, Vienna, public domain. Completed shortly after their marriage, Dürer captured his wife in an unguarded moment. He took care over the curves of her body and contemplated its interaction with her clothing.

potential of the body. Creating a quick ink sketch of his new wife Agnes in 1494 (Figure 3.8), for instance, Dürer observed her posture, as she rests her chin on the back of her hand, as well as the interaction of her body with her dress. He used curved lines at the side of her figure to contemplate how her flesh pressed into her clothing. The image appears full of affection.[56] Seeming to capture his wife in an unguarded moment, Dürer's drawing suggests an intimacy which goes beyond his inscription of *mein Agnes.* The care that he took over the curves of her body, noticing even such slight details as the folding of her flesh at a seam, demonstrates a closeness which is enhanced through the informal manner of the portrait.

Throughout his career, Dürer used body size and fleshiness to present emotion, reserving the most explicit examples of this for such private drawings. In his portrait of his dying mother from 1514 (Figure. 3.9), for example, Dürer represented feelings

[56] Chipps Smith, *Dürer,* 50–3. Recent scholarship has challenged the view put forward by Panofsky that the Dürer's was a 'loveless marriage'. Panofsky, *Life and Art of Dürer,* 6–7. See Corine Schleif, 'Albrecht Dürer between Agnes Frey and Willibald Pirckheimer', in Larry Silver and Jeffrey Chipps Smith (eds), *The Essential Dürer* (Philadelphia, 2010), 185–205, 267–71.

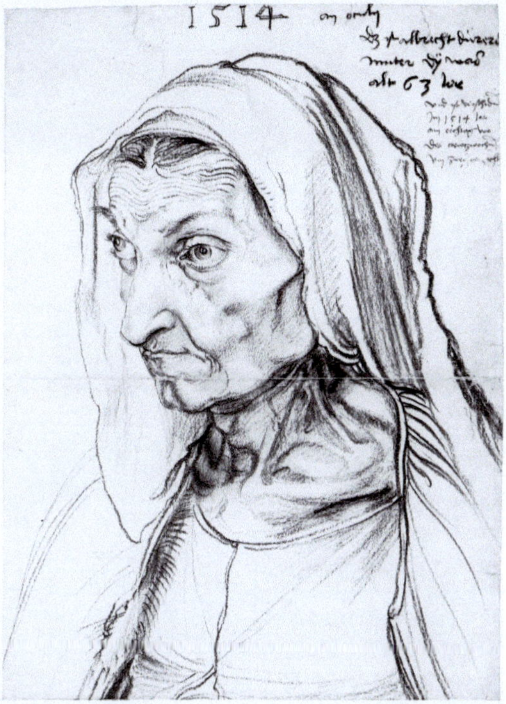

Figure 3.9 Albrecht Dürer, Barbara Dürer, 1514. Charcoal on paper, 42.2 × 30.6 cm. Kupferstichkabinett Berlin, public domain. Dürer depicted the emaciated body of his dying mother in this private drawing.

of grief, loss, and desperation through the depiction of her wasted body.[57] He was concerned to present a naturalistic depiction of her sickness and frailty, yet he also exaggerated his mother's emaciated upper body, showing her face and neck to be gaunt and skeletal.[58] He wrote in his 'Memory Book' (*Gedenkbuch*), 'I feel so grieved for her that I cannot express', and given early modern associations between extreme thinness and unhappiness, suffering and discomfort, his rendering of her emaciated body appears to reflect his emotional description of the 'great poverty, scorn, contempt, mocking words, terrors and great adversities' she suffered in her life.[59] In Dürer's 1524 portrait of Pirckheimer at the age of 53,

[57] Based on this image, it is believed that Dürer's mother suffered from a wasting disease which left her emaciated. Wolfgang Pirsig, 'Dürers Mutter: Aus ärztlicher Sicht', in Michael Roth (ed.), *Dürers Mutter: Schönheit, Alter und Tod im Bild der Renaissance* (Berlin, 2006), 17–22.

[58] See Michael Roth, 'Dürers Mutter in der Bildniskunst Albrecht Dürers', in Roth, *Dürers Mutter*, 129–35, here 132.

[59] Jeffrey Chipps Smith, 'Dürer's Losses and the Dilemma of Being', in Lynne Tatlock (ed.), *Enduring Loss in Early Modern Germany: Cross Disciplinary Perspectives* (Leiden, 2010), 71–101, here 74–5. See also Merback, *Perfection's Therapy*, 178–9. On the connection between thinness, unhappiness, and discomfort see the discussion in Chapter 2.

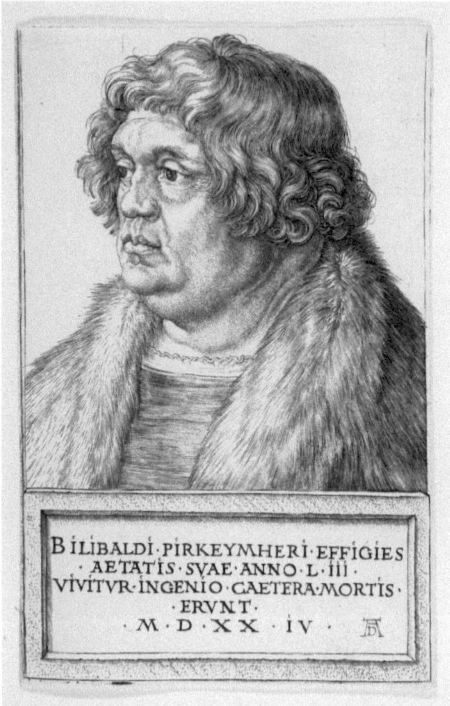
BILIBALDI·PIRKEYMHERI·EFFIGIES
·AETATIS·SVAE·ANNO·L·III·
VIVITVR·INGENIO·CAETERA·MORTIS·
·ERVNT·
·M·D·XX·IV·

Figure 3.10 Albrecht Dürer, Portrait of Willibald Pirckheimer, 1524. Engraving, 18.2 × 11.5 cm. Metropolitan Museum of Art, New York, public domain. In this intimate portrait, Dürer presented his friend with a thick and jowly neck, seeming to reflect on the transformation of his body with age and illness.

his careful and sensitive modelling of his friend's thick and jowly neck is suggestive of the pair's emotional closeness (Figure 3.10). Rejecting the format of idealized portraiture, Dürer paid attention to the fleshiness and bulk of Pirckheimer's body. He seems to reflect on the transformation of his friend's body with age and illness (Pirckheimer was suffering from gout), and thus his consideration of body size adds to the intimacy of this engraving.[60]

Depicting Naked Bodies

Dürer's awareness of the potential for body size and fleshiness to convey meaning and emotion encouraged him to experiment with the production of bodies in a range of forms. His early studies of the naked body show that he was particularly interested in capturing the material texture of different bodies, whether fleshy and

[60] Chipps Smith, *Nuremberg*, 125, no. 30; Rublack, *Dürer's Lost Masterpiece*, 143 and 149.

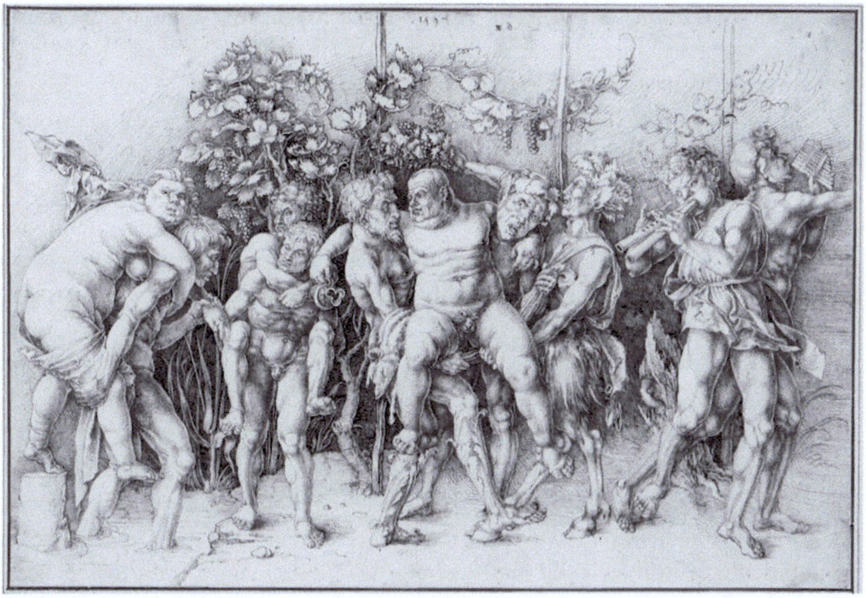

Figure 3.11 Albrecht Dürer, Bacchanal with Silenus, 1494. Pen and ink, 29.8 × 43.3 cm. Albertina, Vienna, public domain. One of two prints by the Italian master Andreae Mantegna which Dürer copied, this is the first image in which Dürer contemplated a variety of differently formed bodies. Dürer enlivened the figures by softening their contours.

soft or firm and muscular. In 1494 he produced copies of two prints by the Italian master Andreae Mantegna: 'Battle of the Sea Gods' and 'Bacchanal with Silenus' (Figure 3.11). In both images, Dürer elevated Mantegna's representation of bodies by softening the contours of the figures, deviating from Mantegna's parallel lines to enliven the flesh.[61] 'Bacchanal with Silenus' is the first image in which Dürer contemplated a variety of differently formed bodies, pre-empting his later interest in the geometrical construction of a wide range of bodily proportions. In doing so, Dürer emphasized the differences between the bodies on show. For the bodies of Silenus, the central figure, and the large woman on the left, Dürer enhanced the rolling qualities of fat, by curving his pen around their bulges and folds.[62] He also presented the softness of these figures by using longer more uniform strokes, creating a sense of expanse which is developed through the presentation of blank

[61] For an overview of the alterations Dürer made to the *Bacchanal* see Andrew John Martin and Christof Metzger, 'Das Ideal der Antike', in Metzger, *Albrecht Dürer*, 192–204, here 198. See also Johann Konrad Eberlein, *Albrecht Dürer* (Reinbek, 2003), 19.

[62] The woman has been identified as the nymph Aegle, who was supposed to be particularly fair and lovely, yet is here transformed into the personification of Gluttony and Sloth. See John Varriano, *Wine a Cultural History* (London, 2011), 116.

space, free of shading and contour. To depict the contrasting, hard and muscular bodies of the other men, Dürer used shorter, more horizontal lines, as well as a greater amount of cross-hatching. Recognizing that the sense of liveliness and frivolity, as well as the debauchery and excess, of this piece was expressed through the fleshiness of the figures as much as their movements and actions, Dürer enlivened their bodies through this attention to bodily form.

Shortly afterwards, Dürer created his own visual scheme to experiment with constructing bodies of varying proportions and in different poses, situating them within the context of the bathhouse. This was the ideal setting in which to explore such variation, since contemporaries understood bathing practices to materially influence the size and form of the body.[63] Dürer produced two such images around the year 1496; the 'Women's Bath' (Figure 3.12) and the 'Men's Bath' (Figure 3.13). These works indicate Dürer's early interest in representing the varying forms that women and men's bodies could take, a fascination which motivated the production of his 'Four Books on Human Proportion'. The two images have notable differences. The 'Women's Bath' was a private drawing, perhaps intended as a model for a future print but which ultimately did not receive wide circulation, while the 'Men's Bath' was a woodcut which was reprinted numerous times. Moreover, the 'Men's Bath' contains greater iconographic complexity. Based on Dürer's connection with the humanist Conrad Celtis, this image has been persuasively interpreted as a humanist allegory, depicting the classical figures of Mercury, Apollo, Bacchus, Socrates, and Plato.[64] The various male figures on display have also been said to represent the different temperaments or complexions of the body, a view which is supported by their position in the bathhouse where people sought to rebalance the humours and restore or promote health.[65] This reading relies on the correlation between humoral complexion and body size which was widely acknowledged in this period and which Dürer himself commented upon.[66] In a 1513 draft of his 'Handbook on Painting' Dürer wrote, 'we have many kinds of human forms, due to the four complexions'.[67]

Such distinctions notwithstanding, the two images share an unquestionable interest in the form of different bodies. Both contain one figure who is notably larger than the others and shown in a seated position. In each case, Dürer considered the materiality of a fat stomach and how it might roll or bunch up in such

[63] See Chapter 2, 46–9.

[64] Thomas Schauerte, *Dürer und Celtis: Die Nürnberger Poetenschule im Aufbruch* (Leipzig, 2015), 103–65.

[65] This argument was first put forward in Edgar Wind, 'Dürer's "Männerbad": A Dionysian Mystery', *Journal of the Warburg Institute* 2 (1939), 269–71. See also Jan-David Mentzel, 'Körper und Welt. Albrecht Dürers *Männerbad* in neuer Deutung', in Thomas Schauerte, Jürgen Müller, and Bertram Kaschek (eds), *Von der Freiheit der Bilder: Spott, Kritik und Subversion in der Kunst der Dürerzeit* (Petersberg, 2013), 58–73.

[66] See Chapter 2, 36–42. On the influence of humoral medicine for Dürer's engraving 'Melencolia I' see Merback, *Perfection's Therapy*, 143–7.

[67] Rupprich, *Dürer*, vol. 2, 119. Aschroft, *Documentary Biography*, vol. 1, 376.

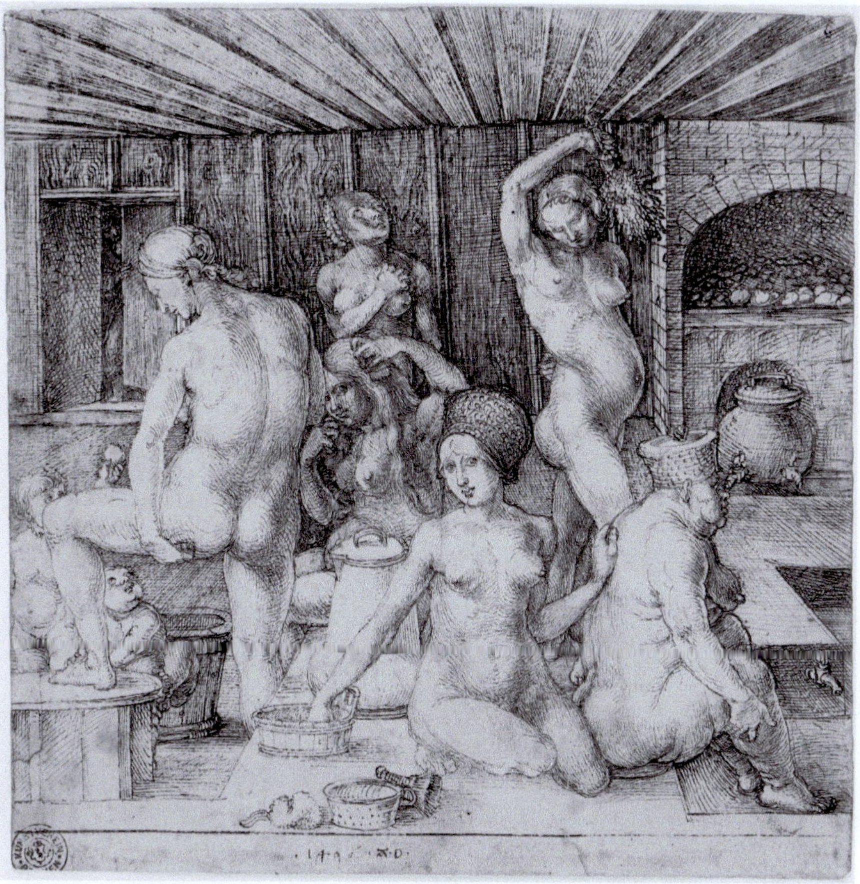

Figure 3.12 Albrecht Dürer, Women's Bath, 1496. Pen and ink, 23.1 × 23 cm. Kunsthalle Bremen—Der Kunstverein in Bremen, public domain. Dürer depicted a range of differently proportioned female bodies in the context of the bathhouse. In the background a clothed voyeur peeks around the open door.

a position. Both figures appear to be influenced by those in Mantegna's engraving but are also distinct. In the 'Women's Bath' in particular, Dürer's presentation of the larger woman's body is softer and more subtle than Mantegna's. The softness with which Dürer renders her body adds to the sensuality of the scene, challenging art historian Kenneth Clark's hostile statement that 'The fat monster on the right confirms [Dürer's] feeling of the obscenity of the whole situation.'[68] There is, certainly, an element of obscenity, as the young child on the left stares directly into the open legs of the standing woman, presenting a confrontation between innocence and sexuality. Yet, the sensitivity with which Dürer renders the women's bodies,

[68] Clark, *The Nude*, 324.

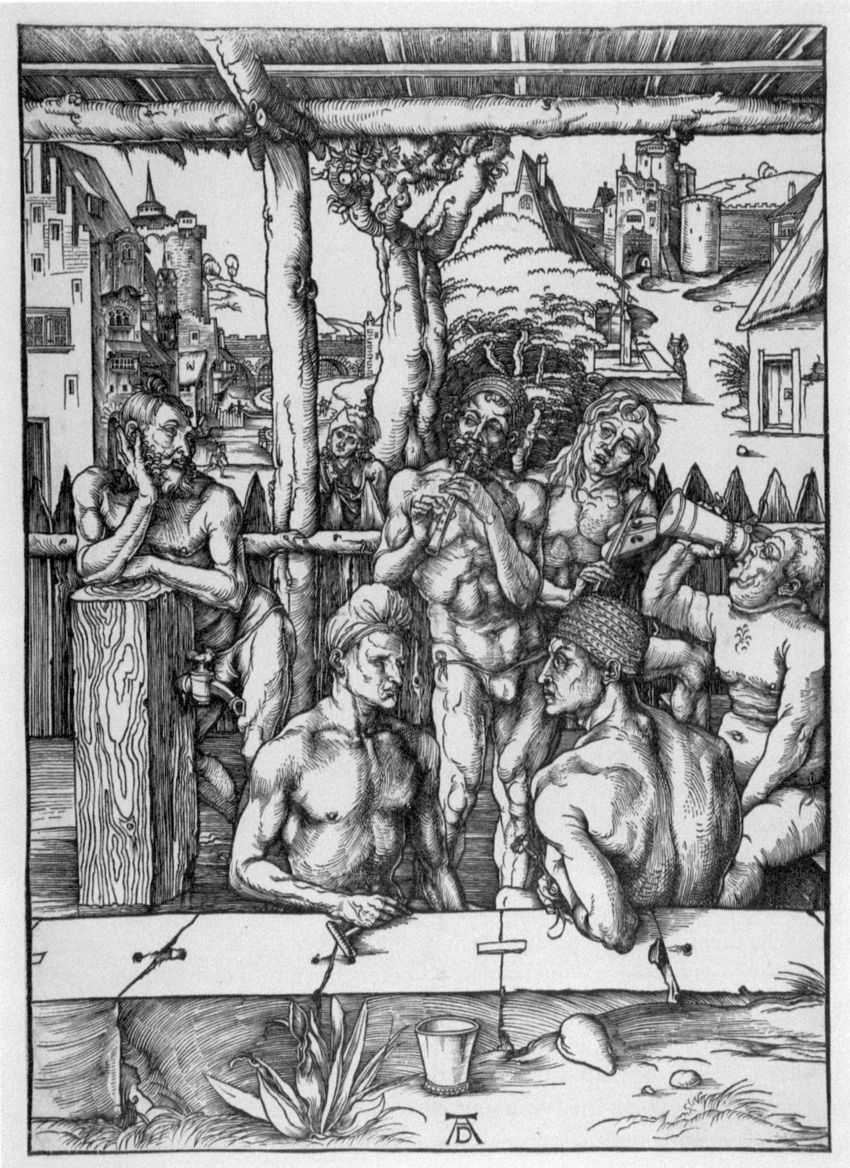

Figure 3.13 Albrecht Dürer, Men's Bath, 1496. Woodcut, 38.7 × 27.9 cm. Metropolitan Museum of Art, New York, public domain. Dürer presented a variety of male figures, possibly intended as a humanist allegory or a representation of the bodily complexions. As in the 'Women's Bath' a dressed observer appears in the background.

as well as the intimacy presented, encourages the view that this is also a celebration and exploration of the female nude. The hand which the central figure places on the back of the larger woman includes her in this sensuality, and there is no reason to believe that she is any less involved in Dürer's wonder and appreciation than the other women depicted.

In both images the other figures, while all being relatively slim, display slight variations in their proportions. Of the two foreground figures in the 'Men's Bath' for instance, the right-hand man has notably broader shoulders than the left-hand figure, while the latter has a somewhat concave belly in comparison to the muscular fullness of the musician above. Similarly, in the 'Women's Bath' the standing figure on the right has a distended belly which contrasts with the seated, centre figure whose body aligns more closely with classical Italian models for the female nude.[69] Both images also show the presence of a clothed voyeur who overlooks the scene. This figure, who in the 'Women's Bath' is disguised behind the partially opened door in the background, is crucial to Dürer's depiction of bodily variety. The inclusion of such a viewer sets up a dichotomy between the dressed and the undressed, the hidden and the exposed. The bathhouse was a key site for the visibility of bodily difference. It was there that the reality of a person's body beneath their clothing would be revealed and both small and great differences between individual bodies could be observed.[70] The Swiss physician Felix Platter, for example, described an acquaintance from Zürich named Hirzel who was the fattest person he had ever seen, and 'when he sat naked in the bathhouse he was an object of wonder for the people who saw his corpulence'.[71] Such wonder was made possible by the context of the bathhouse, and this context likewise enabled Dürer to contemplate a spectrum of bodily forms, culminating in his theorization of human proportion.

Theorizing the Body

Dürer's interest in theories of bodily proportion began with his search for the ideal form for the bodies of Adam and Eve. Their proportions were of particular importance since God had constructed them from the earth in his own image and likeness, understood as both a physical and spiritual resemblance.[72] In Dürer's 1504 engraving, he chose to present Adam and Eve immediately prior to the Fall, and thus in the final instant at which they represented ultimate and

[69] Bonnet, *'Akt' bei Dürer*, 87.

[70] This point is developed in Chapter 5.

[71] Sarah Maria Schober, *Gesellschaft im Exzess: Mediziner in Basel um 1600* (Frankfurt, 2019), 101.

[72] Luther later suggested that it was not a physical resemblance but a spiritual one. See Kathleen Crowther, *Adam and Eve in the Protestant Reformation* (Cambridge, 2010), 66–7.

perfect humanity (Figure 3.5).[73] Dürer sought to convey this perfection through their ideal bodies, which he constructed through geometry following several years of study. Beginning in 1500, Dürer initially focused on the creation of the female body, constructing numerous versions of a nude woman using a compass and measured lines. In doing so he created a range of female forms, varying their size and shape in the search for ideal beauty.

In his resulting engraving, Dürer based his figures on classical forms, reminiscent of the Medici Venus and the Belvedere Apollo, which were familiar to him from Italian prints and drawings.[74] At this point, therefore, he used the classical nude as a model for perfection. Dürer would later write that:

> In the same way that they applied the most beautiful form (*schönsten gestalt*) of man to the proportioning of their idol Apollo, so we will use the same measure for Christ our Lord who is the most beautiful in all the world. And just as they took Venus as the most beautiful woman (*schönste weib*), so we will portray the same fair form (*tzirlich gestalt*) chastely as the purest virgin Mary, mother of God.

In order to 'direct [art] with high honour towards the praise of God', Dürer instructed the reader to use ideal classical proportions for these ideal Christian figures.[75]

Yet when Dürer came to represent Adam and Eve again in 1507 (Figures 3.14 and 3.15), he elongated their proportions, choosing to make their heads one-ninth rather than one-eighth of their overall height. Their bodies thus appear both taller and slimmer in these paintings. Dürer was unable to decide on just one bodily form that he considered to be the most beautiful and this indecision informed his varying presentation of Adam and Eve. While he initially sought a singular ideal for the human body based on classical models, Dürer moved on to the opinion that 'to produce one pattern of human form (*gestalt*) unerringly correctly as being the most beautiful, seems to me impossible'.[76] In part, this difficulty was based on the problem of subjectivity. Earlier Dürer had written that, 'our nature is such that we see one figure or image (*gestalt vnd pildnus*) more gladly than others, even though it is not necessarily better or worse than the rest'.[77] He also recognized that beauty ideals for the body changed over time. Dürer stated, 'certain human forms (*gestalten der menschen*) are more prized and praised at one particular time than at another'.[78] The creation of a beautiful body could, therefore, depend

[73] Ibid. 58–60. See also Koerner, *Moment of Self-Portraiture*, 195.
[74] Chipps Smith, *Nuremberg*, 45.
[75] Rupprich, Dürer, vol. 2, 104. Ashcroft, *Documentary Biography*, vol. 1, 339. I have translated *schönsten Gestalt* as 'most beautiful figure' (Ashcroft translates as 'ideal figure').
[76] Rupprich, *Dürer*, vol. 3, 285. Ashcroft, *Documentary Biography*, vol. 1, 523.
[77] Rupprich, *Dürer*, vol. 2, 113. Ashcroft, *Documentary Biography*, vol. 1, 368.
[78] Rupprich, *Dürer*, vol. 3, 285. Ashcroft, *Documentary Biography*, vol 1, 523.

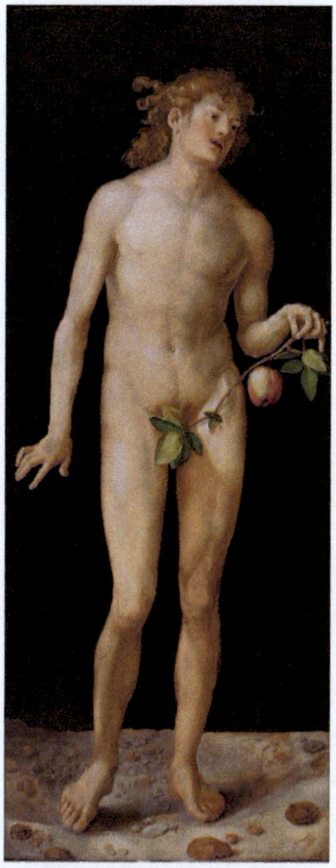

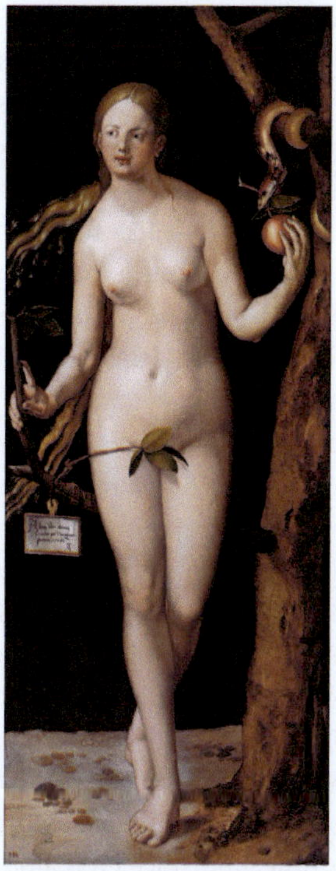

Figure 3.14 Albrecht Dürer, Adam, 1507. Oil on panel, 209 × 81 cm. Prado, Madrid. © Photographic Archive Museo Nacional del Prado.

Figure 3.15 Albrecht Dürer, Eve, 1507. Oil on panel, 209 × 81 cm. Prado, Madrid. © Photographic Archive Museo Nacional del Prado. Dürer's paintings display a different model of bodily perfection from his 1504 engraving—the bodies of Adam and Eve appear taller and slimmer.

on the ideal that was most in favour at a given moment. In a 1512 draft of his 'Discourse on Aesthetics', Dürer claimed that his book could help 'someone who wants to make a portrait based on the general estimation of what people consider beautiful.'[79] By his final draft, however, Dürer wrote 'When we ask, how shall we make a beautiful image, some will say: follow the general taste. Others will not concede that and neither do I.' Dürer understood that 'divine truth alone…contains the secret of what the most beautiful form and measure (*schönste gestalt vnd maß*) of man may be.'[80]

[79] Rupprich, *Dürer*, vol. 3, 275. Ashcroft, *Documentary Biography*, vol. 1, 430. This text has traditionally been termed the 'Aesthetic Excursus' but Jeffrey Ashcroft has suggested it should instead be termed the 'Discourse on Aesthetics' see Ashcroft, *Documentary Biography*, vol. 1, 425.

[80] Rupprich, *Dürer*, vol. 3, 293. Ashcroft, *Documentary Biography*, vol. 2, 875.

This acknowledgement of the limits of human knowledge, as well as a recognition of conflicting ideals both within and across time, encouraged Dürer to argue for a theory of proportions which was not a universal canon but accounted for the differences between bodies. He recognized that multiple bodily forms could be considered equally beautiful, and on this point, he explicitly took the fatness or thinness of bodies into account. He wrote: 'it is quite possible for two different pictures to be painted, neither resembling the other, one fatter and one thinner figure (*ein dickre, ein dünre gestalt*), and for nobody to be able to judge which is more beautiful.'[81] Crucially, therefore, Dürer believed that both fat and thin bodies could be beautiful as long as they were well proportioned. It was important, Dürer stated, that one body part was not 'fleshy' (*fleischig*) while another was 'skinny' (*mager*) but that each part existed in harmony.[82] This was the first time such a conclusion had been reached as part of an artistic theory of ideal proportions.[83]

By the time of his final version of the 'Discourse on Aesthetics', therefore, which was published as part of his 'Four Books on Human Proportion', Dürer no longer described his aim as the construction of definitive beauty. Instead he wrote, 'I do not know how to describe reliably what definitive measure might bring us close to true beauty. Yet I would gladly help as best I know how, to eliminate and avoid the crude deformity (*grobe vngestalt*) of our work except in cases where someone set out deliberately to produce deformity.'[84] Since people's opinions on beauty changed over time, and since God alone knew the ideal proportions for the human body, Dürer suggested that the ultimate aim of his works on proportion was to help artists create images which would please those who commissioned them. The satisfaction of a client deserved praise, Dürer stated, and it also required practical experience. It followed, therefore, that 'no powerful artist should devote himself to one type of subject alone but should be practised and knowledgeable in many different ways and about all types'. This would enable them 'to portray whichever category of image may be demanded', including those which might be considered 'deformed'. Through correct measurement, Dürer's books on proportion would enable an artist to portray 'all the types of human being (*allerley Geschlecht der Menschen*), whether their nature is fiery, airy, watery or earthy', once again connecting body type to humoral complexion.[85]

As promised, the 'Four Books on Human Proportion' included a wide range of figures of varying size and shape (Figures 3.16–3.19). In the first book, Dürer

[81] Rupprich, *Dürer*, vol. 2, 119. Ashcroft translates Dürer's *ein dickre, ein dünre gestalt* as 'chalk and cheese' rather than a literal translation which shows the importance of various sizes of body in Dürer's understanding. See Ashcroft, *Documentary Biography*, vol. 1, 377.

[82] Rupprich, *Dürer*, vol. 3, 285. Ashcroft, *Documentary Biography*, vol. 1, 523.

[83] Fedja Anzelewsky, 'Dürers "ästhetischer Exkurs" in seiner Proportionslehre', in Friedrich Mielke (ed.), *Kaleidoskop. Eine Festschrift für Fritz Baumgart zum 75. Geburtstag* (Berlin, 1977), 70–8, here, 72.

[84] Rupprich, *Dürer*, vol. 3, 293. Ashcroft, *Documentary Biography*, vol. 2, 875–6.

[85] Rupprich, *Dürer*, vol. 3, 296. Ashcroft, *Documentary Biography*, vol. 2, 880.

outlined the construction of five different types of women and men, with ratios of head to overall height varying from one to seven, seven-and-a-half, eight, nine, and ten. These were constructed around a central axis and shown from the front, back, and in profile.[86] In the following books, Dürer presented mathematical systems to diversify these types still further.[87] This included altering the body's form—using 'the reverser', Dürer explained in an earlier draft, 'you may make a thing long or short, fat or thin (*dick oder dün*), broad or narrow (*preit oder schmall*)'.[88] While the correct construction of all such bodies could ensure an image was beautiful and pleasing to a patron, Dürer's description of the figures shows that he

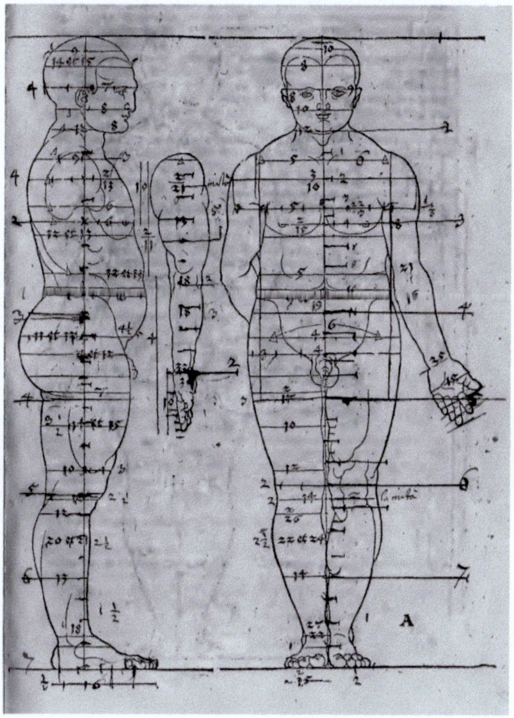

Figure 3.16 Albrecht Dürer, *Four Books on Human Proportion* (Nuremberg, 1528), fol. Avi^{r}. Glasgow School of Art Library, CC BY-SA 3.0. The proportions for a 'thick rustic man' show a solid and broad male figure. The body is not shown to be particularly fleshy, reflecting Dürer's use of the term *dick*. His body is seven times the length of his head.

[86] For an overview of the *Four Books on Human Proportion* see Jaya Remond, 'Albrecht Dürer: *Vier Bücher von menschlicher Proportion* and Proportional Study', in Susan Dackerman (ed.), *Prints and the Pursuit of Knowledge in Early Modern Europe*, exh. cat., Harvard Art Museums (Cambridge, MA, 2011), 236, cat. no. 54.

[87] Rupprich, *Dürer*, vol. 3, 290. Ashcroft, *Documentary Biography*, vol. 2, 872.

[88] Rupprich, *Dürer*, vol. 3, 276. Ashcroft, *Documentary Biography*, vol. 1, 431.

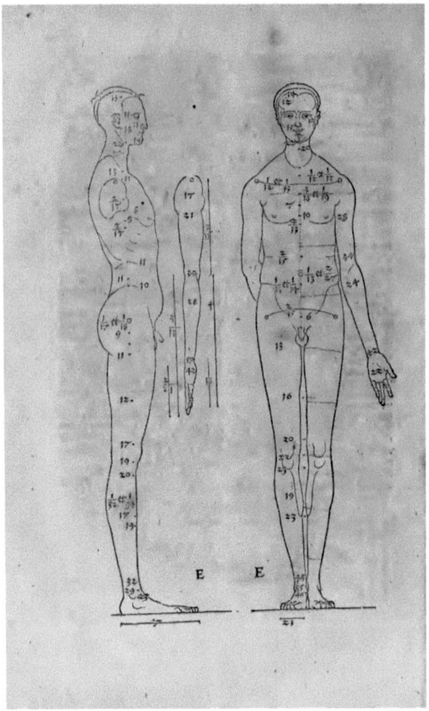

Figure 3.17 Albrecht Dürer, *Four Books on Human Proportion* (Nuremberg, 1528), fol. Diii^v^. Glasgow School of Art Library, licence: CC BY-SA 3.0. Dürer described this figure as a tall, thin man. His body is ten times the length of his head.

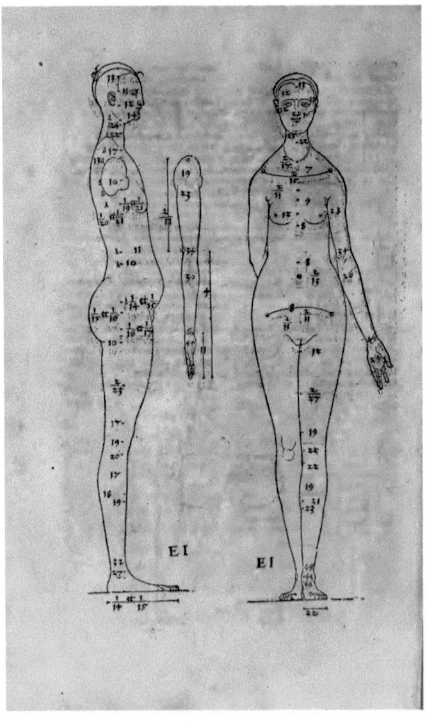

Figure 3.18 Albrecht Dürer, *Four Books on Human Proportion* (Nuremberg, 1528), fol. Dv^v^. Glasgow School of Art Library, licence: CC BY-SA 3.0. This female figure has the same head to body ratio as the previous male figure. This is the thinnest female figure Dürer represented in the text.

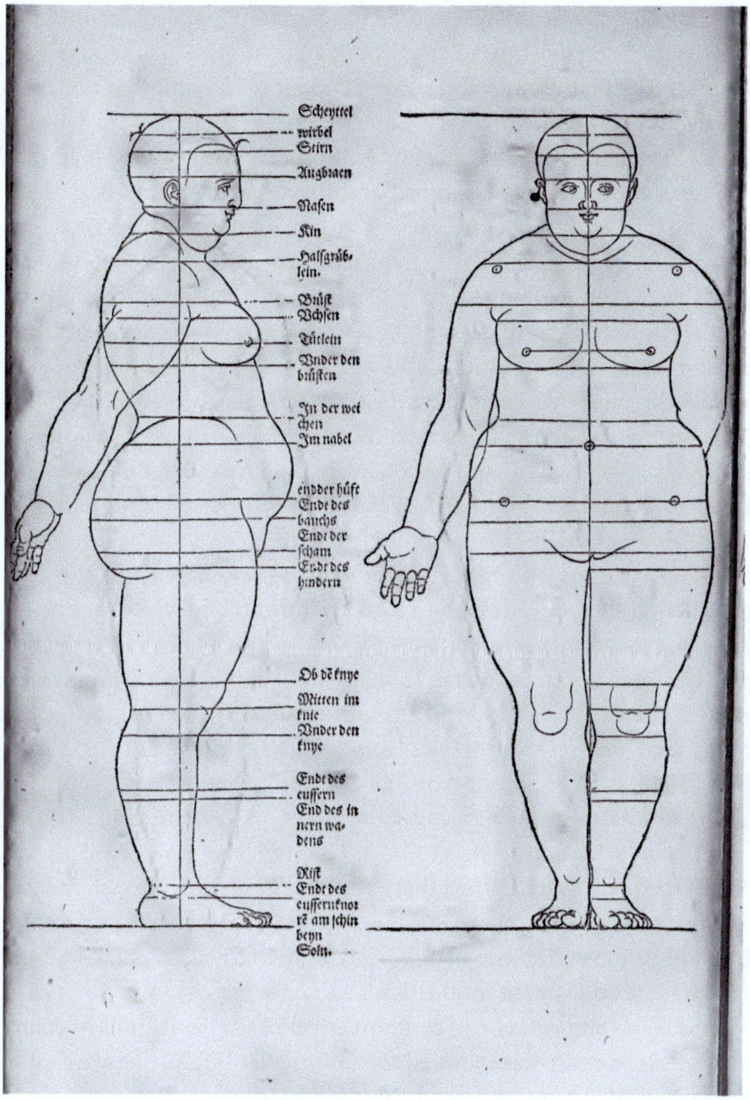

Figure 3.19 Albrecht Dürer, *Four Books on Human Proportion* (Nuremberg, 1528), fol. Rii^{v}. Glasgow School of Art Library, licence: CC BY-SA 3.0. This figure shows the effects of applying Dürer's method of the 'twin pointer' to an existing female figure with a head to height ratio of seven, in order to make her body thicker and wider. This is the largest female figure Dürer included in the book.

attributed certain characteristics to different bodies. He stated, for instance, that his book would teach one how to create both a 'rustic (*pewrisch*) and noble (*adellich*) figure'.[89] The first geometrical construction included in the volume is that of a 'thick rustic man' (*einen dicken bewrischen Man*) (Figure 3.16) which is followed by a 'strong, thick, rustic woman' (*ein starck/dick/bewrisch Weib*).[90] These 'rustic' bodies are represented as broad and strong, while 'noble' bodies are slender, showing how body size could be used to represent the virtues or characteristics of particular social ranks. Dürer depicted such 'rustic' figures in his engraving of a peasant couple dancing from 1514 (Figure 3.20) in which he presented their bodies as heavy and thick, with bulky limbs, creating a sense of clumsiness in their movements. The rustic simplicity of solid, hefty bodies, in contrast to self-consciously cultivated slenderness, became increasingly entwined with conceptions of Germanness across the sixteenth century, encouraging mature German men to present themselves with large and bulky figures. Here, however, Dürer continued to connect nobility with slenderness, likely reflecting late fifteenth-century ideals and possibly his own slim form.

Dürer's instructions on proportion presented seemingly endless possibilities for constructing the body, though to avoid 'deformity' he wrote that one should take care: 'for sometimes one contracts things too much or expands them too far, so that...the body becomes too fat, thin, broad or slim (*zu dick, dünn, breyt oder schmal*)'.[91] Extremes of fatness and thinness were thus understood in terms of 'deformity' by Dürer. He also wrote: 'you can make any nude hard or soft (*hert oder lind*). But it is more appropriate that a strong corpulent nude figure (*ein dick starck nackett pild*) is given a harder stamp...than a delicate, thin, slender nude (*ein subtill dün schwankell nackett bild*)'.[92] Dürer thus considered the textural qualities of the body, and he wrote that one should not do 'too much in the case of any one thing', suggesting that to make a corpulent body 'soft', or a thin body 'hard', would be too extreme to be beautiful. Dürer also wrote, however, that 'one must make some adjustment for the thin and fat (*mägeren vnd feysten*) in images, yet soft and hard (*lind vnd hördt*) can properly be used in all kinds of contrasts as one wishes'.[93] If contrast was required for a particular image, therefore, one could use soft corpulent figures and hard thin bodies, though such contrasts 'do not

[89] Rupprich, *Dürer*, vol. 3, 277. Ashcroft translates these terms as 'rustic' and 'aristocratic', see Ashcroft, *Documentary Biography*, vol. 1, 432.

[90] Albrecht Dürer, *Hierinn sind begriffen vier Bücher von Menschlicher Proportion* (Nuremberg, 1528), fols Aiii^v and B^r.

[91] Rupprich, *Dürer*, vol. 3, 291. Ashcroft, *Documentary Biography*, vol. 2, 872.

[92] Rupprich, *Dürer*, vol. 3, 276. Ashcroft, *Documentary Biography*, vol. 1, 431.

[93] Rupprich, *Dürer*, vol. 3, 295. Ashcroft, *Documentary Biography*, vol. 2, 878. Here I have adjusted Ashcroft's translation of *doch* from 'and' to 'yet'.

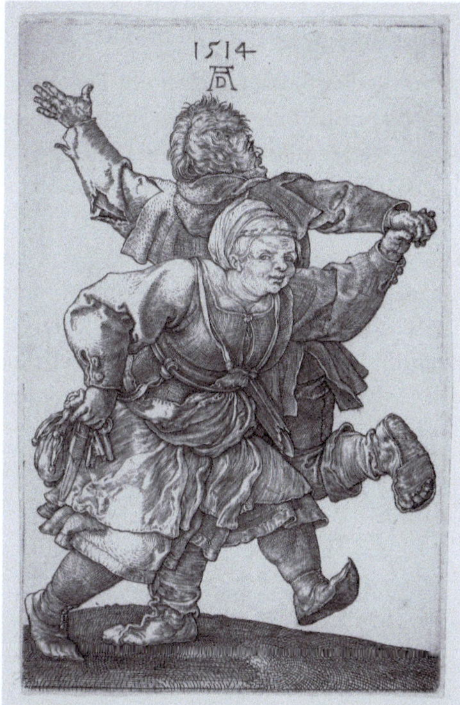

Figure 3.20 Albrecht Dürer, Peasant Couple Dancing, 1514. Engraving, 11.8 × 7.5 cm. Metropolitan Museum of Art, New York, public domain. Dürer presented peasant bodies as broad and bulky, indicating the clumsiness of their movements.

look good if they are wrongly used and do not show a master's touch'.[94] To create pleasing work a painter needed to master the art of proportion and this included the ability to construct bodies of all different sizes and shapes.

Questions of body size, fatness, and thinness mattered to Dürer for creating meaning, beauty, and emotion in his artworks. His theoretical texts presented a broad range of body types which could be constructed using mathematical systems, enabling the creation of a beautiful and well-executed painting. Such precision was necessary to ensure the satisfaction of one's patrons, yet even more importantly, Dürer claimed, 'work well done honours God'. According to Dürer, therefore, it was essential 'for everyone to apply experience and understanding to work that is to be shown in public'.[95] In private, however, he also acknowledged the possibility of crafting bodily forms which resisted theorization altogether.

[94] Rupprich, *Dürer,* vol. 3, 291. Ashcroft, *Documentary Biography*, vol. 2, 873.
[95] Rupprich, *Dürer,* vol. 3, 291. Ashcroft, *Documentary Biography*, vol. 2, 873.

The Fat Female Body

Dürer was privately fascinated by the fat female body. This was a figure which deeply intrigued him, though it appears only rarely in his public works. The variations on this form in his copy of Mantegna from 1494 and the 'Women's Bath' from 1496 were both private drawings rather than prints to be circulated to a wider audience. Probably the largest female body created by Dürer for a public viewership appears in his engraving of 'Nemesis' or 'The Great Fortune' from 1501–2 (Figure 3.21). This image is thought to be Dürer's first printed representation of a constructed figure based, though imperfectly, on Vitruvius's theory of human proportion.[96] Yet her physicality departs from classical models.[97] Her body is weighty, with muscular thighs, rounded buttocks, and a protruding stomach. Her

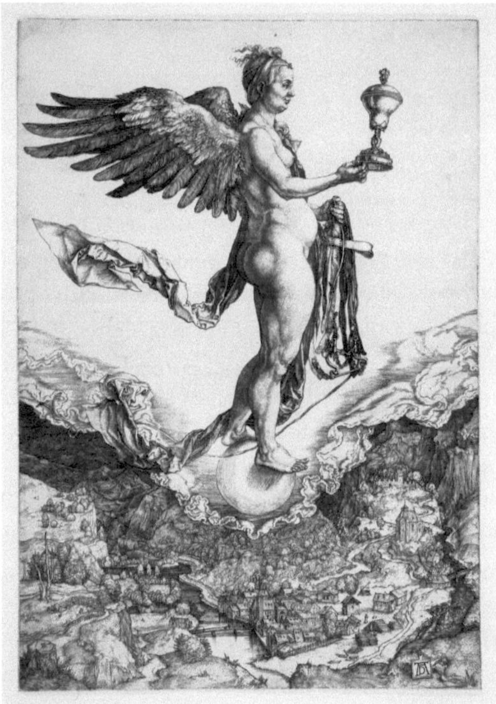

Figure 3.21 Albrecht Dürer, Nemesis, 1501–2. Engraving, 33.3 × 23.1 cm. Metropolitan Museum of Art, New York, public domain. The figure of Nemesis was based on Vitruvian proportion, but her physicality departs from classical models. Her fleshiness emphasizes her perfect balance upon the sphere of Fortuna.

[96] Chipps Smith, *Dürer*, 138.
[97] See Jaya Remond, 'Dürer: Nemesis', in Dackerman, *Prints and Pursuit*, 232.

fleshiness is central to this image which merges the representation of Nemesis, the goddess of retribution, with the figure of Fortuna, the goddess of luck. In the humanist tradition, Fortuna was understood to maintain 'such a steady and unvarying mean in all things that one kind of fortune is unfailingly balanced and interspersed with the other', as described by humanist Helius Eobanus Hessus in 1515.[98] Dürer used the physicality of this female nude to present this perfect balance, showing her weighty body to be delicately poised on a sphere, as was typical of images of Fortuna. The heaviness of her form adds to the seeming impossibility of this position, just as the large and heavy metal cup which rests on her fingertips appears to defy any force of weight or gravity.[99]

Dürer's use of body size in this image becomes even more apparent when we consider the numerous caricatures that emerged based on his famous print. Inverting his presentation of Fortuna as steady and balanced, these caricatures drew instead on the competing image of fortune as a foolish and unreliable woman. In 1513 (Figure 3.22), for example, Urs Graf used the size of her nude body to enhance the presentation of Fortuna's immorality and caprice. Where Dürer's nude stood poised and controlled despite her solid form, Graf's figure appears unable even to lift her large body off the ground. With one foot on the sphere she appears in a classic pose of fickleness, and she looks down to where she has dropped both her lamp and maiden's crown (*Jungfraukranz*) symbolizing a loss of honour in each case.[100] The large size and fleshiness of her figure is central to Graf's presentation of her volatility, seeming to prevent her from balancing on the sphere at all. Her bulk creates, therefore, an image of clumsy heaviness which contrasts starkly with Dürer's perfectly balanced Nemesis.

In his personal drawings, Dürer explored the possibility of presenting larger, fleshier women. Around 1500, Dürer depicted a female nude praying (Figure 3.23), focusing on the curves of her lower body, and using his line strokes to mould her fleshy form. Although highly unusual for nude images, Dürer was fascinated by depicting bodies from behind and he did so on multiple occasions.[101] He repeated this view in 1505, again representing the body of a voluptuous woman. Here he spent time modelling her figure, using colour, highlight, and contour to create

[98] Harry Vredeveld (ed.), *The Poetic Works of Helius Eobanus Hessus*, vol. 3. *King of Poets 1514–1517* (Leiden, 2012), 85.

[99] On the significance of the cup in Dürer's print see Jennifer Spinks, 'Objects in Motion: Albrecht Dürer's *Nemesis*', in Edward H. Wouk and Jennifer Spinks (eds), *Albrecht Dürer's Material World* (Manchester, 2023), 35–47.

[100] Christianne Andersson, 'Jungfrau, Dirne, Fortuna: Das Bild der Frau in den Zeichnungen von Urs Graf', *Kritische Berichte* 16 (1988), 26–35, here 31.

[101] Bodo Brinkmann, 'Liebe von hinten, Liebe von vorn: Dürer und Pirckheimer lesen Lukian. Love from the Back, Love from the Front: Dürer and Pirckheimer Read Lucian', in Bodo Brinkmann (ed.), *Hexenlust und Sündenfall: Die seltsamen Phantasien des Hans Baldung Grien. Witches' Lust and the Fall of Man: The Strange Fantasies of Hans Baldung Grien*, exh. cat., Städel Museum, Frankfurt am Main (Petersberg, 2007), 97–108.

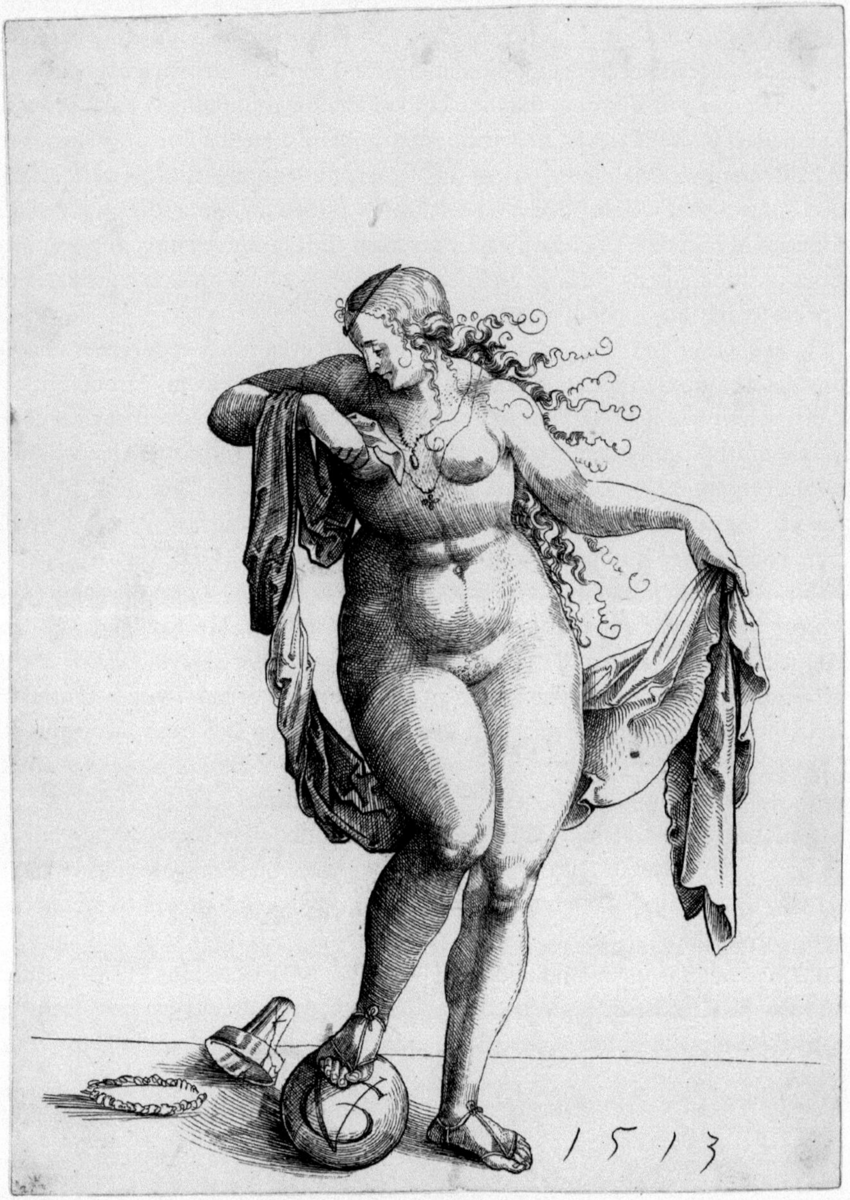

Figure 3.22 Urs Graf, Foolish Young Woman, 1513. Pen and ink, 28.8 × 20.5 cm. Kunstmuseum Basel, public domain. Graf inverted Dürer's presentation of Nemesis as steady and balanced, instead showing the fickleness and volatility of Fortuna who is unable to balance her large body atop the sphere at her feet.

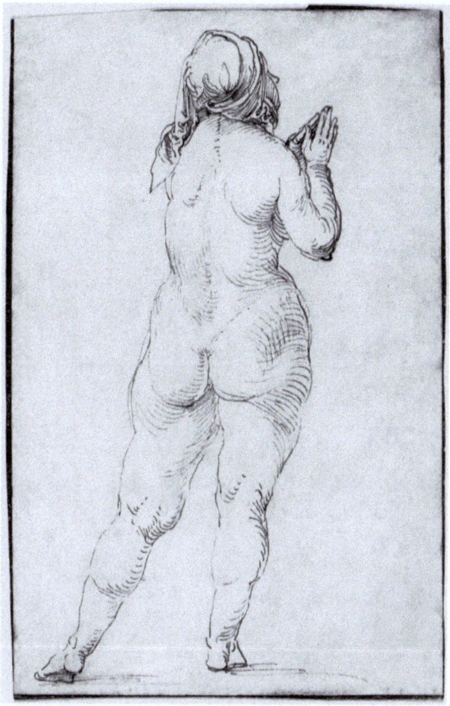

Figure 3.23 Albrecht Dürer, Female Nude Praying, 1500. Pen and ink, 21.5 × 13.6 cm. National Gallery of Art, Washington, DC, public domain. This image is one of several studies completed by Dürer which show fleshy female figures from behind.

this image of soft fleshiness. He focused, for instance, on the rolls of her inner thighs, particularly on the leg which lifts lightly off the floor in a contrapposto stance.[102]

Then, in 1508, Dürer's interest in more extreme versions of the fat female body reached its peak. Dürer focused on constructing a large woman's body in profile, repeating this multiple times on separate study sheets with very slight alterations.[103] In one image, Dürer added a line to the back of the figure, enlarging the buttocks (Figure 3.24), and in other studies, he emphasized the bulges of fat around the woman's neck and legs. As in the numerous drafts of his works on proportion, in these sketches Dürer was developing his ideas and understanding through practice and repetition, yet he struggled to construct the figure he had in mind. Besides one study, Dürer presented the figure seated on a small stool (Figure 3.25). As for the large figure in his 'Women's Bath' Dürer thus experimented with the effects of posture on the fat body, showing her belly to bunch up through the

[102] 'Une grosse femme nue, de dos' (A Large Nude Woman from behind), 1505, Louvre, Paris, Inv. No. 18609, recto.

[103] Anne-Sophie Pellé, 'Mesurer l'excès: Albrecht Dürer et la figure obèse', *Histoire de l'art* 70 (2012), 1–10, here 4.

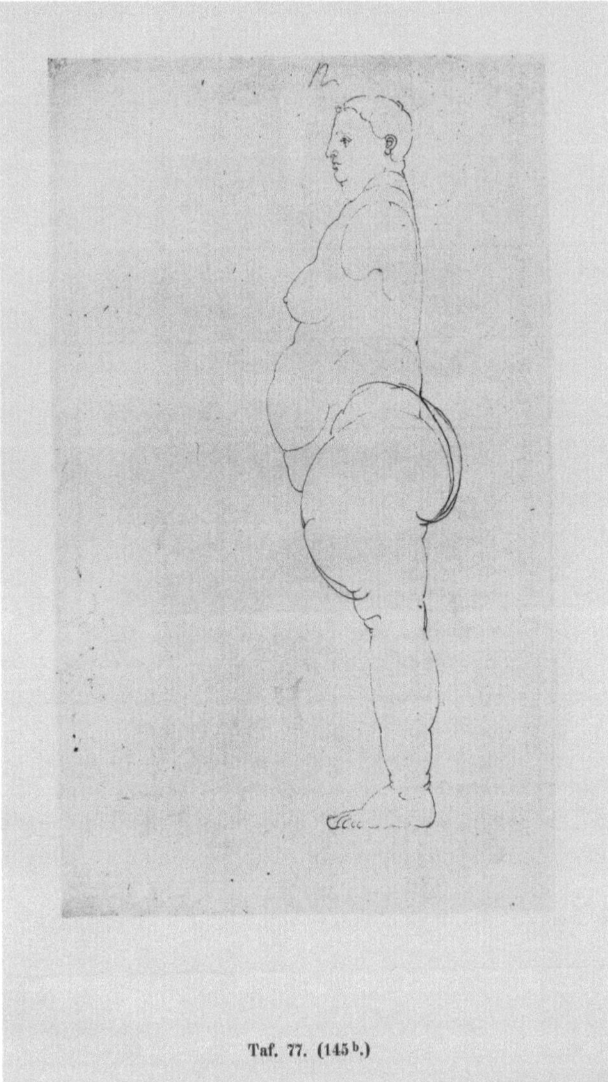

Figure 3.24 Albrecht Dürer, Stout Woman in Profile, 1508. From *Das Skizzenbuch von Albrecht Dürer in der Königl. Öffentl. Bibliothek zu Dresden* (Strassburg im Elsass, 1905), figure 77. Sächsische Landesbibliothek, Dresden, public domain. Dürer experimented with constructing a fat female form, beginning with a profile view. Several lines have been added to enlarge the woman's buttocks and thigh.

compression of sitting and leaning forward. He was particularly intrigued by the effects of this position, as he then created another study of the woman's body in blocks, showing her standing and sitting and considering how the building blocks of her form, and the curves of fat attached to them, would shift and fold through movement.

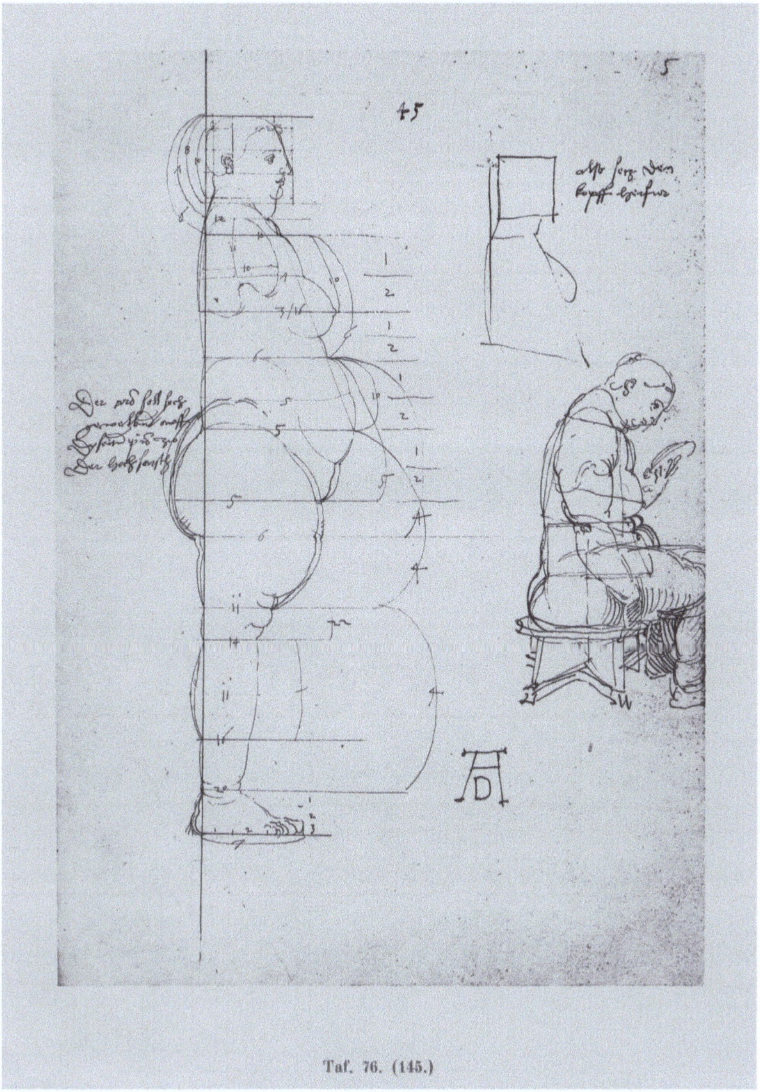

Figure 3.25 Albrecht Dürer, Stout Woman in Profile and Seated on Stool, 1508. From *Das Skizzenbuch von Albrecht Dürer in der Königl. Öffentl. Bibliothek zu Dresden* (Strassburg im Elsass, 1905), figure 76. Sächsische Landesbibliothek, Dresden, public domain. Dürer was interested in the effects of posture on the body and by showing this figure on a small stool, he contemplated how her fat would roll and bunch up when seated.

Dürer also presented this figure from the front (Figure 3.26). Perhaps due to his uncertainty, Dürer repeatedly overdrew the outline of her body, attempting to position the belly, limbs, and chin in the correct place. Through these reworked lines, Dürer appears to reflect on degrees of fatness and even the process of accumulating fat on the body. Examining the belly, for instance, the three lines of its

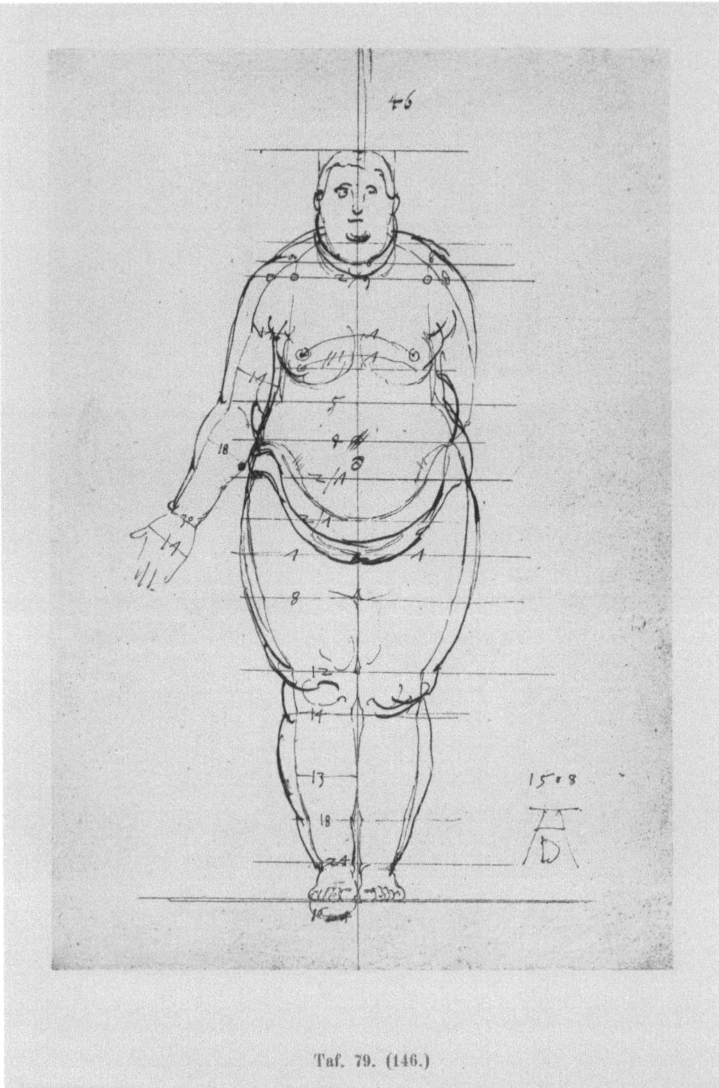

Figure 3.26 Albrecht Dürer, Stout Woman from the Front, 1508. From *Das Skizzenbuch von Albrecht Dürer in der Königl. Öffentl. Bibliothek zu Dresden* (Strassburg im Elsass, 1905), figure 79. Sächsische Landesbibliothek, Dresden, public domain. Dürer presented the same figure from the front. He overdrew the lines of her form, appearing to reflect on degrees of fatness or even the accumulation of fat on the body.

positioning seem to show the various places in which such fat could rest depending on the extent of the body's size. These lines also evoke the materiality of fat, showing it to bulge and hang from the body in a manner which Dürer's later models of larger women, included in his 'Four Books on Human Proportion', did not replicate.

In another version of this figure, Dürer covered his study in text, going into great detail concerning its construction, and clearly struggling to describe this process concisely and systematically. He wrote for instance that 'the curves of the flesh should descend from the hips to the level of the groin, so that the body is a little wider where the belly ends than at the hips'.[104] Rather than measured calculation, the prominence of the belly depended on the painter's judgement. Dürer thus appears unable to rationalize these proportions through arithmetic construction.[105] He was also unable to fully represent these figures with their fleshy curves and hanging, heavy bellies in the geometrically constructed figures that he included in the third section of his 'Four Books on Human Proportion'. The figures in his published theoretical works were deliberately simplified, enabling readers to create the basic outlines of bodies to which they would then add detail as they completed the painting. Yet in these earlier drawings we see Dürer attempting to theorize the details of the fat body and contemplating the materiality of fat which rolled, folded, and bulged, and did not fit easily within any systematic method of constructing the body. Despite his repeated efforts to construct such figures, he was never satisfied with the result. Above one image he wrote 'this is accomplished', yet he subsequently returned to the subject, focusing specifically on the parting between the woman's legs where flesh accumulated and pressed together, thus evoking its essential materiality.[106] Not believing himself able to construct this figure with the 'experience and understanding' he insisted on, Dürer would never replicate such figures in images for public circulation.

Dürer had an intense interest in the flesh which manifested in a private fascination with the fat female body. That Dürer focused his exploration of fat, which could not be regulated or theorized, on the construction of women's bodies is of the utmost significance. This may have been encouraged by humoral understandings of the gendered body, according to which women's bodies were colder and moister and therefore softer and fleshier than men's bodies. Yet associations between women, flesh, and fat also went beyond humoral theory. Fatness and the flesh could depict the sensuality, seduction, and even the threatening nature of women, as Dürer explored in his drawing of the 'Women's Bath'. Body size and particularly fatness could also be associated with care and nurture, comfort, and health, understandings which were frequently associated with women who, as mothers and wives, took responsibility for maintaining the bodies of their families. Finally, fat could also be viewed as something to be controlled and contained, particularly on the bodies of women which were consistently idealized for their slenderness and grace despite the increasing praise for large bodies among German men in this period.[107] Clothing contained German women's flesh, lacing

[104] Strauss, *Complete Drawings*, vol. 5, 2438, no. HP: 1508/10.

[105] Pellé, 'Mesurer l'excès', 3.

[106] Strauss, *Complete Drawings*, vol. 5, 2439, no. HP: 1508/11.

[107] On the significance of enclosing and controlling the female body for early modern gender ideologies see Laura Gowing, *Common Bodies: Women, Touch and Power in Seventeenth Century England* (New Haven and London, 2013), 7.

it into tight-fitting bodices which displayed the control and moderation of the wearer. Depicting the rolling flesh of a fat, undressed, and thus uncontained woman, whose body further defied the constraints of mathematical proportion, Dürer presented an image which was starkly opposed to such control. Dürer's challenge was to master, through his theoretical understanding of proportion, a body which epitomized the uncontrolled and was the very opposite of his own lean, male figure. His repeated studies suggest that he recognized his own inability to standardize the fat female body, reflecting his wider acknowledgement of the unstable and unconscious elements of his life which did not fit neatly within theoretical models.

Beyond Dürer

Dürer had a deeply personal interest in the form of the human body which was shaped by his own embodied experience and subjectivity. While concerns about body size were becoming increasingly prevalent throughout sixteenth-century Germany, therefore, Dürer's example is an important reminder of the personal significance that body size assumed in dialogue with social and cultural conceptions of the body. This is particularly evident when his exploration of body size is compared with the study of the body by his contemporary Cranach the Elder. Despite the significant overlap in their lifespans, representations of nude bodies by Cranach, court painter to the electors of Saxony in Wittenberg, indicate a notably different approach to body size and proportion than those of Dürer.[108] Cranach did not share Dürer's interest in anatomy and constructed proportion, but was motivated by his own understanding of the beauty to be found in the human form.[109] In contrast to Dürer's view that beauty existed in bodies of various sizes and shapes, Cranach developed a consistent presentation of an idealized, beautiful body, most notably in his depiction of female nudes.

Like Dürer, Cranach had a particular interest in the naked female body. In addition to his paintings of Adam and Eve (Figure 3.27), of which his workshop produced over fifty examples, Cranach was famed for his nude portrayals of classical figures such as Venus (Figure 3.28), Lucretia (Figure 3.29), and Diana.[110]

[108] For a brief biography of Cranach, including his interactions with Dürer, see Caroline Campbell, 'The Artist Known as Lucas Cranach', in Caroline Campbell (ed.), *Temptation in Eden: Lucas Cranach's Adam and Eve*, exh. cat., Courtauld Institute of Art (London, 2007), 12–17. Gunnar Heydenreich has uncovered technical evidence that the two artists shared material expertise. See Gunnar Heydenreich, 'Adam and Eve in the Making' in Campbell, *Temptation in Eden*, 19–33, esp. 19–21, and *Lucas Cranach the Elder: Painting Materials, Techniques and Workshop Practice* (Amsterdam, 2007), 315–18.

[109] Heydenreich, 'Adam and Eve', 25. See also Thomas Kren, 'Lucas Cranach the Elder: Adam and Eve', and 'Lucas Cranach the Elder: The Temptation of Adam and Eve', in Burke et al., *Renaissance Nude*, 34–6, cat. nos. 1 and 2.

[110] Campbell, 'Artist Known as Cranach', 17. Cranach's focus on classical figures reflected a shift in his output with the Reformation. See Andreas Tacke, 'Winners and Losers: The Impact of the Reformation on the Art Market', in Kayo Hirakawa (ed.), *Sacred and Profane in Early Modern Art* (Kyoto, 2016), 37–58.

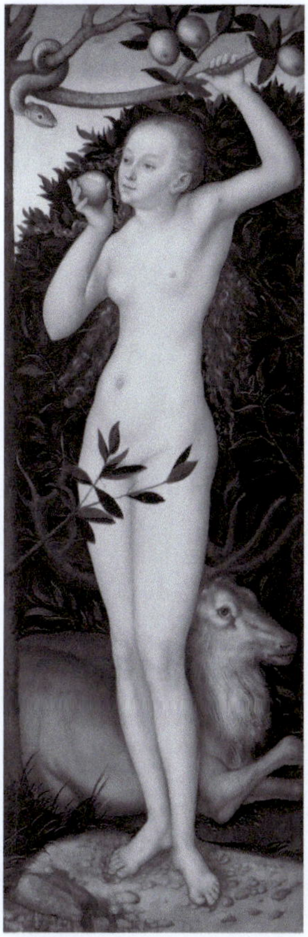

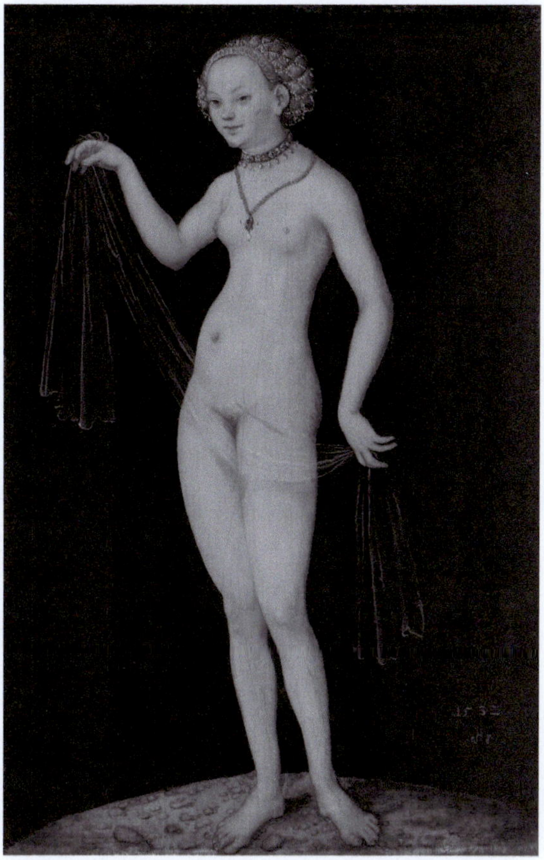

Figure 3.27 Lucas Cranach the Elder, Eve, 1533–7. Oil on beech, 107.6 × 36.4 cm. Art Institute of Chicago, public domain. One of over fifty paintings of Eve produced by Cranach's workshop. Eve's figure displays an elongated slenderness.

Figure 3.28 Lucas Cranach the Elder, Venus, 1532. Mixed technique on beech, 37.7 × 24.5 cm. Städel Museum, Frankfurt am Main, public domain. Cranach was famed for his depiction of classical figures, particularly Venus, of whom his workshop produced over seventy paintings. Venus's proportions are notably similar to those of Eve in the previous figure.

Regardless of whether he was representing Eve or Venus, however, Cranach's nude female figures are virtually indistinguishable in terms of their body types. While Cranach's early depictions of Venus from the first decade of the sixteenth century appear slightly more rounded and voluptuous, with prominent bellies and larger breasts, his later examples all replicated a slender, streamlined silhouette, with small breasts, long limbs, and just a slight curve at the belly and hips.[111]

[111] Earlier, fleshier examples of Venus include Cranach's woodcut 'Venus and Cupid' from 1508–9 in the British Museum, London, AN49475001, and his painting 'Venus and Cupid', from 1509 in the Hermitage Museum, St Petersburg, ГЭ-680.

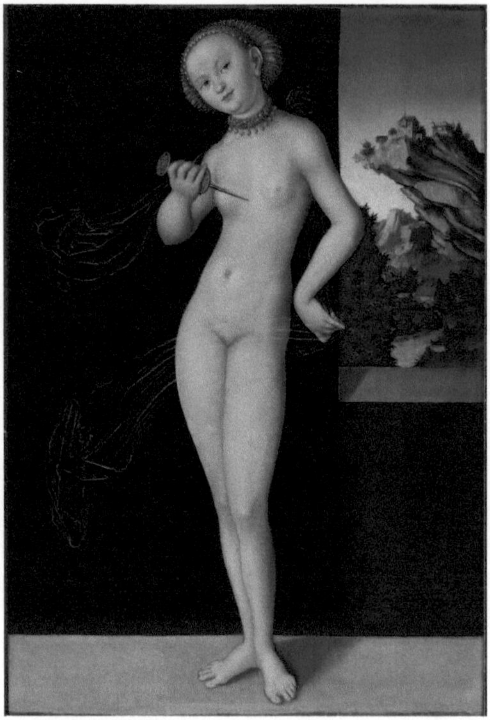

Figure 3.29 Lucas Cranach the Elder, Lucretia, 1528. Oil on panel, 57 × 38 cm. National Museum, Stockholm, public domain. Lucretia's body is virtually indistinguishable from Cranach's depictions of Eve and Venus. The vast majority of Cranach's nudes share this slender, streamlined silhouette, with small breasts and long limbs, often in very similar poses.

This type of figure became a kind of signature for Cranach, making his paintings of the female nude instantly recognizable.

Cranach's consistent vision of beauty as embodied in the slender female figure had practical motivations. Cranach's workshop was prolific, creating over seventy paintings of Venus alone. To increase his productivity, Cranach worked alongside numerous assistants and apprentices, dividing the workshop's labour through the delegation of particular tasks. To maintain the quality of his images Cranach developed painting techniques which his assistants could replicate, which likely informed the consistency in the presentation of female bodies emerging from his workshop.[112] Keeping the proportions of the body the same, while altering the facial features or background scenery, allowed the fundamental structure of the body to be easily copied. Cranach's personality also shaped such practices,

[112] See Heydenreich, 'Adam and Eve', 26–8; Heydenreich, *Lucas Cranach*, 289–90.

as favouring speed over preparation, he did not complete detailed studies for his paintings as Dürer did, instead merely doing quick sketches and outlines.[113]

Yet issues of practicality do not explain Cranach's preference for this particular slender, female form. As a court painter, Cranach was frequently engaged in producing portraits of elite women, whose bodies typically present little individualization but instead reproduce the fashionable silhouette for German women during this period, consisting of sloping shoulders, slender arms, and a narrow waist (Figure 3.30). These figures appear as the dressed equivalent of Cranach's nude paintings, which thus appear to reproduce 'the general estimation of what people consider beautiful', a definition of beauty which Dürer had considered in 1512 but later rejected.[114] Cranach to a greater extent than Dürer, therefore, seems to have

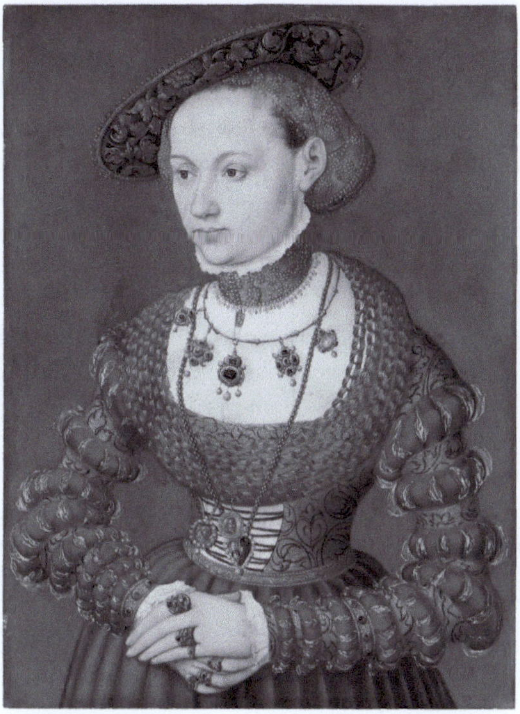

Figure 3.30 Lucas Cranach the Elder, Portrait of Agnes von Hayn, 1543. Oil on beech, 59.5 × 43.5 cm. Staatsgalerie Stuttgart, public domain. Cranach's portraits of elite women present them in figures which appear as the dressed equivalent of his nude paintings. These images reproduce the slender fashionable ideal for German women across the sixteenth century.

[113] Heydenreich, 'Adam and Eve', 25.

[114] Anne Marie Bonnet suggested that Cranach's nudes presented autochthon German bodies in contrast to Dürer's. See Anne-Marie Bonnet, *Der Akt bei Dürer und die Rezeption durch zeitgenössische Künstler* (Habilitationsschrift, Munich, 1992) 262. See also Anne-Marie Bonnet, 'Der Akt im Werk Lucas Cranachs: Bedeutung und Spezifität der "nacketen Bilder" innerhalb der deutschen Renaissance-Malerei', in Claus Grimm, Johannes Erichsen, and Evamaria Brockhoff (eds), *Lucas Cranach: Ein*

modelled his image of beauty upon the popular ideal for the female body in the German-speaking lands which remained fairly consistent throughout the sixteenth century, in contrast to the dramatic development of a bulky silhouette among German men. Cranach's preference for the popular, slender female figure may thus have reflected his grasp of the commercial potential of his seductive female nudes, which were intended to hold broad appeal among elite male society.[115] His preference for this form was likely also shaped by his own personal desires. In 1520, Cranach joked that his paintings of Venus were produced through his 'foam', referencing the story of Venus's birth, which was said to have been caused by Saturn throwing the genitals of his father Uranus into the sea. Cranach's 'foam' was the pigments used to create his paintings, yet here he connected these materials to his virility.[116] Cranach thus presented the centrality of his body for the construction of his female nudes, not merely through the physical act of painting, but also the sexual desire and potency which drove their conception.[117]

While Dürer's investigation of diverse bodily proportions was motivated by personal fascination and was not replicated by contemporaries such as Cranach, his theorization and presentation of bodies of various sizes had lasting consequences for the depiction of bodies in early modern German art. Through his workshop instruction, his theoretical writings, and the widespread dissemination of his prints, Dürer inspired a subsequent generation of German artists to pay attention to body size.

Hans Baldung Grien, one of Dürer's most talented pupils, was deeply influenced by his master's approach to the body; he regularly used the body's fleshiness to create meaning in his artworks and enliven his figures.[118] In his 1523 painting of 'Two Witches' (Figure 3.31), for example, Baldung presented two female bodies of notably different shape and proportion. The seated figure has a fleshy, hanging belly, while the standing nude is slender. In their proportions, they correspond roughly to the basic types outlined in Dürer's books on proportion, measuring

Maler-Unternehmer aus Franken, exh. cat., Haus der Bayerischen Geschichte, Augsburg (Regensburg, 1994), 139–49. See also Christian Schoen, *Albrecht Dürer: Adam und Eva. Die Gemälde, ihre Geschichte und Rezeption bei Lucas Cranach d. Ä. und Hans Baldung Grien* (Berlin, 2001), 195 and 209–10.

115 Thomas Kren, 'Lucas Cranach the Elder: Venus Standing in a Landscape', in Burke et al., *Renaissance Nude,* 139, cat. no. 41.

116 Pfisterer, 'Personalizing the Nude', 311.

117 On the coupling of artistic creation and sex in this period see for instance Maria Ruvoldt, *The Italian Renaissance Imagery of Inspiration: Metaphors of Sex, Sleep and Dreams* (Cambridge, 2004), 110.

118 On Baldung's relationship to Dürer see Chipps Smith, *Nuremberg,* 136. Koerner, *Moment of Self-Portraiture,* 250. For Baldung's biography see also Giulia Bartrum, *German Renaissance Prints 1490–1550* (London, 1995), 67–8. On the influence of Dürer's study of the body on Baldung see Bodo Brinkmann, 'Die Hexe als Aktmodell: Künstlerstreit um Körperformen. The Witch as a Nude Model: The Artist's Debate on Body Forms', in Bodo Brinkmann (ed.), *Hexenlust und Sündenfall. Witches' Lust and the Fall of Man,* exh. cat., Städel Museum, Frankfurt am Main (Petersberg, 2007), 74–96, esp. 78–80, and Berthold Hinz, 'Baldung und Dürer: Nackte Figuren und ihre Bildgelegenheiten. Baldung and Dürer: Nudes and the Occasions for Depicting Them', in Brinkmann (ed.), *Hexenlust und Sündenfall: Witches' Lust and the Fall of Man,* 203–33.

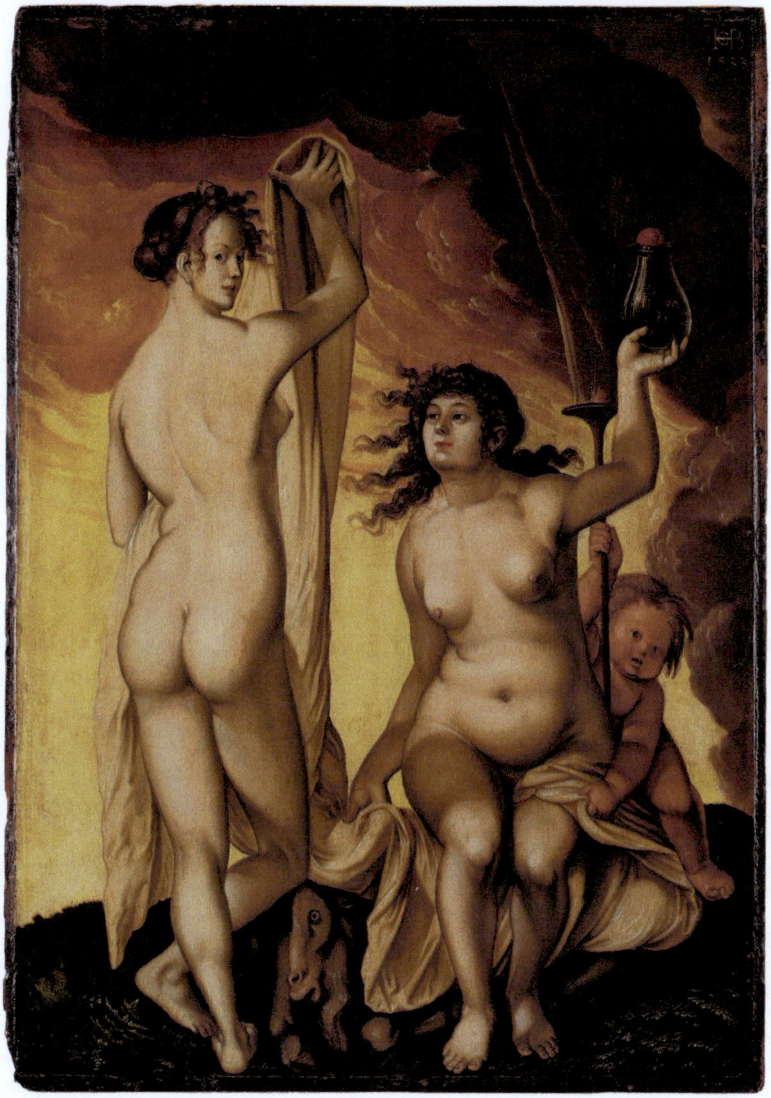

Figure 3.31 Hans Baldung Grien, Two Witches, 1523. Mixed technique on limewood, 65.4 × 45 cm. Städel Museum, Frankfurt am Main, public domain. The two women are shown with notably different figures which correspond to two of the basic types contained in Dürer's *Four Books on Human Proportion*. The corporeality of the witches appears as the source of their power.

approximately seven and eight heads in height respectively.[119] Moreover, the curving belly of the seated figure echoes Dürer's private sketches of the large female body from 1508, in which he meditated upon the placement of the belly's

[119] Brinkmann, 'Die Hexe als Aktmodell. The Witch as a Nude Model', 95.

contours. With their contrasting bodies, Baldung seems to draw on Dürer's teaching that fat and thin 'can properly be used in all kinds of contrasts as one wishes' and that 'no powerful artist should devote himself to one type of subject alone'.[120] Through his focus on their naked, fleshy bodies, Baldung shows the corporality of the witches to be the source of their power.[121]

Indeed, Baldung frequently used voluptuous female bodies to present the potential for women to hold power over men.[122] His many well-known prints of witches attending Sabbath gatherings are typically populated by women with notably fleshy bodies. In his 1510 print of witches arranged around a cauldron (Figure 3.32), for example, Baldung put care into creating the women's curves and contours which he emphasized through chiaroscuro and the use of short curving lines to construct the rounded forms of their bodies. Equally, Baldung's use of shading and contour moulded the haggard body of the central witch who is identifiable as an older woman in part through her leaner and less fleshy form.[123] Baldung again used contrast, therefore, presenting bodies of varying size and form. Nevertheless, when depicting the power of women's bodies, Baldung most often tended towards fleshiness and fatness in his nude figures. When he depicted Phyllis riding Aristotle in 1515, Baldung emphasized the fleshy belly of Phyllis and thus the power of voluptuous femininity over male intellect.[124] For Baldung, fatness and the flesh presented an image of uncontrolled womanhood, echoing Dürer's exploration of the fat female form.

The brothers Sebald and Barthel Beham, who likely also trained in Dürer's workshop, were similarly fascinated by fleshy female bodies.[125] In Sebald's 'Three

[120] Rupprich, *Dürer*, vol. 3, 295 and 296. Ashcroft, *Documentary Biography*, vol. 2, 878 and 880. See pp. 86 and 90 of this chapter.

[121] On the significance of women's bodies in images of witchcraft see Charles Zika, *The Appearance of Witchcraft* (London, 2007), 70–98. On this image specifically see 84. See also Heiner Borggrefe, 'Anatomie, Erotik, Dissimulation. Nackte Körper von Dürer, Baldung Grien und den Kleinmeistern', in Andreas Tacke and Stefan Heinz (eds), *Menschenbilder. Beiträge zur Altdeutschen Kunst* (Petersberg, 2011), 33–55, esp. 41.

[122] On the association between fatness, power, and eroticism in early modern art see Alexander Pyrges, 'Frühneuzeitliche Verbildlichungen von Beleibtheit: Versuch einer körper- und kunsthistorischen Einordnung', in Michael Stolberg (ed.), *Körper-Bilder in der Frühen Neuzeit: Kunst-, medizin- und mediengeschichtliche Perspektiven* (Berlin, 2021), 103–25, esp. 109–15.

[123] On the representation of age through thinness see Fletcher, 'Age, Gender and the Body'.

[124] Diane Wolfthal, 'From Venus to Witches: The Female Nude in Northern Europe', in Burke et al., *Renaissance Nude*, 81–91, here 88. See also Diane Wolfthal, 'Hans Baldung (Grien): Aristotle & Phyllis', in Burke et al., *Renaissance Nude*, 103, cat. no. 30. This image is held in the British Museum, London. Museum number: 1872,1012.903.

[125] On the Beham brothers see Alison Stewart, 'Sebald Beham and Barthel Beham' in *The Dictionary of Art*, ed. Jane Turner (New York, 1996), vol. 3, 505–8; Herbert Zschelletzschky, *Die 'Drei gottlosen Maler' von Nürnberg* (Leipzig, 1975). On Sebald specifically see Alison Stewart, 'Sebald Beham: Entrepreneur, Printmaker, Painter', *Journal of Historians of Netherlandish Art* 4 (2012), 1–25; Alison Stewart, *Before Bruegel: Sebald Beham and the Origins of Peasant Festival Imagery* (Aldershot, 2008). On the contribution of the Behams to early modern German printmaking see Jürgen Müller and Thomas Schauerte (eds), *Die gottlosen Maler von Nürnberg—Konvention und Subversion in der Druckgrafik der Beham-Brüder*, exh. cat., Albrecht-Dürer-Haus (Nuremberg, 2011); Bartrum, *German Renaissance Prints*, 99–100 and 122–3.

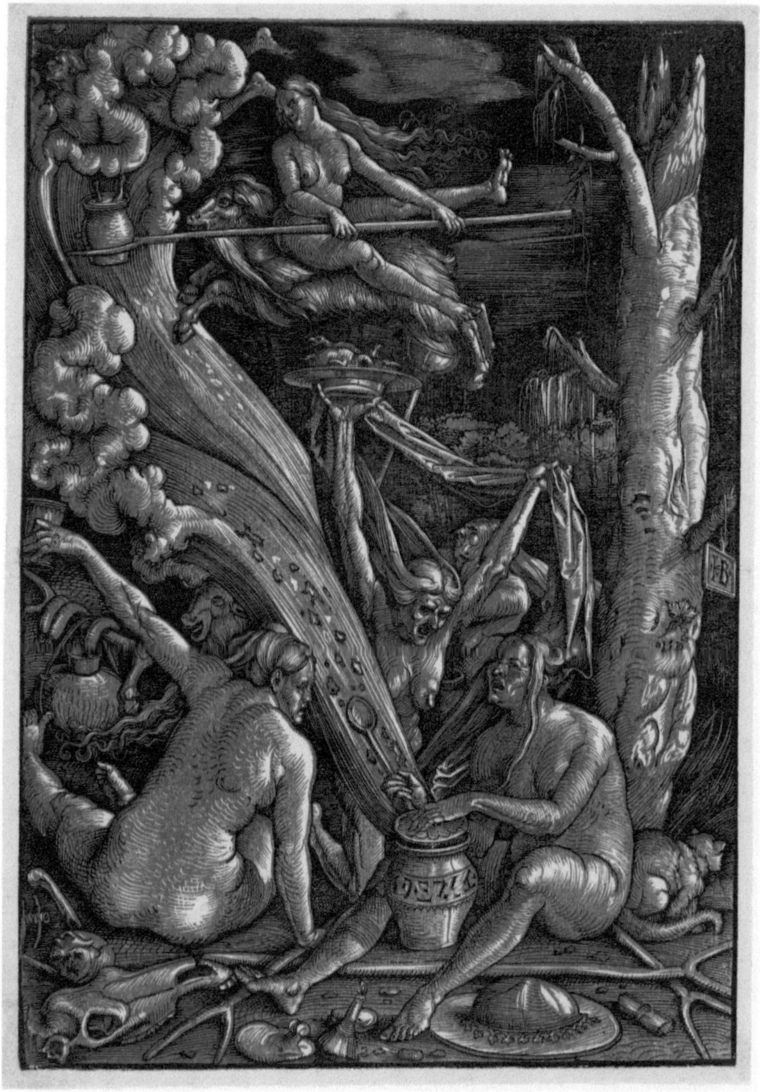

Figure 3.32 Hans Baldung, The Witches, 1510. Chiaroscuro woodcut, 38.9 × 27 cm. Metropolitan Museum of Art, New York, public domain. Baldung used curving lines to present the rounded forms of the younger women's bodies. The central figure is shown as lean and haggard and is thus identified as an older woman.

Women Bathing' (Figure 2.2), which was based on a print by his brother Barthel, he chose to present the women with rolling curves of fat on their stomachs and limbs. The fatness of these figures appears central to the eroticism they portray, evoking both the carnal and sensual elements of their interactions and associating them firmly with the desires of the flesh.[126] Body size is also central to the print 'Death and Three Nude Women' (Figure 3.33), which was again created by Barthel and copied by Sebald.[127] Barthel deliberately presented the two central women with notably fleshy bodies, particularly the woman shown from behind whose rounded bottom spans almost half the width of the print. He took care depicting the curves and folds of the two younger women's bodies and, by contrast, used concave shading lines on the older woman's thighs to indicate the empty, boniness of her figure. Significantly, when Sebald reproduced this image, he reworked his brother's printing plate, adding shading to the women's bodies which further emphasized the volume and fleshiness of their figures. For Sebald in particular, therefore, the corporality of the younger women was essential to this image as it heightened the contrast between their bodies and the figures of the old woman and death. The significance of contrast for this print is clear from the image's physical scale since it measures just 78 by 54 millimetres. In this format the large size of the central women's bodies appears as an intentional and humorous contrast to the miniature scale of the print itself.[128]

Sebald's interests in measurement and scale encouraged his production of a treatise on proportions which was intended for young painters and goldsmiths and focused on the representation of horses. Appearing in 1528, shortly after Dürer's death yet before his 'Four Books on Human Proportion' had been published, the volume resulted in accusations of plagiarism, as Sebald was said to have included material from Dürer's unpublished work.[129] Sebald was forced to flee Nuremberg and settled in Frankfurt. Later he would republish this treatise within a broader manual on measurement which first appeared in 1546 and entered eight editions until 1605.[130] As well as his interest in proportion theory, Dürer's influence on the young artist is particularly evident in his depiction of peasant festivals.[131] Sebald may have copied Dürer's own depictions of peasants (Figure 3.20) during his time as an apprentice, and he replicated the heavy-set bodies of such figures

[126] On the eroticism of the brothers' prints see Janey L. Levy, 'The Erotic Engravings of Sebald and Barthel Beham: A German Interpretation of a Renaissance Subject', in Stephen H. Goddard (ed.), *The World in Miniature: Engravings by the German Little Masters, 1500–1550*, exh. cat., Spender Museum of Art (Lawrence, KS, 1988), 40–53.

[127] David Bardeen, 'Barthel Beham: Death and Three Nude Women', in Burke et al., *Renaissance Nude*, 178–9, cat. no. 54. See also Janey L. Levy 'Barthel Beham and Sebald Beham: Death and the Three Nude Women', in Goddard (ed.), *World in Miniature*, 183–4, cat. nos. 49A and 49B. On the repurposing of Barthel's plates by Sebald see Kurt Löcher, *Barthel Beham: Ein Maler aus dem Dürerkreis* (Munich, 1999), 53.

[128] On the measurements of this image see Bartrum, *German Renaissance Prints*, 125. This small size was typical of prints produced by the group of young artists from Dürer's circle, including the Behams, who became known as the 'Little Masters'. See Stephen H. Goddard, 'The Origin, Use and Heritage of the Small Engraving in Renaissance Germany', in Goddard, *World in Miniature*, 13–29.

[129] Sabine Peinelt, 'Der Verleger als Vollender? Zum "Kunst und Lehrbuchlein" von Sebald Beham', in Müller and Schauerte, *Die gottlosen Maler*, 136–8. See also Stewart, 'Sebald Beham', 4; Bartrum, *German Renaissance Prints*, 104.

[130] Chipps Smith, *Nuremberg*, 196, no. 95.

[131] Sebald produced many images of the peasant festival 'Kermis'. See e.g. 'The Village Fair', 1535, British Museum, London, 1895,0122.303.

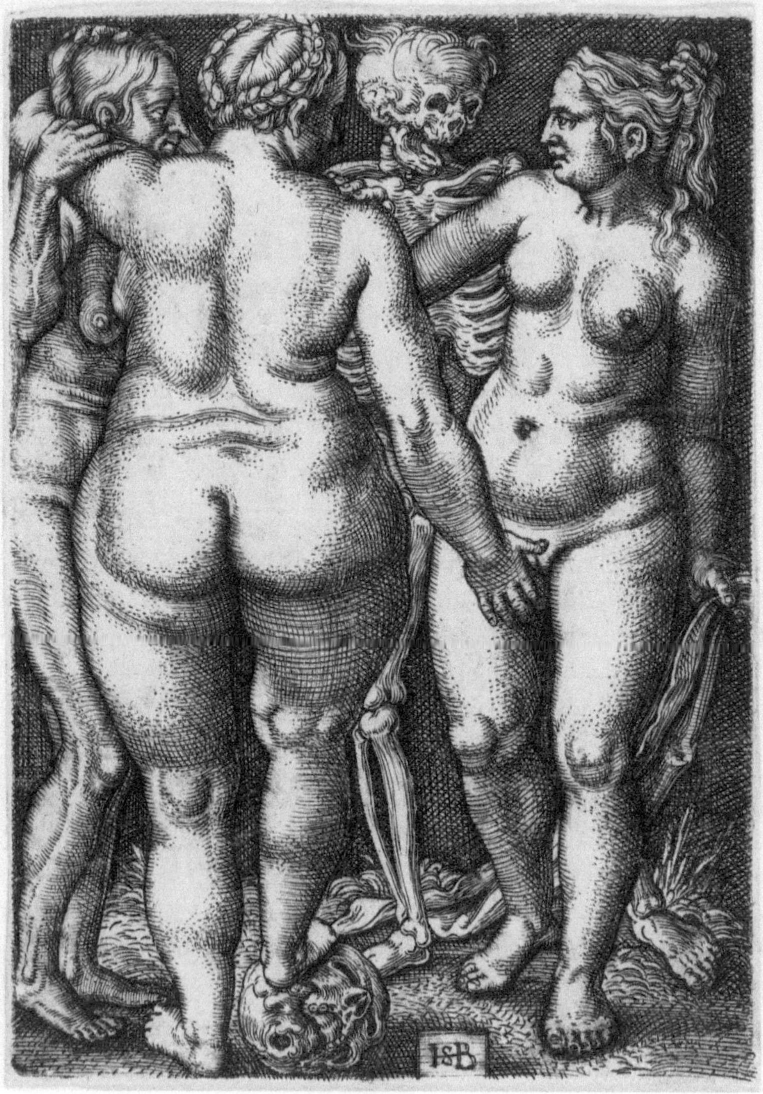

Figure 3.33 Sebald Beham, Death and Three Nude Women, 1525–7. Engraving, 7.3 × 5.4 cm. National Gallery of Art, Washington, DC, public domain. The two central women are shown with notably fleshy bodies in contrast to the figures of death and the older woman. In this reworking of his brother's print, Sebald added to the shading on the women's bodies to emphasize their corporality.

(including those of Dürer's proportion studies) in his presentation of the lack of bodily control exhibited during peasant festivities.[132] Despite overflowing with bodily excretions as a result of excessive consumption, in these prints peasant

132 Stewart, *Before Bruegel,* 50.

bodies are depicted as solid and sturdy, appearing as the epitome of the simple, robust German body which took pleasure in eating, drinking, and sexuality.[133]

Both Sebald and Barthel had previously been banished from Nuremberg in 1525 for advocating radical religious views, and while Sebald returned to the city, Barthel settled in Munich, eventually entering the service of the Dukes of Bavaria.[134] In this setting, Barthel concentrated on paintings, including around a dozen portraits of the Wittelsbach family. Among these were portraits of Ottheinrich, Elector of the Palatinate, who possessed a large and imposing body, the rounded corporeality of which Barthel took care to present in his paintings (Figure 5.14). Barthel became a key figure in the production of portraits which depicted the bulky masculinity of sixteenth-century German men. He was joined in this endeavour by another of Dürer's purported students, Georg Pencz. Along with the Beham brothers, Pencz had been banished from Nuremberg for radical statements made against the church, yet he returned shortly afterwards and later became the official painter to the city.[135] Pencz produced numerous large-scale portraits of Nuremberg citizens which display a powerful corporeality and show the particular attention Pencz paid to the modelling of his sitters' figures (Figure 1.4).

After Dürer's death, a woodcut portrait produced by Erhard Schön presented Dürer too with a relatively bulky and solid form (Figure 3.34). In contrast to his previously lean and youthful body, the mature Dürer is shown with a thick neck, sloping chin, and an expansive upper body in his gown. By the age of 56, Dürer's figure had assumed the robust proportions of mature German manhood. Schön, who was likely a pupil of Dürer's, became the most prolific designer of woodcuts in Nuremberg after Dürer and was clearly influenced by his predecessor's style.[136] In 1538, Schön produced a treatise on bodily proportion in which he taught the reader how to model bodies in various postures and stages of movement. In his preface, Schön stated that the text was intended to convey the art of proportion and measurement, as imparted by Dürer and Vitruvius, in the simplest possible terms for the apprentice painter.[137] For Schön, simplifying bodily proportions

[133] For interpretations of these images see Stewart, *Before Bruegel,* esp. 148–58; Keith Moxey, *Peasants, Warrior and Wives: Popular Imagery in the Reformation* (Chicago, 1989). On patriotism in relation to the Behams' work see Levy 'The Erotic Engravings', and Jessica Buskirk, "Man tragt nit schwer an guter kunst": Das Goldene Zeitalter der Kunst und des Patriotismus' im Nürnberg des 16. Jahrhunderts', in Müller and Schauerte, *Die gottlosen Maler,* 56–63.

[134] On their banishment see Herbert Zschelletzschky, *Die 'Drei gottlosen Maler'*; Gerd Schwerhoff, 'Wie gottlos waren die "gottlosen Maler"? Zur Rekonstruktion des Nürnberger Verfahrens von 1525 und seiner Hintergründe', in Müller and Schauerte, *Die gottlosen Maler,* 33–48; Theodor Kolde, 'Zum Prozess des Johann Denck und der "drei gottlosen Maler" von Nürnberg', in *Kirchengeschichtliche Studien Hermann Reuter zum 70. Geburtstag gewidmet* (Leipzig, 1888), 228–50.

[135] Bartrum, *German Renaissance Prints,* 115. On Pencz see Katrin Dyballa, *Georg Pencz: Künstler zu Nürnberg* (Berlin, 2014).

[136] Bartrum, *German Renaissance Prints,* 92. On the possibility that Schön was in Dürer's workshop see Chipps Smith, *Nuremberg,* 46.

[137] Erhard Schön, *Unnderweissung der Proportzion vnnd Stellung der Possen* (Nuremberg, 1540, first publ. 1538) fol. Aii^r. See Chipps Smith, *Nuremberg,* 173, no. 71.

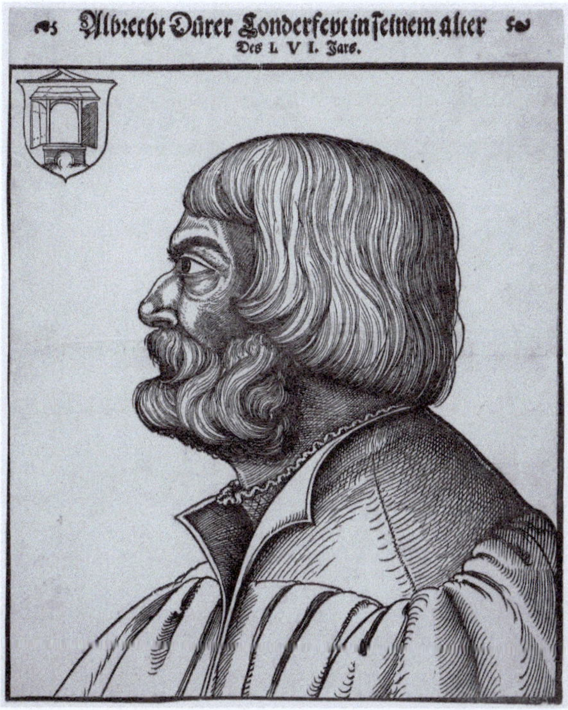

Figure 3.34 Attributed to Erhard Schön, Portrait of Albrecht Dürer, c.1538. Woodcut, 32 × 25.7 cm. Metropolitan Museum of Art, New York, public domain. This portrait, completed shortly after Dürer's death, shows Dürer at the age of 56. As a mature man, Dürer's figure is shown as more solid and bulky than his youthful form.

included the curious construction of bodies through solid blocks or cubes, which were rendered in three dimensions and set within a perspectival box (Figure 3.35). Once such blocks had modelled the correct volume and posture of the body, their straight edges could be softened and details be added to transform it into a human form.

Schön's conceptualization of the body in terms of these cube-like shapes likely stemmed from the use of a wooden mannequin. The title of his work describes it as a 'Manual of Proportion and the Positioning of *Possen*'. The term *Possen* might simply refer to the models represented in Schön's woodcut, but it has also been persuasively interpreted as a direct reference to the jointed mannequins which were used in artists' workshops to assist with the study of bodily proportion and posture.[138] Through their jointed limbs these figures necessarily divided the body into connected blocks or sections, though they generally took the form of

[138] See Walter Strauss (ed.), *The Illustrated Bartsch* (New York, 1981), vol. 13, 139; Arpad Weixlgärtner, 'Dürer und die Gliederpuppe', *Beiträge zur Kunstgeschichte: Franz Wickhoff gewidmet* (1903), 80–90, esp. 90; Leo Baer, 'Vorwort', in Erhard Schön, *Unterweisung der Proportionen und Stellung der Possen,*

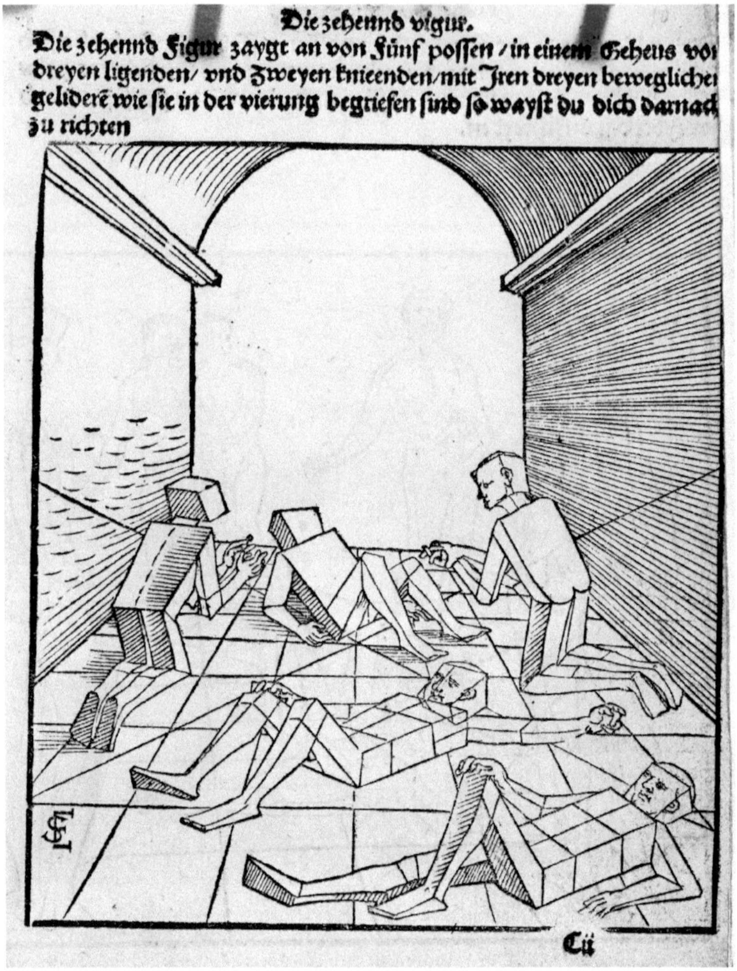
Die zehennd vigur.
Die zehennd Figur zaygt an von Fünf possen / in einem Geheus vo
dreyen ligenden / vnd zweyen knieenden / mit Jren dreyen beweglicher
gelideré wie sie in der vierung begriefen sind so waysst du dich darnach
zu richten
Cii

Figure 3.35 Erhard Schön, woodcut from *Underweissung der Proportzion und stellung der possen*, 1538, fol. Cii^r^. Woodcut, 17.7 × 13.7 cm. Metropolitan Museum of Art, New York, public domain. Schön's treatise on proportions includes the construction of the figure through cuboid shapes within a perspectival box. His conceptualization of the body in these terms may have resulted from his use of an artist's mannequin.

naturalistic nude bodies. Surviving mannequins from this period are typically slender, and in Schön's study of proportion, his cuboid bodies do not noticeably differ in size or shape.[139] Yet these figures, and Schön's drawings, offered a basis

Nuremberg 1542, facsimile ed. Leo Baer (Frankfurt am Main, 1920), n.p.; Markus Rath, *Die Gliederpuppe: Kult, Kunst, Konzept* (Berlin and Boston, 2016), 345.

[139] For a surviving mannequin see Skulpturensammlung und Museum für Byzantinische Kunst, Staatliche Museen zu Berlin, Inv. No. 2167.

from which a variety of bodies could be constructed through the manipulation of this essential human form. The growing use of mannequins in artists' workshops in sixteenth-century Germany reflected the increasing interest in the representation of human bodies in Renaissance art, and following Dürer, this included bodies of diverse proportions. Schön's manual, which entered five editions between 1538 and 1561, was indebted to Dürer's theorization of the human figure.[140] Dürer's fascination with body size and proportion thus lived on in German art throughout the sixteenth century.

'Doing Body Size' in German Visual Culture

While each of the artists discussed above 'did' body size in different ways, the body and its form were central to their work. The prominence of bodies of various sizes within the artworks of Dürer's contemporaries and pupils, as well as Dürer's own project of theorizing the proportions of the body, is testament to the increasing consciousness of the body size within German society and culture from the turn of the sixteenth century. Contemporary representations of bodies necessarily took questions of size and fleshiness into account, since these were increasingly recognized to shape the meaning and emotional resonances contained in an image. While Cranach favoured a more uniform approach, reflecting his workshop practice and personal preferences, a later generation of artists inspired by Dürer rejected such uniformity, instead foregrounding contrasting bodies in their images. Gender was of crucial significance for the use of body size. These male creators were often particularly fascinated by representing female bodies and, with the notable exception of Cranach, such representations were often characterized by fleshiness. This fascination with fleshy and fat female figures reflected the significance of body size within a contemporary gender ideology which prioritized the control of women's bodies. Yet it perhaps also reflects the significance of the artist's body for their creations, as these early modern men explored the representation of overflowing female fatness from the perspective of their own male bodies, understood to be hotter, drier, more solid, and muscular than the women they portrayed.

Certainly, Dürer's embodied subjectivity shaped his approach to the body, as he recognized that body size, form, and fleshiness could convey complex emotional significance. Given his attentiveness to the affective potential of the flesh, Dürer's efforts to geometrically construct ideally proportioned bodies at the beginning of the sixteenth century assume particular significance, appearing as an attempt to regulate such meaning through the construction of perfected bodies. Dürer's

[140] On Schön's editions see Chipps Smith, *Nuremberg*, 173, no. 71.

inability to decide on one ideal female or male form encouraged him to include bodies of diverse sizes within his canon of proportions, yet privately he continued to grapple with the depiction of bodies which resisted this theoretical framework.

The impact of Dürer's approach to the body is demonstrated through the publication of texts such as Schön's and Sebald Beham's, as well as the paintings and prints of Dürer's students and successors who continued to draw on his conceptualization of the body and the flesh. Dürer's works dynamized the investigation of bodily form in early modern German visual culture and contributed towards the growing significance of body size within contemporary German society more broadly.

Body Size in Early Modern Germany. Holly Fletcher, Oxford University Press.
DOI: 10.1093/9780198972983.003.0003

4
Body Size and Reformation

In Johannes Agricola's collection of 750 German proverbs, completed in 1534, the Protestant reformer included the phrase: 'He becomes fat from that' (*Er wirt feyßt darvon*). In outlining its meaning, Agricola described how, 'perhaps due to the reason that what the people curse is blessed by God', it often happens that a person becomes fat from the curses of others, and he used the following as an example:

> In the monasteries, the fathers and highest ranks always have fat stomachs (*feyste beuche*), due to the reason, one says, that the common brothers begrudge the fathers their good food, and murmur about their good life. As the fathers sit on soft cushions in their parlour, the poor brother must sit in the chancel and he often reads a wicked verse during the *Vesper* since he knows that the fathers are having a good life and he must freeze. Due to this wicked verse, the fathers become fat (*feyste*).[1]

On the surface, the passage presents fatness as a sign of prosperity, of living a 'good life', and even as a 'blessing' by God. The proverb reads as a message not to resent or curse the good fortune of others; they will only 'become fat' from such bitterness. That this was a common enough phrase for Agricola to include it in his collection indicates a cultural perception of fatness in sixteenth-century Germany as representing luxury and comfort.

Yet Agricola's explanation also needs to be viewed in light of his position as a reformer.[2] With this passage, Agricola reinforced a long-standing tradition which presented the Catholic clergy as fat and intemperate. While the attribution of the fathers' fatness to the bitterness of the monks seems to remove the responsibility for their size from the clergy themselves, their lives are nevertheless shown to be luxurious. The monks' behaviour is also criticized, for not only do they curse or damn the fathers, but they actively lust after their good food, easy lives, and soft cushions, an image of hypocrisy for these supposedly godly men who have taken vows of poverty. Agricola thus described a divided monastery, where the excessive lives of some are symbolized by their fatness, while others hypocritically lust after

[1] Johannes Agricola, *Die Sprichwörtersammlungen*, ed. Sander L. Gilman, 2 vols (Berlin, 1971), vol. 1, 411.

[2] Sander Gilman suggests that Agricola politicized many previously neutral proverbs. Sander L. Gilman, 'Nachwort', in *Die Sprichwörtersammlungen*, vol. 2, 370. See also Robert Scribner, *Religion and Culture in Germany (1400–1800)*, ed. Lyndal Roper (Leiden, 2001), 32.

the luxuries they are denied. This image reflects a view of the Catholic Church propagated by Lutheran reformers who criticized both the gluttons and the ascetics they identified within it. Instead, Luther instructed evangelicals to 'steer a middle course, lest we become either Epicureans and dissolute, or hypocrites and gloomy monks'.[3] Whilst fatness and bulk was often employed in a positive sense in early modern Germany, showing the wealth and power of elite men for example, here fatness is a critique, with such positive connotations invalidated by the monastic setting. Agricola's illustration of the proverb thus demonstrates how body size could hold particular meaning in a religious context, especially in view of the Reformations.[4]

The sixteenth century was a period of immense religious upheaval as Luther's critique of the papacy radically transformed Christianity across Germany and beyond. Reformation debates concerning the body integrated questions of body size. Lyndal Roper's ground-breaking study of Martin Luther's body has shown that his stout and bulky form was linked to 'his character, his views of the devil and the emerging identity of Lutheranism'.[5] Embedded within the Reformation movement, therefore, was an awareness of Luther's own physical heft and what it represented, namely the reformer's embrace of the earthly appetites and his rejection of Catholic teachings concerning fasting and celibacy. Yet the significance of Luther's large body points to a bigger story about body size in the Reformations, and in German culture more broadly. This was a society in which ideas about body size were becoming increasingly prominent, gaining greater attention, and taking on new meaning. The Lutheran Reformation elevated religious discussions concerning the flesh and the earthly appetites, connecting these specifically to images of fatness and the belly. These debates contributed towards the growing cultural significance of body size throughout German society, with consequences reaching across confessional divides. Body size was embedded in fundamental discussions of sin and salvation which sat at the very heart of the Reformation. As the century progressed and Christendom splintered into diffuse factions, body size thus became a recurring motif in arguments against the toleration of opposing groups whose sinfulness was shown to be embodied.

The significance of body size in the Reformations built upon the existing role of embodied piety in medieval theology. Caroline Walker Bynum has shown that the body acquired new religious meaning in the period between 1200 and 1500, as bodiliness increasingly provided access to the sacred through self-inflicted suffering

[3] 'Vorlesungen über 1. Mose Kap. 24', in Martin Luther, *D. Martin Luthers Werke: Kritische Gesamtausgabe* [hereafter *WA*], 120 vols (Weimar, 1883–2009), vol. 43, 334. Translation from the Latin in Martin Luther, *Luther's Works* [hereafter *LW*], 55 vols (St Louis, 1955–86), vol. 4, 277.

[4] On the similar use of fatness to criticize Hutterite Anabaptists see Holly Fletcher, 'The Fat World of the Hutterites: Food and Fatness in the Criticism of Hutterite Anabaptists in Early Modern Moravia', *Food and History* 21 (2023), 173–200.

[5] Lyndal Roper, 'Martin Luther's Body: The "Stout Doctor" and his Biographers', *American Historical Review* 115 (2010), 351–84, quotation, 352.

and other forms of bodily manipulation.[6] Medieval female spirituality in particular was markedly somatic and the lives of female saints were characterized by 'food metaphors, food miracles and food practices' which were entwined with the body.[7] In Germany, a new spirituality of suffering characterized by extreme fasting and bodily mortification was especially prevalent among female mystics, for whom physical and spiritual suffering was a prerequisite of mystical union with God.[8] In the tradition of ascetic piety, therefore, spiritual figures were marked by the thinness of their bodies, as their emaciation underlined their indifference to the temptations of the flesh. Luther challenged this image of spirituality through his bodily form, as well as in specific discussions regarding the bodily appetites and the need for moderation. The Lutheran Reformation was thus a key factor in the transformation of ideas about body size in this period. Luther was certainly not the first to critique excessive ascetism; an anti-ascetic discourse had been growing since the eleventh century, particularly in Germany, which centred on concerns about external displays of piety through bodily mortification.[9] This message was taken up by reformers and had considerable consequences for spiritual conceptions of body size.[10] This chapter focuses on Lutheran discussions of body size, fatness, and the belly which, it suggests, made bodily form an increasingly pressing matter for believers of various confessions across the sixteenth century.

Body Size at the Bodily Resurrection

The doctrine of the bodily resurrection, which asserted that the dead would rise again to face the Last Judgement, was explicitly used by Luther to reinforce the relationship between faith and the Christian body. In his sermons on 1 Corinthians 15

[6] Caroline Walker Bynum, *Fragmentation and Redemption: Essays on Gender and the Human Body in Medieval Religion* (New York, 1992), esp. 181–238.

[7] Caroline Walker Bynum, *Holy Feast and Holy Fast: The Religious Significance of Food to Medieval Women* (Berkeley-Los Angeles, 1987), here 129. Rudolph Bell anachronistically characterized the extreme fasting of medieval religious women as 'holy anorexia', suggesting how such practices may have shaped the bodies of those who followed them. Rudolph Bell, *Holy Anorexia* (Chicago, 1985). For an in-depth discussion of the issues involved in applying the medical term 'anorexia nervosa' to the behaviour of medieval religious women see Bynum, *Holy Feast*, 194–207.

[8] Ronald K. Rittgers, *The Reformation of Suffering: Pastoral Theology and Lay Piety in Late Medieval and Early Modern Germany* (Oxford, 2012), 64. On German mysticism see Elizabeth Andersen, Henrike Lähnemann, and Anne Simon (eds), *A Companion to Mysticism and Devotion in Northern Germany in the Late Middle Ages* (Leiden, 2014). See also Bynum, *Holy Feast*, 150–88.

[9] On anti-asceticism see Giles Constable, *Attitudes toward Self-Inflicted Suffering in the Middle Ages* (Brookline, 1982); Giles Constable, 'Moderation and Restraint in Ascetic Practices', in Haijo Jan Westra (ed.), *From Athens to Chartres: Neoplatonism and Medieval Thought* (Leiden, 1992), 315–27. For the German context see Bernhard Schmeidler, 'Anti-asketische Äusserungen aus Deutschland im 11. und beginnenden 12. Jahrhundert', in *Kultur und Universalgeschichte: Walter Goetz zu seinem 60. Geburtstag* (Leipzig and Berlin, 1927), 35–52. On concerns for the physical health of monks and nuns see Gerd Zimmermann, *Ordensleben und Lebensstandard: Die Cura corporis in den Ordensvorschriften des abendländischen Hochmittelalters* (Münster, 1973), esp. 147, 215–16, 234–5, 459.

[10] See Rittgers, *Reformation of Suffering*, 83. Rittgers argues that Protestants sought to bring about profound change in the doctrine of suffering, which remained largely unchanged in early modern Catholicism.

he suggested that belief in the bodily resurrection was fundamental to Christianity itself. The belief that all humans would rise physically from the dead rested on the certainty that Christ himself has been resurrected, and since Christ's bodily resurrection was central to true Christianity, to deny the doctrine of resurrection was to deny Christ's resurrection, and ultimately to reject the true faith. For Luther, therefore, the doctrine of resurrection held profound implications for what it meant to be a Christian, and within this teaching, body size had long held significance.[11]

Medieval discussions about the bodily resurrection had been preoccupied with issues of bodily continuity.[12] Debates navigated the tension between individuality and glorification, as it was claimed that all would rise again with their own individual bodies but that these would become incorruptible and heavenly.[13] Body size was included in such concerns, as it was questioned to what extent bodies would return with the same shape and form they possessed on earth. Issues of fatness and thinness were explicitly discussed in relation to Augustinian teachings on the harmony of the resurrected body. The twelfth-century German chronicler Otto I, Bishop of Freising, for example, wrote 'we must not suppose that…the fat or the thin [are brought back] in their superabundance or their lack of flesh, to a life which ought to be free from every blemish and every spot'. Moreover, he quoted Augustine's teaching that, 'there will be no deformity…and what is less than is seemly shall be supplied from a source known to the Creator, and that which is more than comely shall be removed, though the integrity of the matter is preserved'.[14] Taken as a whole, Otto's text suggested that the resurrected body would be the same as the earthly body, the parts of which would be reassembled following the same structure.[15] Here it appears clear, however, that this reassembling could include an elevation of the body, enabling it to gain a more beautiful form. Following Augustine, whose teachings on the resurrection maintained their authority among reformers, it was understood that there would be no fat or thin bodies in heaven, since such bodies would be perfected through either the removal or supply of bodily matter.

In the sixteenth century, theologians continued to discuss the question of how the dead and decaying body could rise, what it would look like, and, crucially, what form it would take. Whilst Lutheran theologians generally took the view that resurrected bodies would be glorified, the tension between identity and glorification remained. In 1544, Luther himself emphasized change in the body in

[11] Erin Lambert, 'The Reformation and the Resurrection of the Dead', *Sixteenth Century Journal* 47 (2016), 351–70, esp. 355–7.

[12] Caroline Walker Bynum, *The Resurrection of the Body in Western Christianity, 200–1336* (New York, 1995), 11. See also Caroline Walker Bynum, 'Material Continuity, Personal Survival, and the Resurrection of the Body: A Scholastic Discussion in its Medieval and Modern Contexts', *History of Religions* 30 (1990), 51–85.

[13] Bynum, *Resurrection*, 59–60.

[14] Otto, Bishop of Freising, *The Two Cities: A Chronicle of Universal History to the Year 1146 A.D.*, tr. Charles Christopher Mierow, ed. Austin P. Evans and Charles Knapp (New York, 1928), 470.

[15] See Bynum, *Resurrection*, 183.

a sermon on 1 Corinthians 15, when he wrote that it would 'lose its figure (*Gestalt*), that one will see neither a human body nor bodily figure (*weder Menschlichen Leib noch Leibes Gestalt*) and therefore a more beautiful, clearer, lovelier and more joyful body (*Leib*) will rise, in another nature and life'.[16] Yet in the same text he stated, 'it will be wholly the same body (*derselb Leib*) of a person, as it was created, though it will be another figure or usage of the body (*ein ander Gestalt und Brauch des Leibes*)'.[17]

Similarly, a verse from Nikolaus Hermann's song on the resurrection written in 1550 recorded,

> So the earthly body (*irdisch Leyb*) is buried in the grave and will turn to ash and dust, and from that will grow a body clear (*ein Cörper klar*), which will live with God for evermore…And what one sees in mortality, that will rise in splendour, and what is buried without power, that will stand in great strength.[18]

In the first half of the verse, we gain a sense of a new body rising from the dust of the previous one, and the statement that 'a body' grows seems to suggest it is not *the* body. This distinction is reinforced by a shift in vocabulary—while the earthly body is referred to with *Leyb*, *Cörper* is used for the heavenly body. In the second half, however, it is 'what' was buried that will return in splendour, thus suggesting that the body that arises is the same body that was buried. As singers sang such verses, feeling the vibration of the music and drawing breath for each new line, they would have been intensely aware of their own bodies.[19] With voice and vocal tone being intimately connected to age and gender, as well as to body shape and size, the individuality of the body would have been presented to them through this act of singing, perhaps increasing a sense of confusion that this individual body would return and yet it would not be the body as they knew it.

The difficulty of believing in the resurrection of the body, with all the contradictions it contained, was acknowledged by Luther, who wrote, 'Reason says: How can I believe that I will return from the earth? When I die, I putrefy and become nothing.' In response he insisted, '[we] should not continue to dispute questions such as, how the dead will be resurrected and with which bodies they will come', but should trust in almighty God and the power of Christ.[20] By this

[16] 'Die Ander Predigt Von der Todten Aufferstehung', *WA*, vol. 49, 427. Unless otherwise stated, where the original texts from the *WA* are in German, translations are my own.

[17] Ibid. 429. These comments are made with reference to the metaphor of the seed for the resurrection body, in which the heavenly body is understood to be 'the same' as the earthly body inasmuch as a plant is 'the same' as the seed from which is grows. The metaphor of the seed is the dominant metaphor for the resurrection body in 1 Cor. 15 and, Bynum states, the oldest Christian metaphor for resurrection. See Bynum, *Resurrection*, 3.

[18] Nikolaus Herman, *Ein new geistliches Lied von der Aufferstehung der Toten und dem ewigen Leben* (Nuremberg, 1560), fol. 3^{r}.

[19] Erin Lambert, *Singing the Resurrection: Body, Community and Belief in Reformation Europe* (New York, 2017), 15.

[20] 'Die Erste Predigt Von der Todten Aufferstehung und letzten Posaunen Gottes', *WA*, vol. 49, 410–11.

time, however, Luther himself had repeatedly discussed the details of the resurrection body—he gave seventeen sermons on the doctrine across the years 1532 and 1533 and returned to the subject again in 1544/5 in which these comments appear.[21] In these sermons, Luther explored the ways in which a Christian's contemplation of the resurrected body might both challenge and undergird their faith.[22] Questions concerning the glorification of the flesh which were central to considerations of the resurrected body were also key to Reformation discussions about the Real Presence in the Eucharist, an issue which dominated Luther's thinking in this later period and which ultimately split the Reformation.[23] Of the major reformers, Luther alone insisted on the ongoing, incarnate Christ following his death and resurrection, and thus for Luther, Christ had to be both spiritually *and* physically present in the bread and wine, a topic which has been explored extensively by Reformation scholarship.[24] The intertwining of questions of glorification with discussions about the size and shape of the body suggests how complex ideas about fatness and thinness fed into crucial issues of Reformation theology, granting them real significance for reformers.

One of the most extensive treatises to consider the form of the resurrected body in the sixteenth century was a work by Michael Fabri, superintendent of the Sayn region (part of today's Rheinland-Pfalz), titled 'On the Common Resurrection of the Dead', which was published in Frankfurt am Main in 1564.[25] In a volume of over three hundred folios, Fabri answered questions such as whether we will recognize each other in the next life, will those of different skin colours return with the same colour, and 'whether we will rise just as big as we are here, just as long and wide, or how else will we rise'.[26] The questions he included are telling, reinforcing that concerns about glorification and identity in relation to body size continued in this period. In answer to this last question, Fabri quoted Augustine:

[21] See 'Das 15. Capitel der Ersten Epistel S. Pauli an die Corinther' Nr. 1–17, *WA*, vol. 36, 478–696 and 'Vier Predigten Von der Todten aufferstehung und letzten Posaunen Gottes Aus dem 15. Capitel der 1. Epistel S. Pauli an die Corinther: Gepredigt durch den thewren Mann Gottes, D. Mart. Luther zu Wittenberg Anno M. D. XLIIII. und XLV', *WA*, vol. 49, 395–414, 422–41, 727–46, and 761–80.

[22] Lambert, 'Reformation and Resurrection of the Dead', 356–7.

[23] Lyndal Roper, *Martin Luther: Renegade and Prophet* (London, 2016), 15. Roper also suggests that Luther's own physicality and his generally positive attitude towards the physical were linked to his position on the Real Presence. See Roper, 'Martin Luther's Body', 380.

[24] See for instance: Susan C. Karant-Nunn, 'The Mitigated Fall of Humankind: Martin Luther's Reconciliation with the Body', *Past and Present* 234 (2017), 51–66, and Lee Palmer Wandel, *The Eucharist in the Reformation* (Cambridge, 2006).

[25] Little is known about Fabri other than what he informs us in his text which he dedicates to Count Adolph of Sayn. He states he is from 'Megeßheim bei Oetingen' and gives his position as 'Saynischer Superintendens', a role of considerable power and responsibility. The Sayn region is part of today's Rheinland-Pfalz. For more on Fabri see Erin Lambert, 'New Worlds, New Images: Picturing the Resurrection of the Body in Sixteenth-Century Germany', in Anne Eusterschulte and Hannah Wälzholz (eds), *Anthropological Reformations: Anthropology in the Era of Reformation* (Göttingen, 2015), 533–40.

[26] Michael Fabri, *Von der Allgemeinen Aufferstehung der Todten* (Frankfurt am Main, 1564), fol. 319^{v}.

> It does not follow... that the size of those rising back to life will be different, just because one is bigger than another (*eine grosser gewesen dann der ander*) in this life, or that the thin will come back to life with the same thinness (*die magern eben mit derselben magerheit*), or the fat with the same fatness (*die fetten mit derselben fette*). But as it stands with the Creator, each shall retain his special characteristics and the recognizable equality of his figure (*gleichheit in seiner gestalt*), in other conveniences (*kommligkeiten*) of the body, however, everyone will be the same, in the same way the matter (*Materi*) of each will be measured so that nothing of it shall be lost, and He will supply anything that may be missing.[27]

This passage returns to the contradictions of continuity and beautification, for although an individual will retain a 'recognizable equality of his figure', mysteriously in other aspects their body will become the same as all other bodies, presenting a certain flexibility in ideas of 'equality'.

In another passage Fabri also included the quotation from Augustine which Otto of Freising had used in the twelfth century. He wrote:

> the thin or fat (*die magern oder fetten*) need not fear that there they must also be that to which they were here resigned but did not want... what is too small will be changed, what is too few will be substituted... and for that which is too much, the matter (*Materi*), whilst preserving the integrity (*vollkommenheit*) of the body, will depart.[28]

Basing his answer on Augustine, Fabri too concluded that there would be no fat or thin bodies in heaven.[29] Yet how could Fabri reconcile this alteration of body size with the conflicting notion of a 'recognizable equality' of figure? Whilst the endurance of discussions on continuity suggests confusion, such statements may not have appeared so contradictory to early modern commentators. Whether there was an exact image of the body, which could be lost through perfecting and beautification, must be questioned. In this period, bodies were understood to possess a 'natural' or innate form which was nevertheless flexible, changing under the influence of external factors such as the six non-naturals, as well as embodied processes of ageing, illness, or pregnancy.[30] Such contemporary medical understandings of the body may well have assisted with the conceptualization of a resurrected body which was both the same as, yet different from, the earthly figure.

[27] Ibid., fols 319^{v}–320^{r}. See 'Kommlich', *Grammatisch-kritisches Wörterbuch der Hochdeutschen Mundart. Nach der Ausgabe letzter Hand, Leipzig 1793–1801* (*Adelung*) digital edition: www.woerterbuchnetz.de/Adelung/

[28] Fabri, *Von der Allgemeinen Aufferstehung*, fol. 320^{r}.

[29] Augustine himself, however, was inconsistent on the question of whether one would retain the same size and shape as one had on earth. See Bynum, *Resurrection*, 98.

[30] This 'natural' bodily form is discussed in detail in Chapter 2.

The lengthy and complex discussions of bodily resurrection provide a sense of the layers of meaning that ideas about body size and shape could contain, both for this issue and more broadly in this period. Combined with an awareness of natural and unnatural bodies, questions of continuity and glorification in the resurrection suggest that, while body size could function as a marker of identity in early modern Germany, this identity was not necessarily fixed. Furthermore, Fabri's statement that the fat and thin are resigned to bodies they do not want reinforces a contemporary ideal of medium proportion. In stating that they should not worry about having such unwanted bodies in heaven, Fabri presented an image of blessed, glorified bodies as fulfilling such ideals.

Heavenly Bodies

The image of the middling heavenly body suggested by Fabri is also present in a sermon on 1 Corinthians 15 by Lutheran reformer Johannes Mathesius which was published posthumously in 1587.[31] The majority of texts on the resurrection are not as explicit in their discussion of fat and thin bodies as Fabri's, but as Mathesius's work demonstrates, expectations for the resurrected body can be revealed as part of other discussions. In his explanation of the continuity of the body, Mathesius noted that the bodies of all people in this world are from the same flesh and are subject to sin, yet there remain distinctions between them (just as heavenly bodies will be the same as earthly bodies yet will also be superior). He stated, 'one has a beautifully formed, well-proportioned and noble body (*ein schönern geformirtern, wol proporcionirtern vnnd Adelichern leyb*), whilst the other is born for servitude', reflecting the hierarchical model of the *Ständelehre*, by which society was divided into class-based 'estates', or *Stände*.[32] This teaching was reinforced by Lutheranism, and here Mathesius grants it an embodied dimension, suggesting such divisions were innate rather than socially constructed. He continues: 'When God wants to use one person for government or great things, he gives them greater gifts, in bodily power, understanding, heart and bravery, just as virtue shines more brightly and is more majestic in a beautiful and upright (*geraden*) body, as Saul had, than in Marcolpho or a natural fool.'[33] In stating that the resurrection body will be superior to the earthly body in the same way that noble bodies are better formed than those intended for servitude,

[31] Mathesius had been a student of Luther's, attending his lectures in Wittenberg from 1529 and later contributing to the publications of his *Tischreden* (Table Talk). He was ordained by Luther in 1542 and worked as a pastor in the Bohemian town of Joachimsthal. For a brief biography see Robert Rosin, 'Johannes Mathesius (1504–1565)', in Hans J. Hillebrand (ed), *The Oxford Encyclopedia of the Reformation* (Oxford, 1996).

[32] Johannes Mathesius, *Leychpredigten: Auß dem fünfftzehenden Capitel der I. Epistel S. Pauli zun Corinthiern* (Nuremberg, 1565), fol. Xiv^r.

[33] Ibid., fol. Xiv^v.

Mathesius suggests that the heavenly body will contain features he identifies as noble and virtuous. Body size is brought into this image with his mention of 'Marcolpho', a figure from the story of Solomon and Markolf which was popular in Germany, in which the figure of Markolf was typically presented as short and fat. In a Shrovetide play by Hans Sachs, for instance, a market stall holder compares the ugliness of another character, Esopus, with that of Markolf, who 'has a large mouth, swollen jowls (*aufgschwollen packen*)...a big swollen belly (*grosen aufgschwollen pawch*)...with bandy legs, fat and short (*krumen schenckeln, dick vnd kurcz*)'.[34] In comparison to such bodies of 'natural fools', the blessed body will be like that of Saul, described in the Bible as tall and handsome (1 Sam. 9: 2).

In addition to their beauty, the strength of heavenly bodies was repeatedly emphasized. In Luther's sermons on 1 Corinthians 15 from 1533, he stated that the heavenly body 'will be so strong that with one finger it will be able to carry this church, with one toe it will be able to move a tower and play with a mountain as children play with a ball...For then the body will be sheer strength (*eitel kraft*) (as it is now sheer feebleness and weakness)'.[35] Mathesius connected this strength of the heavenly body directly to its size when he stated: 'from this slender (*schmachtigen*), wretched body which is wasting away, a stronger, more powerful, more solid and healthier body will grow'.[36] The blessed body is thus glorified in comparison not only to the shortness and fatness of Markolf, but also to weak and feeble bodies. Mathesius's use of *schmachtigen*, a variant of the modern German term *schmächtig*, is a specific reference to body size; the word was used to mean 'delicate', but in the sense of slender, slight, or slim.[37] Following both Fabri and Mathesius, therefore, the bodies of the blessed would be neither thin nor fat, but rather, well-proportioned, strong, powerful, and solid, reinforcing characteristics of the male ideal for earthly bodies.

Although strong and solid, heavenly bodies were understood to be weightless. This book avoids discussing body size in terms of weight, as is common in a modern context, since bodies were not regularly weighed in early modern Europe and thus fatness and thinness were not generally conceived of in terms of heaviness or lightness.[38] This is a particularly pertinent point when considering heavenly bodies. In Mathesius's text, for instance, he describes how the bodies of the blessed will 'float in the air like the birds of heaven and the angels'.[39] Luther too described them as being 'so light and nimble (*leicht und behend*) that [they] will soar both

[34] Hans Sachs, *Sämmtliche Fastnachtspiele*, ed. Edmund Goetze, 7 vols (Halle, 1887), vol. 7, 144.

[35] 'Das 15. Capitel der Ersten Epistel S. Pauli an die Corinther', *WA*, vol. 36, 657.

[36] Mathesius, *Leychpredigten*, fol. dv^r.

[37] In the *Deutsches Wörterbuch von Jacob Grimm und Wilhelm Grimm* '*schmächtig*', of which Mathesius used a variant, is defined in terms of the verb *schmachten* and therefore as 'suffering from hunger' and 'in need of food', thus directly suggesting thinness. Digital edition: www.woerterbuchnetz.de/DWB/

[38] See Introduction, 12–13.

[39] Mathesius, *Leychpredigten*, fol. ci^r.

down here on earth and up above in the heavens in a moment' and he repeatedly stated the body would be 'as light as the air'.[40] Sander Gilman has used such descriptions of the lightness of heavenly bodies to argue that they were understood as 'perfectly light and slim', and he therefore proposes that 'Luther's text [on 1 Corinthians 15 from 1533] depicts only fat bodies this side of heaven'.[41] Yet this notion of the weight of the body in heaven was not necessarily intended as a comment on body size, as ideas about the weight and size of the body were not inherently connected in this period.

Images of the Last Judgement did occasionally present differences in weight between the blessed and damned in terms of fatness and thinness. In Stefan Lochner's painting (Figure 4.1), for instance, we see a clear distinction in which those bodies destined for heaven are shown as slender, with long and narrow limbs, whilst the hellish are shown with rotund bellies. While hellish bodies were considered the only resurrected bodies that held weight, both heavenly and

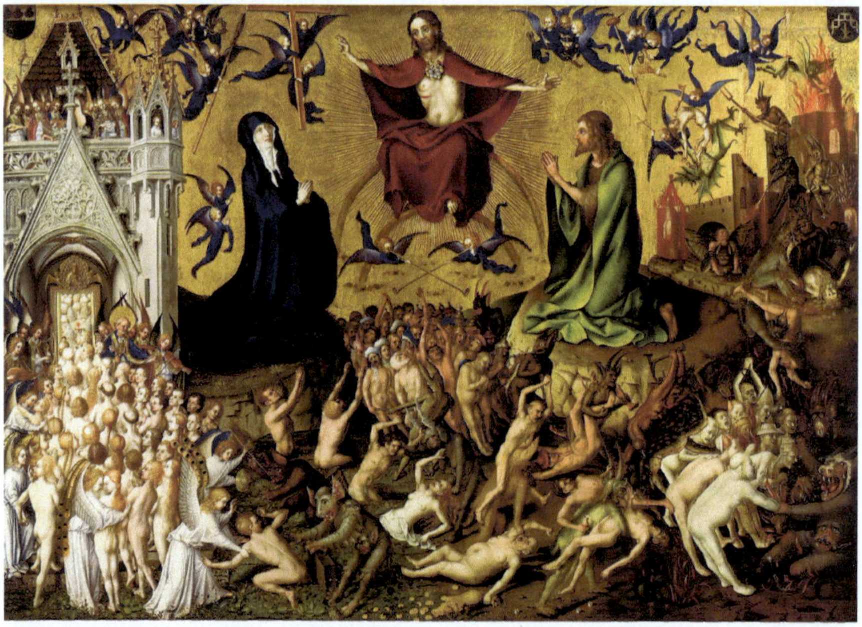

Figure 4.1 Stefan Lochner, Last Judgement, c.1435. Tempera on oak, 124.5 × 173 cm. Wallraf-Richartz Museum, Cologne. Photo © Rheinisches Bildarchiv Köln, Michael Albers, rba_d029131_01. The bodies of those destined for heaven on the left of the image all appear to be slender and elongated. Meanwhile several of those being dragged to hell, in the centre and right-hand side of the painting, possess fleshy, rotund bellies.

[40] 'Das 15. Capitel der Ersten Epistel S. Pauli an die Corinther', *WA*, vol. 36, 657; For instance: *WA*, vol. 36, 660 and 671.

[41] Sander L. Gilman, *Fat Boys: A Slim Book* (Lincoln, NE, 2004), 52 and 55.

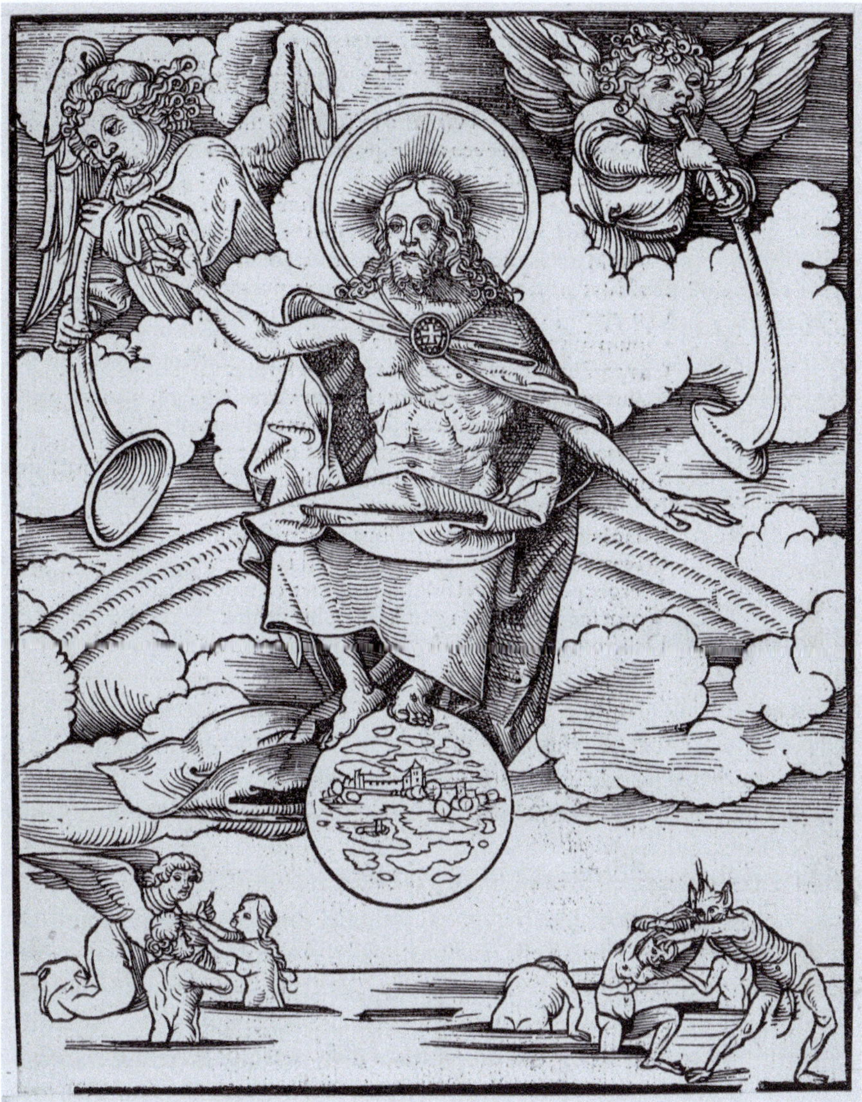

Figure 4.2 Hans Wächtlin, Last Judgement, 1508. Woodcut, 16.7 × 21.4 cm. British Museum, London. © The Trustees of the British Museum. The bodies of those going to heaven and hell do not appear to be notably different in their size and shape but are differentiated in terms of their weightiness. Those meeting the angel of heaven hover effortlessly from their graves, while those destined for hell must push or be pulled up from the ground.

hellish figures were, however, often depicted as the same size, with the distinction in weight indicated by other means. In Hans Wächtlin's woodcut of the Last Judgement from 1508 (Figure 4.2), the bodies of the damned and the blessed appear to be the same size, but they are differentiated by their weightiness. Those rising to meet the angel of heaven hover effortlessly from their graves, whilst those destined for hell are shown as either needing to be pulled up by a demon, or as having to push themselves up from the ground, which appears to require great effort and thus indicates their heaviness.

Weight also had a particular meaning in images of the Last Judgement, as this traditionally involved the weighing of souls. In Rogier Van der Weyden's painting (Figure 4.3), the two figures on the scales appear the same size, but the body of the damned soul weighs down the scales, perhaps presenting this notion of the weighted bodies of sinners. By contrast, in Hans Memling's image from the 1460s (Figure 4.4), the blessed figure is shown as weighing more, although again their bodies appear of equal size, probably because in the Catholic tradition the act of weighing was understood as an assessment of the good works of an individual—weighing more was a measure of having performed a greater number of good works.[42] Whilst these paintings are both fifteenth-century examples, with their contradictory presentations of weight in relation to judgement, they suggest that equating weight (as a measure of heaviness) with ideas of fatness and thinness in this context is problematic.

The distinction between heavenly and earthly bodies was not simply one of thin versus fat; lightness was not necessarily an indication of thinness. Moreover, Luther specifically stated that the heavenly body would 'no longer hunger or thirst, become tired or decrease in size (*abnemen*)', indicating that only earthly bodies were at risk of becoming thin. Indeed, Luther never referred to the earthly body as fat, but rather he referred to the belly of the earthly body, describing how 'we must bear this heavy, indolent paunch (*wanst*) about with us, lift it, and have it led'.[43] In an earlier sermon he stated that in heaven it will be wholly different and beautiful, 'otherwise what would God really have accomplished, if things would not be different, if man would always have to bear his paunch (*wanst*) and sack of stench (*stancksack*) with him and eternally stuff himself and eliminate'.[44] This large and heavy belly is to be read metaphorically, as a reference to the appetites and bodily processes to which we are all subjected. Luther certainly embraced earthly appetites, but his concern here is that, in heaven, man will not 'eat, drink, or do what follows', meaning the processes of digestion and excretion.[45] In contrast to the heavenly nourishment of God, on earth the needs of the stomach are a burden, like a sack or paunch which one must bear on the body. On earth one cannot escape the belly's needs, an idea that accords with Luther's understanding of human nature as inherently sinful following the Fall. The paunch or sack-like

[42] Craig Harbison commented on a decline in the presentation of the scales of judgement in images of the resurrection in the sixteenth century, as the reference to good works became merely symbolic, intended to indicate that 'Christ's justice and fairness now count more than the careful weighing of specific and select aggregates of good and evil acts'. Craig Harbison, *The Last Judgment in Sixteenth Century Northern Europe: A Study in the Relation between Art and the Reformation* (New York, 1975), 132.

[43] 'Das 15. Capitel der Ersten Epistel S. Pauli an die Corinther', *WA*, vol. 36, 671.

[44] Ibid. 635. [45] Ibid. 633–4.

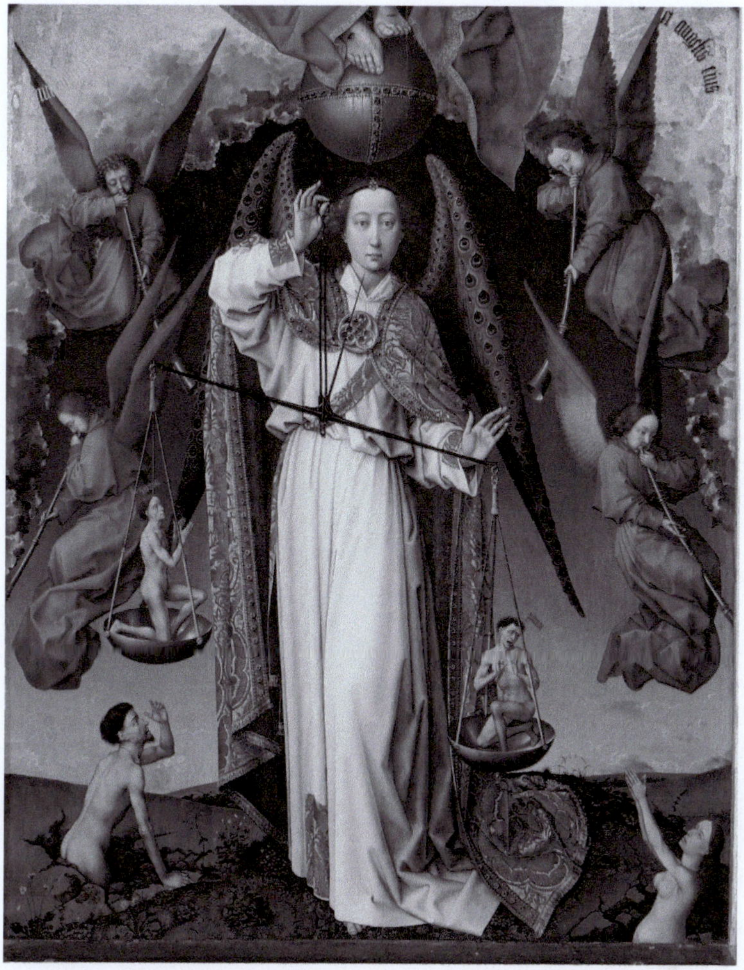

Figure 4.3 Rogier van der Weyden, Central Panel of The Last Judgement Altarpiece, c.1445–50. Oil on oak, 220 × 548 cm. © Hospices Civils de Beaune. The damned soul on the right weighs down the scales though their bodies are not noticeably different in size.

stomach of the earthly body therefore did not merely represent fatness; it had for Luther a deeper meaning associated with appetites and bodily processes, as well as with human sinfulness.

Such discussions within Lutheranism about the form of the resurrected and heavenly body became increasingly relevant with the growth of apocalypticism in the later sixteenth century, for resurrection would take place at the end of the world. The relationship between body size and sinfulness was reinforced in the context of apocalyptic belief, as fatness resulting from the deadly sin of gluttony took on particular meaning as a sign of the coming apocalypse.

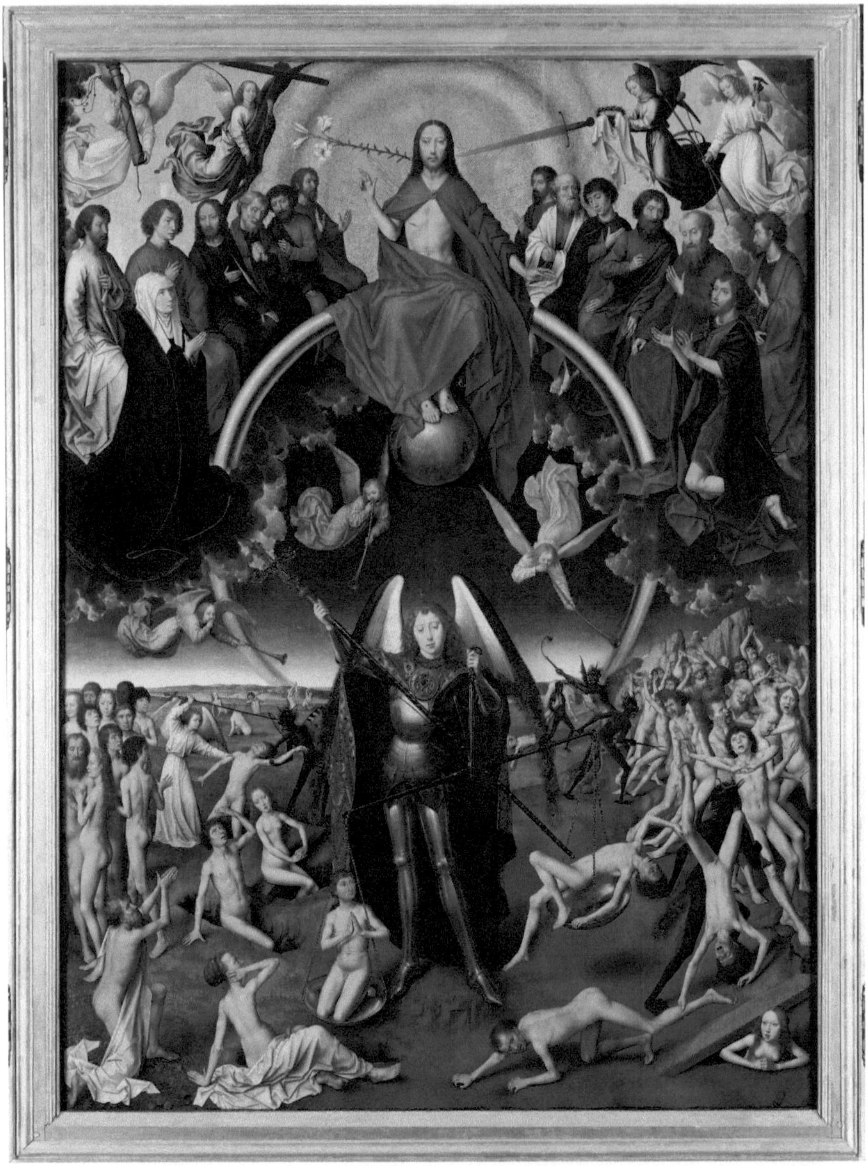

Figure 4.4 Hans Memling, Central Panel of The Last Judgement, 1467–71. Oil on panel, 224 × 162 cm. © National Museum in Gdańsk, Poland. In this painting, the blessed figure on the left is shown to weigh more than the damned, perhaps reflecting the Catholic tradition in which the act of weighing at the Last Judgement was a measure of the good works of an individual.

Gluttony and the Apocalypse

Following Luther's death in 1546, there was a rapid rise in the number of apocalyptic warnings published in Lutheran regions which insisted that the world would soon end.[46] Luther himself had made numerous prophetic statements, and his worldview was fundamentally shaped by anticipation of the apocalypse.[47] In the tumultuous aftermath of the reformer's death, the End of Days seemed increasingly imminent for his followers who had long believed that the biblical signs of the apocalypse were being fulfilled, most prominently with the presence of the Antichrist in the form of the pope (or the papacy in general). In his volume on the coming apocalypse, containing a foreword by Philipp Melanchthon, Johann Funck stated that the whole of Christendom had become subject to the papal Antichrist who was 'lord above Emperor, King and mighty Prince'.[48] For the theologian Nicolaus von Amsdorf, the first Lutheran bishop in the Holy Roman Empire, the false teachings of the pope included the forbidding of 'marriage and food' for his clergy 'under the guise of piety', which, von Amsdorf wrote in 1554, was 'alone enough through which one should recognize the Antichrist'.[49] By denying the appetites of the clergy, the papacy had left God's kingdom behind, as the true church was 'not grounded in eating [and] drinking... but in the power of the spirit, belief and love'.[50] The association of the denial of bodily appetites with the Antichrist thus implicated the body in the belief that the apocalypse was imminent.

A further sign of the end of the world was the proliferation of gluttony and drunkenness.[51] Using Luke 21: 34, 'Be careful, or your hearts will be weighed down with carousing, drunkenness and the anxieties of life, and that day [the Day of Judgement] will close on you suddenly like a trap', commentators claimed that the excessive eating and drinking of contemporary society proved that the world would soon end. Writing of this passage during Advent in 1522, Luther had proposed that 'from these words it is clear that the people will give themselves to gorging and guzzling (*fressen vnd sauffen*) and temporary nourishment beyond all moderation'.[52] Luther related this excess to his own era, writing, 'such sumptuous and various food and drink has... never been so common as it is now'.[53]

[46] Robin B. Barnes, *Prophecy and Gnosis: Apocalypticism in the Wake of the Lutheran Reformation* (Stanford, CA, 1988), esp. 60–99.

[47] Ibid. 36–53.

[48] See Johann Funck, *APOCALYPSIS: Der Offenbarung Künfftiger Geschicht Johannis, Von widerwertigkeit vnd verfolgung der waren Christlichen Kirchen sind der Apostel zeit, bis an der welt ende, Auslegung*, ed. Zacharias Engelhaubt (Wittenberg, 1560), fol. cciii^r.

[49] Nicolaus von Amsdorf, *Fuenff fuernemliche vnd gewisse Zeichen aus heiliger gottlicher Schrifft/so kurtz vor dem Juengsten tag geschehen sollen* (Jena, 1554), fol. Bii^r.

[50] Ibid., fol. Aiii^v.

[51] Volker Leppin, *Antichrist und Jüngster Tag: Das Profil apokalyptischer Flugschriftenpublizistik im deutschen Luthertum 1548–1618* (Gütersloh, 1992), 118.

[52] 'Evangelium am andern sontag im Advent', *WA*, vol. 10/i/2, 94.

[53] Ibid. 95.

At the end of the century, Lutheran churchman, homiletician, and Gnesio-Lutheran official, Gregor Strigenitz, connected these two signs of the apocalypse in his collection of sermons published in 1598.[54] The denial of appetites propagated by Catholicism had prompted such excesses he claimed: 'Because they were so broken by the godless and idolatrous torture-fasts of the Pope, [people] thought…they could reach heaven through gorging and guzzling (*fressen vnd sauffen*).'[55] Unable to maintain moderation, they 'feasted from morning till late at night', which Strigenitz linked directly to the coming apocalypse: 'Then we see before our eyes, that it is happening just as the Lord Christ said, that the last belly-world (*Bauchwelt*) can no longer eat, but gorge, no longer drink, but guzzle.'[56]

What were the implications of such gluttony and drunkenness, and of the coming apocalypse, for the body? One clue can be found in Strigenitz's comparison of contemporary gluttony with the biblical tale of the Israelites, who after their escape from Egypt forgot the struggles they had faced there and became complacent and gluttonous. Strigenitz draws a comparison in noting that 'nowadays we should also not forget the darkness in which our forbearers were placed under the Papacy'—freedom from fasting must not be allowed to lead to gluttony.[57] The story from Exodus was a common trope in tracts against gluttony. Sebastian Franck used the tale in a text from 1531, describing how Moses stated to the Israelites, 'You have become fat, wide and smooth (*feyst, dick vnd glat*), and when one is so fat and full (*feyßt vnd satt*)…he forsakes the God who made him and follows false idols.' Here the idol is the stomach, for Franck wrote, '[those who are] full, call their belly God', using the notion of the 'belly-worshipper' or 'belly-servant' (*Bauchdiener*).[58] In making this comparison to the Israelites, Strigenitz presented the reader with an image of the gluttonous, apocalyptic body as 'fat, wide and smooth', with 'fatness' thus presented as a direct sign of sin.

Contemporary medical and culinary texts typically understood gluttonous eating to result in a fattening of the body (though not all fat bodies were necessarily understood to have resulted from gluttony).[59] Images of gluttons similarly

[54] Strigenitz (1548–1603) worked as a court preacher in Weimar and then as a superintendent in Jena and Orlamünde. In 1593 he was appointed as superintendent in Meissen, where he stayed until his death. He may be considered 'one of the most important Lutheran theologians of the second half of the sixteenth century outside the academic context'. Johann Anselm Steiger, 'Strigenitz, Gregor' in *Neue Deutsche Biographie* 25 (2013), 556–7.

[55] Gregor Strigenitz, *IEIVNIVM, Das ist: Vom Fasten/Einfeltiger vnd gruendlicher bericht* (Leipzig, 1598), fol. 2^{v}.

[56] Ibid., fols 2^{v} and 46^{r}. Philip Soergel has written of Christoph Irenaeus's consideration of the biblical Flood and all subsequent floods as being caused by gluttony and drunkenness, as 'the surfeit of water…resembled the overdrinking that produced intoxication and by extension overindulgence in all things'. Philip M. Soergel, *Miracles and the Protestant Imagination: The Evangelical Wonder Book in Reformation Germany* (Oxford, 2012), 135–40.

[57] Strigenitz, *Vom Fasten*, fol. 44^{r}.

[58] Sebastian Franck, *Von dem grewlichen laster der Trunckenheit so inn disen letzten zeytenn erst schier mit den Frantzosen auffkommen* (Augsburg, 1531), fol. Giii^{r}. The notion of the 'belly-worshipper' is explored in detail later in this chapter.

[59] See Chapter 2, 34, 36–42.

presented them with rotund and expansive bodies and moralizing works reinforced this connection.[60] In a sermon published in 1584, for instance, Mathesius stated that the glutton 'fattens (*mestet*) himself like a pig in a sty'.[61] Similarly, the edited volume of reformer and theologian Matthias Erb on the vices of gluttony and drunkenness included the statement: 'we should not fatten (*mesten*) the body like a pig'.[62] The pig was a common symbol of gluttony, and its recognized fatness was part of this association.[63] Tied to the urgent threat of the coming apocalypse, therefore, was a sense that people's bodies were changing physically; that they were growing fatter as gluttony became more frequent.

For some, the increasing number of Germans who possessed large bodies from the early sixteenth century onwards would have reinforced this narrative. While the large bodies of elite men could represent wealth and power, in the context of apocalyptic belief, fatness resulting from gluttony was associated with a weakening of the earthly body.[64] The impending end of the world was connected to a sense of earthly deterioration. In 1595, for instance, Lutheran pastor Daniel Schaller argued that the earth itself was ageing, causing light to become darker, and stones and iron to become less solid.[65] Through excessive eating and drinking, the human body was likewise implicated in this sense of decline as people lost the ability to control their bodily appetites, overfilling their bodies and fattening themselves like pigs. In advance of the end of the world, therefore, humans were thought to be giving in to animal impulses with physical consequences.

Fatness and the Belly

Fatness took on new religious significance with the Reformations, particularly among Lutherans. Luther's own conception of fat centred on a distinction between fatness in general and the specific fatness of the belly.[66] For Luther, fatness could be connected with fruitfulness and prosperity. At the same time, however, he consistently used the image of a fat belly to present the figure of the

[60] On images of gluttons see pp. 133–6 below.

[61] Johannes Mathesius, *Postilla: Das ist, Außlegung der Sontags vnnd fürnembsten Fest Euangelien, über das gantze Jar* (Nuremberg, 1584), fol. 144r.

[62] Matthias Erb (ed.), *Von sauffen vnd fressen: Den zweyenn greülichen Lasteren wie die durch den heiligen Chrysostomum Hieronymum vnd Basilium Magnum vnd anderen Vätteren vor tausent Jaren in jren predigen sind gestraafft worde(n)* (Mülhausen, 1559), fol. 16r.

[63] Alison Stewart, 'Man's Best Friend? Dogs and Pigs in Early Modern Germany', in Pia F. Cuneo (ed.), *Animals and Early Modern Identity* (Farnham, 2014), 19–44.

[64] See also Chapter 3, 58–9.

[65] Thomas Kaufmann, '1600: Deutungen der Jahrhundertwende im deutschen Luthertum', in Thomas Kaufmann (ed.), *Konfession und Kultur: Lutherischer Protestantismus in der zweiten Hälfte des Reformationsjahrhundert* (Tübingen, 2006), 413–64, here 420–3.

[66] This challenges Sander Gilman's argument regarding Luther's attitude towards fat. See Sander L. Gilman, *Diets and Dieting: A Cultural Encyclopaedia* (Abingdon, 2008), 166–7. See also Holly Fletcher, '"Belly-Worshippers and Greed-Paunches": Fatness and the Belly in the Lutheran Reformation', *German History* 39 (2021), 173–200, here 183.

'belly-worshipper' (*Bauchdiener*), who worshipped the belly, and its needs, over God. These various meanings of fatness entered into Luther's thinking as he translated the Bible into German, an effort motivated by his belief that the word of God should be read and heard by ordinary people.[67]

A distinction between different forms of fat is discussed by Luther, for instance, in connection to his translation of Psalm 92, which states that the righteous shall flourish like a palm tree. Explaining his process of translation in 1531, Luther first quoted the Psalm as he had translated it: 'When you become old, you will nevertheless blossom and remain fruitful and fresh'. He then clarified his choice of language,

> We know well that word for word it says: 'you will still bloom with grey hair, and be fat (*fett*) and green'. Yet what is really being said? The Psalm compared the Righteous with the trees, both palm tree and cedar, which do not have grey hair, and are also not fat (*fett*) (which a German will understand as lard and think of a fat belly (*einen feisten bauch*)). But the prophet wants to say, the Righteous are such trees, which continue to blossom, remain fruitful and fresh, despite becoming old, and they remain so eternally.[68]

Fatness in this Psalm, Luther suggested, represented fruitfulness and prosperity. Yet this was not fatness as Germans understood it—it did not mean 'a fat belly'—and so he removed any reference to fat in his translated version.

A similar process of translation took place for Psalm 63: 5.[69] While a literal translation of the Psalm states 'let my soul become full, as with lard and fat, that my mouth shall praise with joyful lips', Luther's translation reads: 'this would be my heart's joy and bliss, if I could praise you with a joyful mouth'. Luther justified this choice with a fascinating explanation:

> Because no German understands this [first version] we let go of the Hebrew wording (lard and grease (*schmaltz und fett*), with which they express joy, just like a healthy, fat (*fett*) animal is happy, and in turn a happy animal becomes fat (*fett*), a sad animal becomes smaller and grows thin (*abnimpt und mager wird*), and a thin (*mager*) animal is unhappy), and we have given this clarity in German.[70]

Luther's explanation suggests that ideas about the intertwining of animal emotional states with fatness and thinness were widespread, but that the Hebrew association between lard and joy in this Psalm would not be understood among

[67] Roper, *Martin Luther*, 207–8.
[68] 'Summarien über die Psalmen und Ursachen des Dolmetschens', *WA*, vol. 38, 14–15.
[69] On Luther's translation of the Bible see Eric W. Gritsch, 'Luther as Bible Translator' in Donald K. McKim (ed.), *The Cambridge Companion to Martin Luther* (Cambridge, 2003), 62–72.
[70] 'Summarien über die Psalmen und Ursachen des Dolmetschens', *WA*, vol. 38, 10.

Germans. Fatness certainly could be associated with happiness and comfort for early modern Germans, and it seems likely that Luther was also reflecting on potential confusion at the idea of the soul itself being full of greasy fat.[71] Luther's statement with regard to Psalm 92—that a 'German' understanding of lard was connected primarily to the fatness of the belly—suggests that his decision to cut out references to fat also drew on the contemporary association between a fat stomach and excess.

Primarily, a fat belly was understood as a sign of gluttony and drunkenness since the fattening caused by these vices was said to be isolated to the stomach. Gregory the Great had stated in his 'Pastoral Care' that, 'when the belly is distended through gluttony, the virtues of the soul are ruined by impurity', identifying the fatness of gluttony as the fatness of the belly.[72] Similarly, Matthias Erb's volume described how, with gluttony and drunkenness, the stomach expands to the point where it 'wants to rip with the weight of food' and becomes 'stretched like a drum'.[73] Such descriptions offer an image of the glutton's belly as unnaturally large, and these disproportionate bellies can most clearly be seen in several caricatures created by Hans Weiditz around the year 1520.[74] Seven of his woodcuts created in this period contain such figures.[75] Perhaps most notably, in 'Dance Partners' (Figure 4.5), the man's belly is drastically out of proportion in comparison to his limbs. With his chin lifted as though gasping for air, he appears to struggle to move with the weight of his over-extended stomach, even though he pronounces he can dance and skip 'in a courtly manner'. In 'Winebag and Wheelbarrow' (Figure 4.6), the drunkard's belly is so large that he needs a wheelbarrow to trundle it around; he states, 'I am a true winebag, for [I carry] my belly on wheels'. This use of the wheelbarrow appears to have become a common motif and was repeated elsewhere in northern Europe in this period.[76]

The motif of the wheelbarrow also appears in a caricature of Luther from the 1630s (Figure 4.7).[77] Here Luther's distended belly is used to critique the reformer, displaying his indulgence in the earthly appetites. While Luther's large size became part of the positive image of Lutheranism, his opponents repeatedly capitalized upon his stout form to argue against his piety. In 1524, Thomas Müntzer, the radical reformer who became Luther's most hated opponent, described Luther as 'Brother Fattened Pig' (*bruder mastschwein*) and published a refutation

[71] See Chapter 2, 33, 44–5.

[72] Gregory the Great, *Pastoral Care*, tr. Henry Davis (Westminster, MD, 1950), 148.

[73] Erb, *Von sauffen vnd fressen*, fols 40^{v} and 2^{r}.

[74] On Weiditz's images see Sara Benninga, 'The Faces of Fatness in Early Modern Europe', *FKW: Zeitschrift für Geschlechterforschung und visuelle Kultur* 62 (2017), 24–35, 29–33.

[75] Max Geisberg (ed.), *The German Single-Leaf Woodcut 1500–1550* (New York, 1974), vol. 4, 1471–81.

[76] See Book of Hours, 1520s Bruges, Morgan Library, New York, MS M.1175, fol. 191^{r}, and Lorenz Schultes, *The Brotherhood of Bacchus*, in Wilhelm Hollstein, *German Engravings, Etchings, and Woodcuts, c.1400–1700*, 73 vols (Amsterdam, 1954–2007), vol. 52, 241.

[77] On the wider use of this motif see Benninga, 'Faces of Fatness', 32–4.

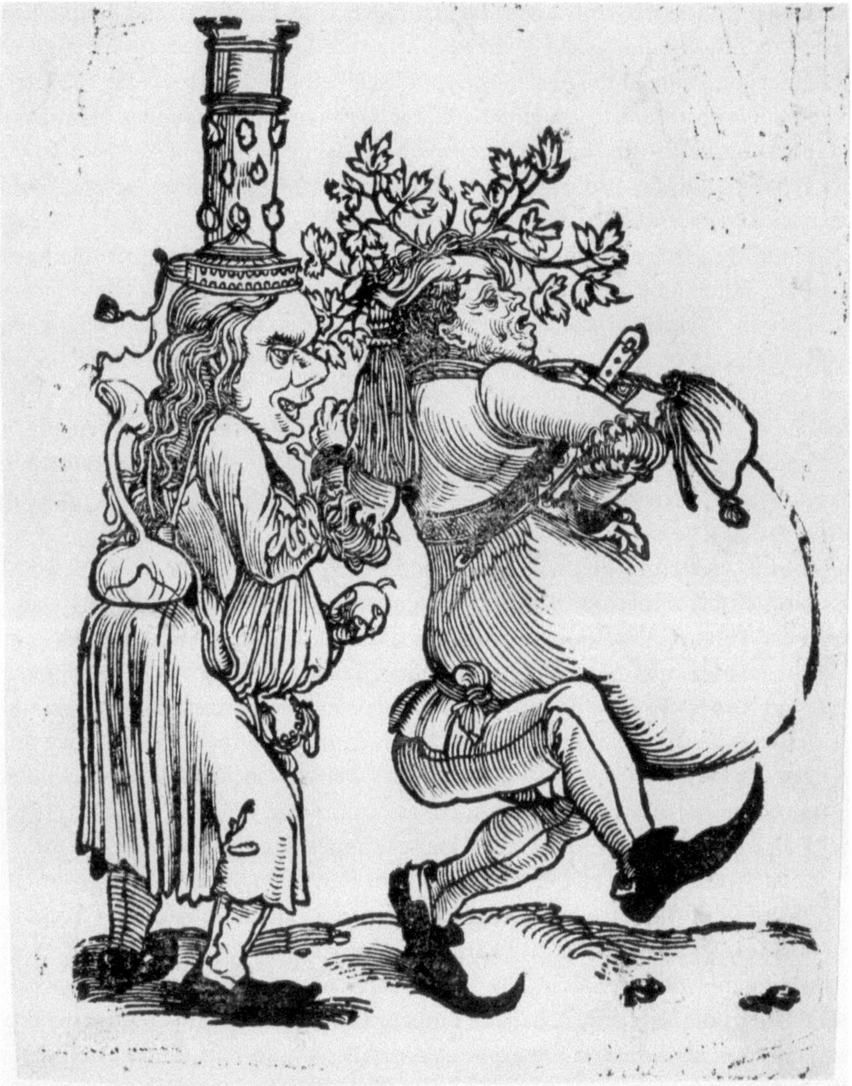

Figure 4.5 Hans Weiditz, Dance Partners, 1521. Woodcut, 28. 6 × 21.9 cm © bpk/ Herzog Anton Ulrich Museum. The glutton's belly is shown to be unnaturally distended. An association with drunkenness is suggested by the winebag on his partner's back.

of 'the Unspiritual, Soft-Living Flesh in Wittenberg' by which he referred to Luther.[78] He used the image of Luther's fleshy, fattened body to mock his 'soft-living', comfort, and wealth.

[78] Thomas Müntzer, *Auszlegung des andern vnterschyds Danielis* (Allstedt, 1524), fol. C^{r}; Thomas Müntzer, *Hoch verursachte Schutzrede und antwort wider das Gaistloße Sanfft lebende fleysch zu Wittenberg* (Nuremberg, 1524). On Müntzer see Roper, *Martin Luther*, 249–51, and Lyndal Roper, *Living I was your Plague: Martin Luther's World and Legacy* (Princeton, 2021), 47–50.

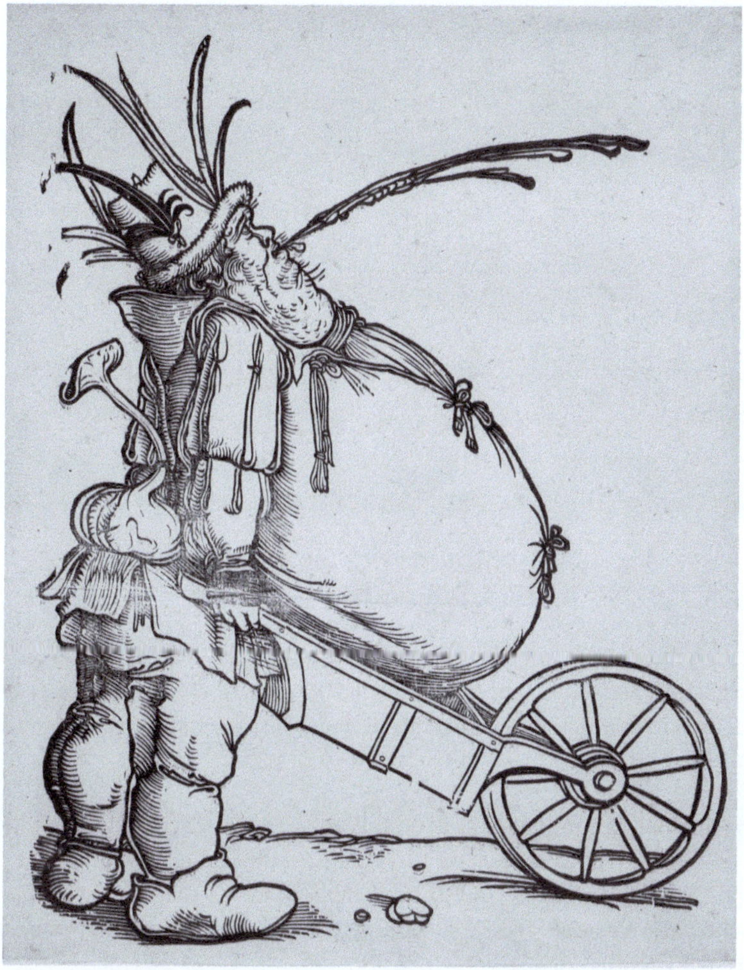

Figure 4.6 Hans Weiditz, Winebag and Wheelbarrow, 1521. Woodcut, 27.7 × 21.2 cm. British Museum, London. © The Trustees of the British Museum. The drunkard's belly is so large that he trundles it around in a wheelbarrow. A winebag is shown attached to his back, the rounded form of which echoes the bulk of his stomach.

Writing about the period shortly before Luther's death, the Catholic humanist Johannes Cochlaeus similarly argued that he had not lived as a true disciple of Christ, stating, 'What kind of sanctity or of a miracle is there in this, that every evening after a supper lavishly prepared and abundantly partaken of, with his belly distended by food and drink, he looked out of the window of his dwelling and prayed for a little while.'[79] Here Cochlaeus did not critique Luther simply by

[79] Johannes Cochlaeus, 'The Deeds and Writings of Martin Luther from the Year of the Lord 1517 to the Year 1546 Related Chronologically to All Posterity by Johannes Cochlaeus', in Elizabeth Vandiver and Ralph Keen (eds), *Luther's Lives: Two Contemporary Accounts of Martin Luther* (Manchester, 2003), 56–355, here 351–2.

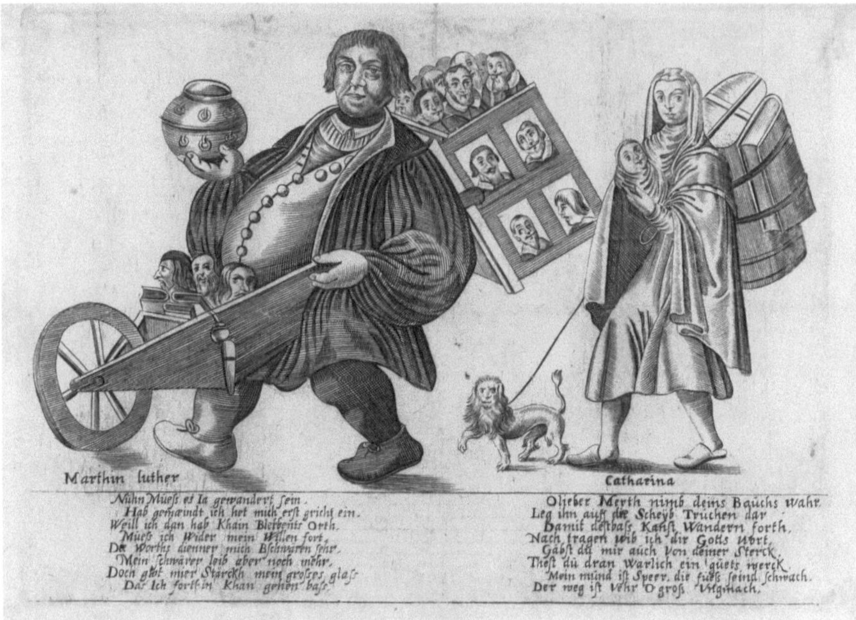

Figure 4.7 Anonymous, Now it Must Have Wandered, 1630–40. Engraving, 17 × 37.5 cm. © Stiftung Luthergedenkstätten in Sachsen-Anhalt. Luther's distended belly is used in this caricature to critique his indulgence in food and drink and mock his expansive body.

calling him 'fat', but rather focused on this enlargement of (just) his belly through food and drink. His emphasis on the isolated largeness of Luther's belly evoked the specific sins of gluttony and drunkenness, while also suggesting Luther was a hypocrite, for he was himself a 'belly-worshipper', the very charge he placed against the Catholic clergy.

Preaching against the monastic vow of chastity in the late 1530s, Luther explicitly described the Catholic clergy as 'vain belly-worshippers [and] greed-paunches' (*bauch diener [und] Geitzwenste*).[80] He characterized the Catholic Church as servants of the stomach, associating Catholicism with the belly, and particularly the fat belly. In 1522, Luther instructed Christians to 'be in the empire of Christ and not of the Pope, for they say they are spiritual but are more worldly than spiritual, they are fat bellies (*mestbeuch*) and remain fat bellies'.[81] This image of the fattened belly of Catholicism presented the gluttony of the Catholic clergy

[80] 'Matthäus 18-24 in Predigten ausgelegt. Das dreiundzwanzigste Kapitel', *WA*, vol. 47, 481.

[81] 'Der dritt predigt Martini Lutheris der selbigen vor genanten wochen am Freittag uff dem schloss gethan', *WA*, vol. 10/iii, 379. On Luther's wider use of invective language see Markus Wriedt, 'Invectives as a Stylistic Device in Martin Luther's Reformation Rhetoric', *Journal of Early Modern Christianity* 10 (2023), 43–71.

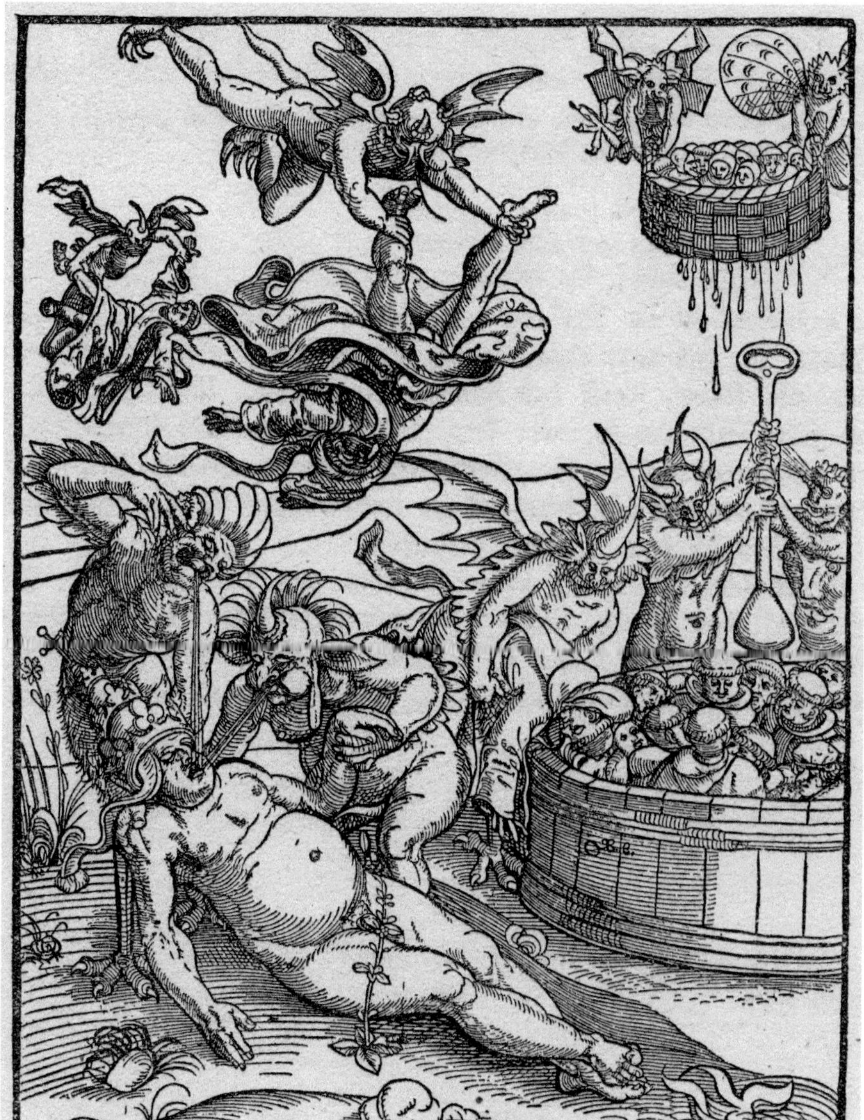

Figure 4.8 Cranach the Elder, From the Origin of the Antichrist, c.1545. Woodcut, dimension unknown. © akg-images. The pope, as the Antichrist, is shown lying nude with a particularly rounded belly.

and thus the hypocrisy of their teachings on fasting. The term *mestbeuch* from the quotations above derives from the verb *mästen*, meaning to fatten, usually in the context of livestock, and thus suggests overfeeding with the intention of becoming fat. In 1527 Luther spoke of preachers who were 'stomach worshippers and gormandizers (*bauchdiener und fresslinge*)' who 'through their preaching seek for nothing other than that they possess enough and may fill their paunches (*wanst*)'.[82] He described the pope specifically as being a 'foul paunch [and] lazy belly (*unfletiger wanst, fauler bauch*)' and the fat belly of the clergy is perhaps best depicted visually in Lucas Cranach's 'Origins of the Antichrist' of 1545 (Figure 4.8), where the pope (as the Antichrist) is shown lying nude, exposing a particularly fat stomach, and thus presented as a worldly belly-worshipper.[83]

Reformers also used this association between the belly and the clergy to present a gendered image of Catholicism.[84] The popular print of the Papal Ass, created by Cranach in 1523 and accompanied by an interpretation by Philipp Melanchthon, depicted a hybrid creature with a rounded belly and breasts that was reportedly found in the River Tiber in 1495 and interpreted as a divine portent.[85] Melanchthon interpreted each body part of the monster as representing a different aspect of the papal regime. In his expanded description of the creature from 1535, he stated that its 'womanly belly and breasts' symbolized the body of the papacy, meaning cardinals, bishops, priests, and monks. These were:

> whorish folk and fattened pigs (*masst sewe*), as their lives are spent in gorging, boozing, all unchasteness/lust and all have good lives on earth, unpunished and with the greatest freedom, that they may live such lives without shame, to the great outrage and corruption of the youth and all the world, just as the Papal Ass bears his womanly belly naked and free.[86]

Echoing Luther's use of *Mestbeuch*, in this passage Melanchthon similarly drew on the verb *mästen* in his description of the clergy as 'fattened pigs'. In connecting the exposed womanly belly and breasts of the Papal Ass with the 'fattened pigs' of the clergy, whom he described as living in lust, unchasteness, gluttony, and drunkenness, Melanchthon thus specifically associated this worldliness and desire with the female body. Melanchthon drew on a broader framing of the sensuous

[82] 'Über das 1. Buch Mose. Predigten. 1527. Kap. 8', *WA*, vol. 24, 191.

[83] 'Papsttreu Hadriani IV. und Alexanders III. 1545', *WA*, vol. 54, 309.

[84] On the significance of gender for the Reformation see Lyndal Roper, *The Holy Household: Women and Morals in Reformation Augsburg* (Oxford, 1989); Merry E. Wiesner, 'Beyond Women and the Family: Towards a Gender Analysis of the Reformation', *Sixteenth Century Journal* 18 (1987), 311–21.

[85] On the context of the print see Lawrence Buck, *The Roman Monster: An Icon of the Papal Antichrist in Reformation Politics* (Kirksville, MO, 2014). On Melanchthon's interpretation see 103–58.

[86] Philipp Melanchthon, *Der BapstEsel durch M. Philippum Melanchthon gedeutet und gebessert* (Wittenberg, 1535), fol. Bi^r.

worship of Catholicism in terms of femininity and female sexuality which was popular among reformers.[87] Joachim von Watt for instance, compared traditional cantors to the sound made by 'hens when they wish to lay' as well as the howling of 'cats in heat'.[88] Reformers also feminized the Catholic Church by connecting it to the 'whore of Babylon' or a harem of courtesans.[89] Strikingly, in the case of the Papal Ass, the body and particularly the belly of the creature becomes the focus for such gendered notions of worldliness. Indeed, when the image was reworked for publication in 1545, Cranach focused his alterations on these areas, enlarging the creature's breasts and the bulge of its 'womanly' stomach which is highlighted through the addition of a prominent belly button.[90]

The use of fatness to denote gluttony and excess in criticisms of the Catholic clergy did not originate with the Lutheran Reformation but had a long tradition across Europe.[91] Boccaccio's *Decameron* from the fourteenth century, for instance, includes a tale about an abbot who on discovering that a monk has a young woman in his cell resolves to sleep with her himself. As he gets onto the monk's bed, however, he decides he cannot lie on top of her for fear of 'hurting her by his excessive weight'.[92] This tale also demonstrates the long-standing connection between overindulgence in food and heightened sexuality, which added a further dimension to the criticism of the clergy's excess. Drawing on medieval critiques, such commentary proliferated in sixteenth- and seventeenth-century Germany. In 1516 Katerina Lemmel, a Birgittine nun in Maihingen, complained that the creator of a new stained-glass window in the nuns' cloister had not done the figure of Christ justice; she stated, 'he sits there like a fat priest!' While Katerina's main concern was that Christ's image would not arouse the same desire and empathy which a bleeding and weakened figure of Jesus would have done (which in itself tells us something about the relationship between body size, suffering, and Catholic piety), since she had previously criticized the behaviour of the secular clergy it seems likely her reference to fat priests drew on negative contemporary associations between fatness and clerical excess.[93]

Monks in particular were often the targets of criticism which was framed in terms of fatness. The chronicle of the Counts of Zimmern (1565–7), for example, contains a tale about a monk who was so fat that he got stuck in a doorway, thus

[87] Jacob Baum, *The Reformation of the Senses: The Paradox of Religious Belief and Practice in Germany* (Urbana, IL, 2019), 115–16.

[88] Joachim von Watt, *Das Büchlein ist genant vom alten vnd neüwen Got, Glauben und Leer* (Strasbourg, 1521), fol. Fii^{v}. Quoted in Baum, *Reformation of the Senses,* 115.

[89] Baum, *Reformation of the Senses,* 115.

[90] See Jennifer Spinks, *Monstrous Births and Visual Culture in Sixteenth-Century Germany* (London, 2009), 77–9.

[91] For the use of fatness as criticism in other religious contexts see Fletcher, 'Fat World of the Hutterites'.

[92] Giovanni Boccaccio, *Decameron,* ed. Cormac O Cuilleanain (Ware, 2004), 47.

[93] Corine Schleif and Volker Schier, *Katerina's Windows: Donation and Devotion, Art and Music, as Heard and Seen in the Writings of a Birgittine Nun* (University Park, PA, 2008), 321 and 325.

preventing 'many honest people' from escaping a fire and thereby causing their deaths.[94] In Julius Zincgref's 'Deutsche Apophthegmata' of 1644, a Carthusian monk is asked why he is so 'very wide and fat (*dick vnd fett*)' when Carthusians 'only eat fish', to which he answers that they make oil from grapes.[95] This tale presents the common accusation that, despite the strict limits on certain foods dictated by Catholicism, the clergy continued to stuff themselves. In his sermon on fasting, Strigenitz stated that, 'The Papacy has not correctly understood the teachings on fasting, and thought that fasting meant when one ate no meat, no eggs nor butter, but continued to eat other food and gorged himself so full on fish, that he wanted to throw-up', and noted that to 'fill oneself so full that the belly groans…that is not what the holy text calls fasting'.[96] Zincgref's anecdote underlines such criticism by suggesting the monk is able to eat so much oil that he can become fat whilst remaining within the supposedly strict diet of the Carthusians.[97]

Luther and his followers took aim at the Catholic papacy through insults about fatness and the belly, yet Catholics were not the only targets of such attacks. Given Luther's influence on the language of both Protestant and Catholic theology, his repeated use of belly-related terms such as *Bauchdiener* (belly-worshipper), *Bauchpriester* (belly-priest), and *Bauchsorge* (belly-cares) became a permanent feature of theological vocabulary.[98] As we have seen, Luther's critics used similar arguments to attack the reformer himself, and his use of the fat belly as theological critique contributed to the wider adoption of fat imagery among polemicists to insult opposing confessions.[99] Menno Simons, for example, the former Catholic priest who became an influential Anabaptist leader and whose followers became known as the Mennonites, used the trope of fatness to criticize evangelical preachers who had no true vocation but merely sought 'praise, money and profit, a soft and easy life'. In 1539 he wrote in his *Foundation of the Christian Doctrine*, 'no doubt it suits perverted fleshly ease to live in luxury here on earth with bodies fat and sleek'.[100]

[94] Froben Christof Graf von Zimmern, *Die Chronik der Grafen von Zimmern: Handschriften 580 und 581 der Fürstlich Fürstenbergischen Hofbibliothek Donaueschingen*, ed. Hansmartin Decker-Hauff and Rudolf Seigel, 3 vols (Sigmaringen, 1972), vol. 3, 70.

[95] Julius Wilhelm Zincgref, *Teutsche Apophthegmata, das ist, Der Teutschen Scharfsinnige kluge Sprüche*, 2 vols (Leiden, 1644), vol. 2, 293.

[96] Strigenitz, *Vom Fasten*, fol. 30^{v}.

[97] On reformers' complaints about fasting regulations see Christopher Kissane, *Food, Religion, and Communities in Early Modern Europe* (London, 2018), esp. 51–104.

[98] See 'Bauch' in Friedrich Lepp (ed.), *Schlagwörter des Reformationszeitalters* (Leipzig, 1908), 131–4. See also Maciej Ptaszyński, 'Theologians and their Bellies: The Erasmian Epithet *Theologaster* during the Reformation', *Erasmus Studies* 41 (2021), 200–29, here 204.

[99] Ptaszyński, 'Theologians and their Bellies', 206.

[100] Menno Simons, 'Foundation of Christian Doctrine', in John Christian Wenger (ed.), *The Complete Writings of Menno Simons: c.1496–1561* (Scottdale, PA, and Waterloo, 1986), 163.

Hutterite Anabaptist leaders were similarly referred to in terms of fatness by Catholic polemical authors who argued against their toleration in sixteenth and seventeenth-century Moravia. Christoph Erhard, a Catholic priest in the town of Nikolsberg, who was a central figure in attempts to re-catholicize Moravia, published a *Short History of the Münster Anabaptists* in 1589 in which he sought to dissuade potential converts to Hutterite communities by stating that they were the direct descendants of the Anabaptists who had led the Münster rebellion in 1534. In arguing that the Hutterites deceived their followers and led them from the correct path, Erhard stated that, 'such people (as the Hutterite brothers of this time) do not serve the Lord Jesus Christ but their own bellies (as nearly all the leaders and principals have fine, good, big, fat bellies (*feine, gute, grosse, faiste Bäuch*) and long beards) and through sweet words and well-spoken speeches...they seduce the hearts of the innocent'.[101] With his image of Hutterite leaders as having fat bellies, Erhard suggested that they were living excessive lives which were marked by gluttony, thus undermining the view of Hutterite communities as providing an alternative, more equal form of society through the practice of a 'community of goods'.[102] The Jesuit priest Christoph Andreas Fischer drew heavily on Erhard's writings in his own text against the Hutterites from 1607 in which he questioned:

> Who lives in greater lust than they?...Truly when nothing other than the luxuriousness of their kings, the servants [of the word/temporal affairs], the householders and other leaders is shown (whereas others sometimes must make do with only cabbage and turnips), alone their protruding, great fat potbellies (*faiste, grosse Schmärbäuche*) and their broad, bloated, fatty faces (*breite, broschete vnd geschmaltzene Gesichter*) betray them because they do not have such things from water and bread, from cabbage and turnips. Is that not called serving the belly?[103]

Fischer too presented the Hutterite leaders as belly-worshippers whose hypocrisy and lack of true piety was symbolized by their potbellies and fat faces. The

[101] Christoph Erhard, *Gründliche kurtz verfaste Historia. Von Münsterischen Widertauffern* (Munich, 1589), fol. 47^r.

[102] See Fletcher, 'Fat World of the Hutterites'. On the Hutterite 'community of goods' see Astrid von Schlachta, *Hutterische Konfession und Tradition (1578–1619): Etabliertes Leben zwischen Ordnung und Ambivalenz* (Göttingen, 2009); Esther Chung-Kim, *Economics of Faith: Reforming Poor Relief in Early Modern Europe* (Oxford, 2021); James Stayer, *The German Peasant's War and Anabaptist Community of Goods* (Montreal, 1991).

[103] Christoph Andreas Fischer, *Vier und funfftzig Erhebliche Ursachen Warumb die Widertauffer nicht sein im Land zu leyden* (Ingolstadt, 1607), 97. *Broschete* is difficult to translate but I have translated it as bloated, following a definition of *broschet* in Josef Pohl, 'Etymologisches über den Namen des Caspar Bruschius', in *Mitteilungen des Vereins für Geschichte der Deutschen in Böhmen*, 76 vols (Prague, 1862–1938 (1913)), vol. 51, 404–6, here 405.

language of fatness and the belly was thus put to use against a variety of communities within an increasingly splintered Christendom.

Beyond Christianity, this rhetoric was used against Jewish communities who were similarly stated to worship the belly. Such discussions of Jewish fatness in this period were invigorated by Luther's writings. In 1528 Luther warned that evangelicals had become complacent and that they needed to pray to God in earnest, so that evangelism could establish itself in Germany and beyond, and thus reach those who had not heard the true word of God. He worried that 'we are doing just the same as the Jews, who pay more attention to the belly than to God, who are more concerned with how they can fill the belly than with how they can become blessed'.[104] Luther's attitude towards Jewish people underwent dramatic changes over his lifetime. In the early days of the Reformation Luther campaigned for toleration of the Jews, yet by the end of his life he displayed a violent hatred towards them which went beyond traditional Christian hostility; he actively adopted and spread premodern antisemitism.[105] Luther insisted that Jews were so dangerous that they must either convert or be expelled, and in his famous 1543 text *On the Jews and their Lies* his arguments for their expulsion integrated imagery of the fat belly. He wrote of Jews as being the house guests of Christians, yet 'they steal from us…the lazy knaves and idle paunches (*wenste*), guzzling and gorging and prospering in our home'.[106] As in Luther's descriptions of Catholics, the image of Jews as being fat-bellies connected them to gluttonous eating which was shown to be at the expense of Christian communities, and thereby fatness was weaponized as an argument against toleration.

Building on such descriptions, sixteenth-century discussions of Jewish eating habits repeatedly suggested that Jews were gluttons who stuffed themselves beyond all limits.[107] In his *Jewish Scourge* from 1598, Ernst Ferdinand Hess suggested that no other people were capable of gorging themselves like the Jews do on Purim, using verbs such as *schlemmen* and *sauffen* to indicate excessive, animalistic consumption.[108] Descriptions of Jewish excess built upon, and encouraged, the long-standing visual representation of Jewish leaders as being fat.[109] Albrecht Dürer, for instance, repeatedly presented the Jewish High Priest Caiaphas with a notably

[104] Martin Luther, *Auslegung der Episteln vnd Euangelien vom Advent an bis auff Ostern* (Wittenberg, 1528), fol. CV^{r-v}. This was one of Luther's numerous advent homilies, listed in *WA*, vol. 10/i/2, XIII–VL, for this text see p. XIX, H.

[105] Thomas Kaufmann, *Luther's Jews: A Journey into Anti-Semitism* (Oxford, 2017). See also Thomas Kaufmann, 'Luther and the Jews', *Antisemitism Studies* 3 (2019), 46–65.

[106] 'Von den Juden und ihren Lügen', *WA*, vol. 53, 529.

[107] Yaacov Deutsch, *Judaism in Christian Eyes: Ethnographic Descriptions of Jews and Judaism in Early Modern Europe* (Oxford, 2012), 223–5.

[108] Ernst Ferdinand Hess, *Flagellum Iudeorum, Juden Geissel, Das ist Ein Neuwe sehr nütze und gründliche Erweisung, daß Jesus Christus, Gottes und der H. Jungkfrauwen Marien Sohn, der wahre verheissene und gesandte Messias sey* (Erfurt, 1598), 104. See Deutsch, *Judaism in Christian Eyes*, 224.

[109] Ruth Mellinkoff, *Outcasts: Signs of Otherness in Northern European Art of the Late Middle Ages* (Berkeley, CA, 1993), 128.

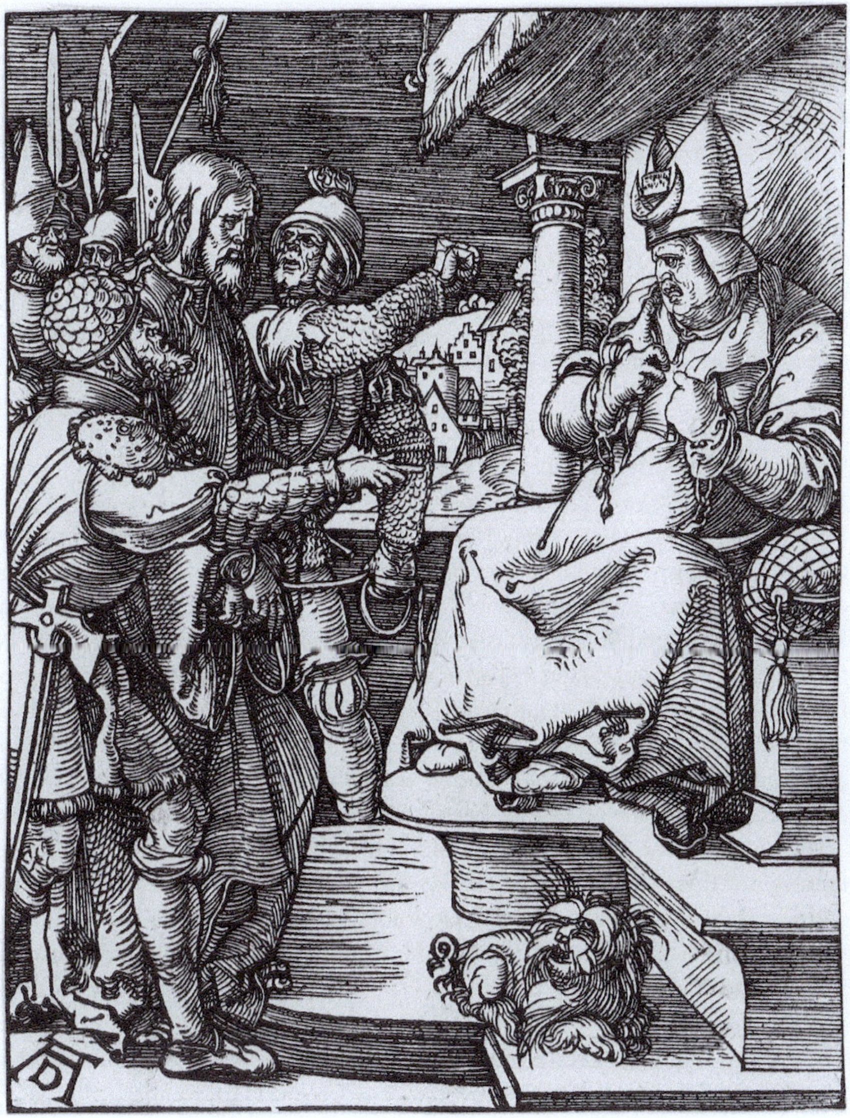

Figure 4.9 Albrecht Dürer, Christ Before Caiaphas from 'The Small Passion', c.1508. Woodcut, 12.7 × 9.7 cm. Metropolitan Museum of Art, New York, public domain. Dürer repeatedly represented the Jewish High Priest in a stout and fleshy body.

stout figure and fat belly (Figure 4.9).[110] Just as Lutherans used fatness to feminize the Catholic Church, it is likely that understandings of Jewish fat likewise drew on associations between fatness and the female body. In this period, Jewish men were frequently described as having a colder humoral complexion than Christian

[110] Dürer presented the High Priest with such a figure in his Small Passion, Large Passion, and Green Passion Series. See also Forth, *Fat*, 128–9.

men, and thus being physically more like women; it was even widely believed that Jewish men menstruated.[111] Since the coldness of female bodies was understood to result in their having fleshier forms, Jewish men would have been understood as naturally fatter than Christian men.[112]

Fatness and the belly became embedded within spiritual arguments against various faiths in the Reformations and Luther played a pivotal role in the proliferation of such imagery. It seems somewhat ironic that the widespread adoption of fatness and the belly in religious criticism stemmed from a figure whose own stout body was central to his image and success. Luther's character and theology was full of contradictions, yet in this case it seems he viewed his own large size in notably different terms to the fatness of which he accused his opponents.

Metaphors of Fat and the Importance of Moderation

Despite characterizing the Catholic clergy as servants of the belly, Luther knew that not all clergy were living lives of luxury; his own monastic experience has certainly not been one of gluttony.[113] Speaking of his time at the monastery in Erfurt, Luther stated, 'I almost fasted myself to death, for again and again I went for three days without taking a drop of water or a morsel of food'.[114] At the time of Luther's disputation with Johannes Eck in 1519, Petrus Mosellanus described the reformer's 'thin body, so exhausted by cares and study that if you look closely you can almost count all his bones'.[115] Luther later reflected that 'being a monk was all about controlling one's diet and sleep, castigating the flesh and fighting sexual urges'; Luther's transformation from monk to reformer was as much physical as theological, therefore, including the expansion of his form into the stout figure with which he became associated.[116] How could Luther reconcile his own experience of monasticism with the critique of Catholicism which presented monks as intemperate 'fat-bellies'?

[111] On Jewish male menstruation see Sander L. Gilman, *Jewish Self-Hatred: Anti-Semitism and the Hidden Language of the Jews* (Baltimore, MD, 1986), 74–75; David S. Katz, 'Shylock's Gender: Jewish Male Menstruation in Early Modern England', *Review of English Studies* 50 (1999), 440–62; Irven M. Resnick, 'Medieval Roots of the Myth of Jewish Male Menses', *Harvard Theological Review* 93 (2000), 241–63; Justin Hastings, 'Hic et Haec: The Feast of Corpus Christi, the Myth of Jewish Male Menstruation, and Allegoresis', *Essays in Medieval Studies* 34 (2018), 39–52.

[112] On the view of Jews as fatter than Christians (mainly in a nineteenth-century context) see Sander L. Gilman, *Fat Boys*, 45–50; Sander L. Gilman, 'Jews and Fat: Thoughts toward a History of an Image in the Second Age of Biology', in Anat Helman (ed.), *Jews and their Foodways* (Oxford, 2016), 218–30. See also Daniel Boyarin, 'Literary Fat Rabbis: On the Historical Origins of the Grotesque Body', *Journal of the History of Sexuality* 1 (1991), 551–84.

[113] See Roper, *Martin Luther*, 56–7, and Martin Brecht, *Martin Luther: Sein Weg zur Reformation, 1483–1521* (Stuttgart, 1981), 70–7.

[114] 'Anton Lauterbachs Tagebuch aufs Jahr 1539', in Martin Luther, *D. Martin Luthers Werke: Kritische Gesamtausgabe. Tischreden* [hereafter *WA TR*], 6 vols (Weimar, 1912–21), vol. 4, 305–6, no. 4422. Translation from Latin in *LW*, vol. 54, 339–40.

[115] Roper, *Martin Luther*, 133. [116] Ibid. 199.

First, Luther recorded that 'only truly afflicted consciences fasted in earnest', suggesting that his asceticism was not the norm in the monastery. He also proposed, however, 'This is the truth: the most pious monk is the worst scoundrel. He denies that Christ is the mediator and high-priest and turns him into a judge'.[117] Luther saw this extreme denial of the flesh, as with good works, as merely an act undertaken to impress Christ, the judge, rather than an act of true belief. This criticism of the fasting of ascetics also suggested their self-denial was intended to impress those around them, as a kind of self-fashioning which allowed them to demonstrate how holy they were through their appearance. Luther thus drew on an existing anti-ascetic discourse which presented extreme fasting as performative.[118] In a sermon from 1532, Luther drew on Matthew 6: 16, 'When you fast, do not look sombre like the hypocrites do, for they disfigure their faces to show others they are fasting', in arguing that such hypocrites fasted only 'to be seen by the people, and to have a name, so that one would wonder and have to say "Oh those are those excellent saints who do not live like common people but dress in grey, hang their heads and look sombre and pale. If they do not reach heaven, where will we be?"' (1530/2).[119] Preaching in Regensburg in 1573, Lutheran theologian Josua Opitz opined that 'this kind [of hypocritical fasting] is also the papist fasting implemented by their idol in Rome' and in recording that such fasting was 'flaunted' before God and the people, Opitz emphasized an element of performance in Catholic fasts.[120] Ascetics were thus shown to act with an audience in mind, undermining their supposed liberation from worldliness since they nevertheless conceived of their fasting in relation to the outside world and the judgement of external observers.[121]

Whether Catholics ignored the restrictions of fasting (either through dispensations or by gorging themselves on permitted foods such as oil or fish) or if they kept a strictly ascetic diet, they could thus still be portrayed as hypocrites by reformers. Returning to Luther's statement that 'they say they are spiritual but are more worldly than spiritual, they are fat-bellies and remain fat-bellies', we recognize that his use of fatness in this context is a reference not merely to gluttony but to worldliness in general. Here he used the notion of the 'fat-belly' or 'paunch' as a metaphor, so even emaciated ascetics could be 'fat-bellies' or 'belly-worshippers', since they acted out of the worldly desire to impress those around them, fashioning their bodies to proclaim their faith. This intentionality is reflected in Luther's

[117] 'Anton Lauterbachs Tagebuch aufs Jahr 1539', *WA TR*, vol. 4, 305–6, no. 4422. Translation from Latin in *LW*, vol. 54, 339–40.

[118] Constable, *Attitudes Toward*, 21–2.

[119] 'Wochenpredigten über Matthäus 5-7', *WA*, vol. 32, 428.

[120] Josua Opitz, *Eine Fastenpredigt von christlichem und antichristischem Fasten: Wider den bäpstischen abgöttischen Fastenteuffel* (Regensburg, 1573), fol. B1r.

[121] On the performativity of asceticism see Christina Johanna Bischoff, 'Ultra Mensuram tendere: Zur Maßlosigkeit mönchischer Askese', in Isabelle Mandrella and Kathrin Müller (eds), *Maß und Maßlosigkeit im Mittelalter* (Berlin, 2018), 29–47, esp. 37.

use of the descriptive term *Mestbeuch*, derived from the verb *mästen* (to fatten up), which suggests *deliberate* fattening.

In the original notion of the belly-worshipper from the Pauline Epistles, Paul did not consider the outward appearance or form of the belly to be a sign of spiritual significance, rather the stomach was a 'codeword' for Paul.[122] The belly represented a life controlled by the desires, and although such desires could involve food or drink, 'belly-devotion' also referred to a 'self-centred attitude aiming at pleasing oneself'.[123] Similarly, Luther's characterization of his opponents as 'fat-bellies' was not merely a criticism of overeating, for Luther also used the belly as a symbol of a life governed by desire. The 'fat belly' could thus be a particularly pertinent term for those who restricted their consumption. When, around 1540, Luther declared, 'It is a religious obligation of the Franciscans not to touch gold and silver with their hands, although in their hearts they foster ravenous hunger, they long for and consume the wealth of the entire world', he was reflecting the idea that those who deny their appetites and desires experience them all the more strongly and are governed by them to a greater extent than those who embrace them.[124]

For Luther, if not for other religious commentators who took up such imagery, both extremes of gluttony and asceticism could be represented by the 'fat-belly', just as in Agricola's explanation for the opening proverb, his portrayal of the monastery criticized both the luxurious lives of the fathers and the jealous lusting of the monks. This duality might help explain how Luther was able to criticize the Catholic clergy as being fat and preach against gluttony and drunkenness whilst embracing the appetites and making his own large body part of his image.[125] It is possible that Luther's indulgent eating may have contributed to a sense of his own sinfulness, perhaps indicating that he was unable to reconcile his criticisms with his own reality.[126] Yet it seems likely that Luther did not view his own large body in the same way as he viewed the 'fat-bellies' of those he criticized. Luther famously described himself as fat in 1546 when he joked that at his death he would 'give the maggots a fat doctor (*einen feisten Doctor*) to eat'.[127] Here Luther used self-deprecating humour to reference his indulgence in food and drink, and the resulting bulk of his body, but this did not mean that he viewed himself as comparable to the fat-bellies of Catholics or Jews.

His was certainly not the fat-belly of the hypocrite, as Luther spoke out against the fasting of Catholicism and embraced the appetites, stating that their enjoyment was admitted by God. In a sermon from 1534, he used the common proverb 'On a full stomach stands a happy head' in noting that eating and drinking 'is a

[122] Karl Olav Sandnes, *Belly and Body in the Pauline Epistles* (Cambridge, 2002), 34.

[123] Ibid. 133–5.

[124] 'Vorlesungen über 1. Mose Kap. 24', *WA*, vol. 43, 332. Translation from Latin in *LW*, vol. 4, 275.

[125] Roper, 'Martin Luther's Body', 381.

[126] Susan C. Karant-Nunn, *The Personal Luther: Essays on the Reformer from a Cultural Historical Perspective* (Leiden, 2017), 41. See also 198.

[127] 'Tischreden aus Johannes Aurifabers Sammlung FB.', *WA TR*, vol. 6, 302, no. 6975.

lovely and necessary work.'[128] His embrace of the appetite for food was linked to Luther's rejection of Catholic celibacy, modifying the medieval connection between appetites whereby indulgent eating suggested lasciviousness.[129] Luther wrote that 'the Pope has as little power to command [chastity] as he has to forbid eating, drinking, the natural movement of the bowels or growing fat (*feyst*).'[130] On eating, Luther insisted that 'abstinence does not please God...He wants us to preserve our bodies, not to kill them. Therefore He has given us food, drink, clothing, the sun, and the moon.' Yet, he was quick to point out, 'It is not our intention to provide a defence of the wicked Epicureans and antinomians in this way. If they hear this, they look for nothing but excessive luxury and gluttony, in which they exceed all bounds and transgress the laws of godliness and respectability.' He emphasized the need to live with humility, stating, 'Hypocrites do not do this. They imagine that they are showing deference to God if they abstain. Nor do gluttons, who imagine that it is godly and permitted to stuff themselves and misuse the creatures of God.' He commanded evangelicals to 'observe moderation' and insisted, 'we ought to steer a middle course.'[131]

This idea of the middle course was a key concept in reformers' understandings of eating and the body.[132] In rejecting the fasting of Catholicism, for instance, in 1523 Luther spoke of the 'Evangelical means of fasting', stating 'this fasting is moderate eating and drinking.'[133] Preaching in 1530, Luther first outlined the fasting of the church fathers who 'did not eat or drink all day and barely slept', then stated, perhaps surprisingly in light of his generally positive attitude towards the body, 'I call that the true fasting of Christians, when one causes pain to the whole body and constrains it with all five senses, and he must reject everything that makes him soft'. He noted, however, 'but I do not trust myself to accomplish such fasting, and I do not want to impose it on anyone else. Everyone must look to themselves and how they feel, because we are not all the same and so there can be no common rule.' He continued, 'as far as there is a common rule for all Christians, everyone is required to remain moderate, sober and virtuous...Although not everyone can keep to the high fasting, they can remain moderate in eating, drinking and all other needs of the body.'[134]

[128] 'Predigt am Gründonnerstag', *WA*, vol. 37, 349. [129] Roper, 'Martin Luther's Body', 380.

[130] 'An den christlichen Adel deutscher Nation von des christlichen Standes Besserung. 1520', *WA*, vol. 6, 442.

[131] 'Vorlesungen über 1. Mose Kap. 24', *WA*, vol. 43, 332–4. Translation from Latin in *LW*, vol. 4, 276–7.

[132] On moderation in Protestant dietary advice see Tessa Storey, 'English and Italian Health Advice: Protestant and Catholic Bodies', in Sandra Cavallo and Tessa Storey (eds), *Conserving Health in Early Modern Culture: Bodies and Environments in Italy and England* (Manchester, 2017), 210–34.

[133] 'Das Siebend Capitel aus der Epistel S. Pauli zu den Chorinthern', *WA*, vol. 12, 103.

[134] 'Wochenpredigten über Matth. 5-7', *WA*, vol. 32, 432–3. These statements may be compared to Luther's stance on celibacy, where he rejected it in general (and for himself), though he stated 'I do not deny that there are several who are able to live without marriage chastely'. He writes that these people 'have a great gift' but that this is not shared by most people. *WA*, vol. 42, 101.

Luther's understanding of the differences between people suggests that the amount of food required to maintain 'moderation' would be dictated by the individual body, just as Strigenitz wrote that one should 'eat [only] as much as was necessary for him to maintain one's body'.[135] This aligns with medical understandings in which each person was believed to possess an innate form, in accordance with their complexion, which would require personalized care to either maintain or alter it.[136] Luther echoed this view when in 1536 he stated of the Elector of Saxony, 'our elector, who is quite a robust man, can stand a great deal of drinking. What he needs to satisfy himself is enough to make his neighbour drunk, for he's a man with a very strong body.' To make allowance for his elector's excessive drinking, Luther presented it as necessary, rather than immoderate, because his body required 'a great deal of drinking' to be satisfied. The eating of a large amount of food by someone of a large body could be similarly justified.

Luther connected the strength of the elector's body with his masculine power, as he followed this comment by writing 'were he given to venery, it would not be a wonder if he worked his young woman to death'.[137] The elector is thus presented as having the potential to be both an excessive drinker and an excessively dominant lover, yet this is balanced against his need to drink a lot because of his large body and his suggested chastity since he is not 'given to venery'. Luther's description evokes the tensions that existed in early modern German conceptions of masculinity, which could involve both the need to prove one's manhood through communal drinking, violence, and sexual prowess, as well as the need to act as the pious head of a godly household, the seat of all order.[138] In this case, such conflicted masculinity is channelled through the bulky size and solidity of the elector's body. While this example presents similar themes to the gendered image of the Catholic Church in the print of the Papal Ass, the elector's powerful, masculine body is not shown to represent his drunkenness, gluttony, and lust in the way that the creature's 'womanly' belly is. While the distinction that Luther made between a fat belly and large size in general was more complicated than simply one of feminine versus masculine fatness, there were clear, gendered dimensions to reformers' use and presentation of body size.

Returning to the issue of personal body size, here might lie an explanation for how Luther's and Philipp Melanchthon's very different bodies could fit into the reformers' teachings about fasting and the body. In contrast to Luther, Melanchthon was frequently presented as thin, wiry, and gaunt, yet Melanchthon's ascetic image could be made acceptable if his thinness was understood simply as his natural body, which he fed with just enough to sustain it, rather than the result

[135] Strigenitz, *Vom Fasten*, fol. 38^{v}. [136] See Chapter 2, 36–42.

[137] 'A. Lauterbachs und H. Wellers Nachschriften', *WA TR*, vol. 3, 338, no. 3468. Translation from *LW*, vol. 54, 206.

[138] See Lyndal Roper, *Oedipus and the Devil: Witchcraft, Sexuality and Religion in Early Modern Europe* (London and New York, 1994), 108–20.

of hypocritical fasting.[139] Of course, the difficulty of judging what was enough to sustain a body would have made the line between eating to support a large body and eating to excess somewhat subjective, complicating definitions of gluttony. In his biography of Luther, Melanchthon wrote that the reformer was 'by nature something I often marvelled at, neither small nor weak in body, though he ate and drank little; I saw him on four consecutive days neither eat nor drink a thing the entire time, yet he remained completely strong.'[140] Here, Melanchthon does not seek to present Luther as a feeble ascetic, as he speaks admiringly of the reformer's strength and largeness.[141] Yet Melanchthon was concerned to clarify that his friend's size was not the result of gluttony; he emphasized that Luther practised moderation and only ate enough to maintain his body, which although naturally large did not require a lot of food.

Just as Luther's size was only a problem if caused by the excesses of gluttony, Melanchthon's thinness could be reconciled with the teachings of moderation and the appreciation of the appetites as long as it was not contrived in order to appear holy. Fasting itself was not rejected by reformers; they set their sights only on fasting as a 'good work'. In 1520 Luther actively encouraged fasting, with the condition that, 'this same work must not occur in the belief that a person will appear pious before God by doing so.'[142] The intention behind eating and fasting were thus of great significance to reformers' discussion of both, and emotional responses could also be significant. Strigenitz wrote: 'If God grants one a good roasted, fat (*fetten*) capon, he should recognize it as a gift of God, and enjoy it and say thanks, and not feel guilty about it.'[143] Luther's distinction between the 'fat-bellies' of the Catholic Church and the prosperous fatness of the righteous, thus had an emotional dimension. In forbidding certain foods at certain times and days through the year, Catholics were creating restrictions which might trouble the conscience, causing a guilt which Luther himself experienced and criticized.[144] God's gifts should be accessed free of such cares or guilt, Luther held, which meant enjoying the 'fatness' of prosperity and fruitfulness denied by Catholicism.

This view too could transcend confessional divides. Despite writing of the life of a Christian as an 'exercise in the mortification of the flesh', the French Protestant

[139] On the relationship between Luther and Melanchthon, including a discussion of their bodies, see Ulinka Rublack, *Reformation Europe* (Cambridge, 2017), 52–5.

[140] Philipp Melanchthon, 'History of the Life and Acts of Dr Martin Luther', in *Luther's Lives*, 15–40, here 17.

[141] This view challenges Roper's interpretation of Melanchthon's comments, see Roper, *Martin Luther*, 304.

[142] 'Von der Freiheit eines Christenmenschen', *WA*, vol. 7, 30. This statement was made whilst Luther's own body appeared thin and he had only recently departed from monasticism, yet even as his body filled out and he began to embrace the appetites more fully Luther never entirely rejected the practice of fasting.

[143] Strigenitz, *Vom Fasten*, fol. 38^r.

[144] Roper, *Martin Luther*, 57. On food and guilt see John Coveney, *Food, Morals and Meaning: The Pleasure and Anxiety of Eating* (London, 2006).

reformer John Calvin had a relatively positive attitude towards eating based on notions of conscience.[145] He wrote of how 'when consciences once ensnare themselves, they enter a long and inextricable maze, not easy to get out of', and therefore 'if any man should consider daintier food unlawful, in the end he will not be at peace before God, when he eats either black bread or common victuals, while it occurs to him that he could sustain his body on even coarser foods'. Calvin thus concluded that 'we should use god's gifts for the use for which he gave them to us, with no scruple of conscience nor trouble of mind'.[146] Calvin did not connect this line of thought to notions of body size, however, but rather such thinking informed distinctly Lutheran approaches to acceptable and unacceptable forms of fatness and thinness.

Making Body Size Matter

Both fat and thin bodies could be accepted and reconciled with Lutheran teachings so long as they were being fed without guilt or pretensions of piety and with the right amount of food to sustain them. Within such an acceptance of various bodily forms, the extremes of fatness and thinness would be rejected if they were a result of departing from the teaching of moderation. In instances of extreme, miraculous fasting which were more typical of medieval mystic devotion yet continued to occur in Reformation Germany, broadsheet authors were thus keen to note that their subjects were not emaciated despite their abstinence. In Lutheran Dortmund, for example, a 1574 broadsheet gave an account of Barbara Kremer, a 10-year-old girl from Unna who had not eaten or drunk anything for months. Despite her fasting Barbara had 'retained all her colour and beauty, in her lips and both cheeks...like a person who has never been ill'.[147] Likewise in 1585 Catharina Binder, who had eaten nothing for years, was described as 'well in body and perfect'.[148] Such young women were understood to have replaced

[145] John Calvin, *Institutes of the Christian Religion*, ed. John T. McNeill, tr. Ford Lewis Battles, 2 vols (Louisville, KY, 2001), 615. On the nuances of Calvin's attitude towards the body and food see Émile Doumergue, 'Calvin: Epigone or Creator?', in William Park Armstrong (ed.), *Calvin and the Reformation* (Eugene, OR, 2004), 1–55, on eating see esp. 48–9, and Margaret Miles, 'Theology, Anthropology, and the Human Body in Calvin's *Institutes of the Christian Religion*', *Harvard Theological Review* 74 (1981), 303–23.

[146] Calvin, *Institutes of the Christian Religion*, 839–40.

[147] '*Eine vberaus Wunderliche Historia vnd Geschichte/ wie Gott der Herr in vorgangnem vnd jetzigem 74. Jare/ ein junges Megdelein/ ohn speise vnd tranck/ etzlige Monden lang/ beim leben erhalten hat vnd noch erhalten thut*' (Dortmund, 1574). Quoted in Waltraud Pulz, 'Innere Schau und/oder Nabelschau—Blicke auf die Nahrungsabstinenten der Frühen Neuzeit', in Waltraud Pulz, Jan Marco Sawilla, and Dieter R. Bauer (eds), *Zwischen Himmel und Erde: Körperliche Zeichen der Heiligkeit* (Stuttgart, 2012), 101–21, here 102.

[148] '*Gründtlicher Bericht vnd Anzeig Einer warhafften Histori/ welcher massen zu Schmidtweyler... ein Mägdlin siben Jahr lang weder gessen noch getruncken*' (Heidelberg, 1585). Quoted in Pulz, 'Innere Schau und/oder Nabelschau', 102.

earthly sustenance with spiritual nourishment, which maintained and replenished their bodies in place of food and drink.[149] Crucially, therefore, their fasting was not described in the same manner as ascetics who caused their bodies to suffer hunger for the appearance of piety. When the medical doctor and famous opponent of the persecution of witches, Johann Weyer, examined Barbara Kremer, he presented a very different picture.[150] He described her as 'very thin and sunken', as though 'her navel and spine had grown together'.[151] Rather than being nourished by God, Weyer suspected that Barbara was starving herself. Observing her for several days, Weyer eventually exposed Barbara as a fraud, and he drew on both contemporary medical and theological understandings for his explanation. He suggested that Barbara had been able to survive for so long with little food due to her moist female body, but he also discussed her deception as signalling the intervention of the devil. For both Weyer and the anonymous pamphleteer, the size and condition of Barbara's body mattered. For her fasting to be acceptable to a Lutheran audience, her body needed to appear well-nourished to show that she was indeed being sustained by God, rather than proclaiming her piety through bodily mortification. In this context, the unnatural thinness observed by Weyer would be unjustifiable, as it indicated either deliberate deprivation or devilish deception.

Body size, fatness, and thinness were made to matter in the Reformations. The size and shape of the body held meaning for reformers in settings ranging from apocalyptic belief and debates surrounding the resurrection of the body to Luther's criticism of the Catholic Church, all of which contributed to fundamental understandings of what it meant to be a Lutheran. A focus on the belly ran through these framings of fatness, with the belly that was a burden weighing down the earthly body, the 'last belly-world' of the apocalypse, and the fat belly of Catholicism as identified by Luther. For Luther in particular, the belly was a source of nuance. His understanding of the belly in relation to fatness is indicative of the complexity of differentiating between fat and thin bodies, for 'fat' could be employed as a metaphor or symbol regardless of actual physicality. The reformers' emphasis on moderation was nuanced in turn, permitting the incorporation of various body types.

149 Pulz, 'Innere Schau und/oder Nabelschau', 105. See also Waltraud Pulz, *Nüchternes Kalkül—verzehrende Leidenschaft: Nahrungsabstinenz im 16. Jahrhundert* (Cologne, 2007), esp. 66–83.

150 Weyer's own religious convictions are unclear and have been the subject of considerable debate. Hans de Waardt suggests that he was neither Catholic, Lutheran, Calvinist, nor Mennonite but a spiritualist who opposed the fragmentation of Christendom. Hans de Waardt, 'Witchcraft, Spiritualism, and Medicine: The Religious Convictions of Johan Wier', *Sixteenth Century Journal* 42 (2011), 369–91, here 373.

151 Johannes Wier, *De lamiis: Das ist: Von Teufelsgespenst Zauberern vnd Gifftbereytern/kurtzer doch gründtlicher Bericht... Samt einem angehängten kleinen Tractätlein von dem falschen vnd erdichten Fasten* (Frankfurt am Main, 1586). Quoted in Pulz, 'Innere Schau und/oder Nabelschau', 113.

It was not only Lutherans who deployed the imagery of fatness and the belly, or for whom body size became important in this period; the significance of body size was trans-confessional, though interpretations of fatness and thinness could differ according to confessional beliefs. It was Luther's writings, however, which elevated the significance of fatness and belly-worship within Christian theology. The Reformation transformed Christianity in Germany and beyond, and the significance of body size within Luther's reform movement both reflected and reinforced a broader contemporary landscape in which body size was taking on new meaning.

Body Size in Early Modern Germany. Holly Fletcher, Oxford University Press.
DOI: 10.1093/9780198972983.003.0004

5

Dress and Undress

In Friedrich Dedekind's *Grobianus*, first published in Latin in 1549, a fictional master Grobian advised his 'apprentices' on how best to behave.[1] With his name deriving from the German term *grob*, meaning coarse or uncouth, this was no typical conduct book, however, and Grobian's comical advice inverted that of traditional conduct literature as he revelled in boorish behaviour. Instructing readers on dinner table etiquette, Grobian stated 'first take off your gown' so that 'everyone can see, who does not already know it / whether you are thin or fat (*mager oder feist*). Go before the table in your doublet and hose'.[2] As Grobian's statement indicates, early modern clothing could conceal or reveal one's body size, forming a crucial part of the presentation of one's own body, as well as the assessment of the bodies of others. Garments like the doublet and hose, which were tight-fitting and tailored to the contours of the body, enabled the display of bodily form, while looser fitting gowns could disguise the body and construct alternative silhouettes. Grobian's instruction also suggests how the relationship between clothing and body size could be understood in terms of acceptability and proper bodily comportment. It would be inappropriate, it seems, to openly display the fatness or thinness of one's body at the dinner table. On the other hand, contemporary moralizers warned against moulding the body into unnatural forms, and thus using clothing as a tool for deception.

Dress played a crucial role in extending bodily experience, thereby shaping perceptions of body size, fatness, and thinness. The body was literally extended through clothing, understood as 'the body's body', which expanded the body's form, increasing one's height or width, or exaggerating particular areas of the body.[3] Dress mediated the relationship between the body and its external world. Clothing formed a porous boundary through which external influences needed to pass in order to infiltrate the body, meanwhile bodily excretions such as sweat would be wicked away from the skin through the textiles worn upon it.[4] As the

[1] The text was first translated into German by Caspar Scheidt in 1551 and later updated by Wendelin Helbach in 1567. See Kat Hill, 'Fun and Loathing in Later Lutheran Culture', *Past and Present* 232 (2017), 67–89, here 67–8.

[2] Friedrich Dedekind, *Grobianus und Grobiana: Von unfletigen, groben, unhöflichen Sitten, und Bäwrischen Gebärde*, tr. Wendelin Helbach (Frankfurt, 1572), fol. 45v.

[3] Erasmus wrote of clothing as 'the body's body', see Erika Rummel (ed.), *The Erasmus Reader* (Toronto, 1990), 108.

[4] See Georges Vigarello, *Concepts of Cleanliness: Changing Attitudes in France since the Middle Ages*, tr. Jean Birrell (Cambridge, 1988), 58–60.

physician Georg Pictorius noted, dress and the materials of its construction could even hold the capacity to physically alter the body and its size.[5] As well as influencing the balance of the humours, clothing shaped the body through padding and tailoring, cinching in or draping loosely over the figure. Such moulding of the body's form might be temporary, lasting only as long as such clothing remained on the body, yet dress could also have a more permanent impact on the body's posture, movements, and development. Body size was so intimately connected to dress in this period that it could be difficult to determine a person's bodily form without taking clothing into account.

This argument draws on those of dress theorists such as Joanne Entwistle who has gone so far as to write that 'human bodies are *dressed* bodies', since most bodies are dressed in some sort of clothing most of the time.[6] In early modern Europe in particular, dress was key to extending the wearer's bodily experience. From the late medieval period onwards, fitted clothing became increasingly popular, encouraged by new methods of tailoring and of fastening clothes to the body.[7] As Ulinka Rublack writes, therefore, in the early modern period 'men in particular were confronted with an intense sense of shape and body weight' due to the tighter fitting construction of their clothes, as well as the popularity of features such as the codpiece and peas-belly which exaggerated the natural shape of the body.[8] Such tailored clothing thus posed a new awareness of bodily form, as well as the appropriate posture and behaviour of the body. These garments would also have made changes in the size and shape of the body more immediately apparent to the wearer. In a period before the widespread weighing of bodies, practices of dress, through which the changing fit of clothing could be sensed, enabled alterations in body size to be registered and even measured. Moreover, since the majority of early modern garments would be cut and fitted on and for particular bodies, early modern people had an acute awareness of the size and form of their own bodies through processes of making and altering clothing. Dress practices were thus integral to conceptions of body size among early modern Germans.

The Dressed Figure

In 1574, Cologne townsman Hermann von Weinsberg noted in his memory book that 'when someone is painted or counterfeited, not only does the head and body

[5] See Chapter 2, 50.

[6] Joanne Entwistle, *The Fashioned Body* (Cambridge, 2015), 6. Emphasis from original source. See also Joanne Entwistle and Emma McClendon (eds), 'The Body: Fashion and Physique', special issue of *Fashion Theory* 23 (2019).

[7] Odile Blanc, *Parades et parures: L'invention du corps de mode à la fin du Moyen Age* (Paris, 1997); Naomi Tarrant, *The Development of Costume* (Edinburgh, 1994), 16–22; Ulinka Rublack, *Dressing Up: Cultural Identity in Renaissance Europe* (Oxford, 2010), 16–17.

[8] Rublack, *Dressing Up*, 18.

need to be depicted but also his clothes'.[9] Weinsberg thus indicated the importance of a person's clothing to their appearance, particularly with his use of the term 'counterfeit'. This described a type of portrait, popular in northern Europe, which was meant to convey the truth of a particular person or event.[10] Weinsberg shows that clothing was integral to the truth of a person's external form. In describing his own figure, therefore, Weinsberg outlined the various layers of dress that made up his appearance. He wrote for instance, about his shirts with pleated collars which reached to his ears and were left open at the front so that his beard hung between the edges. Under a long gown lined with marten or fox fur, he wore a *Samarie,* a loose fitting gown, which he stated reached from his neck to just below his knees. He would wear doublets which were 'tight around the arms', and a gown which reached almost to his feet.[11] Weinsberg thus described and measured his clothing in relation to his body.

Similarly, Nuremberg tailor's son, Hieronymus Köler, considered clothing to be an essential part of his appearance which he described in an illuminated manuscript detailing his life and travels from 1537. In outlining the various outfits he wore at different times in his life, Köler viewed his clothes as inseparable from his figure or shape (*Gestalt*). He wrote, for instance, 'When serving a merchant, on work days my figure (*gstalt*) was: a shorn head, in a grey woollen gown with velvet, on which were wide sleeves which reached to my hands. They had a long slit in them. Green trousers and high shoes.' On holidays his *Gestalt* was instead: 'a big widespread yellow beard, a dark brown woollen gown with a strip of velvet around the edge. The sleeves reach to my hands with a diagonal cut. White trousers and cut-out shoes.'[12] While fatness and thinness could take on different resonances depending on one's confessional beliefs, Köler, a Lutheran, described the material experience of his body in relation to particular garments in similar terms to Weinsberg, a Catholic.

The primary meaning of the term *Gestalt* in this period was that of shape, figure, or stature, and throughout his text Köler used this term to describe the form granted to his body through clothing. His use of *Gestalt* in this way was not exceptional, as Matthäus Schwarz, the Catholic chief accountant to the Fugger, likewise described his clothing as representing his *Gestalt.* He stated for instance that as a child his father 'clothed us all [his siblings] in this figure (*gstalt*)'.[13] He also wrote of mourning his father 'in four *gstalt*' including an image of himself in

[9] Hermann Weinsberg, *Buch Weinsberg,* transcribed by Abteilung für Rheinische Landesgeschichte, Universität Bonn. Digital edition: www.weinsberg.uni-bonn.de, vol. 1, fol. 667^{v}.

[10] Peter Parshall, 'Imago Contrafacta: Images and Facts in the Northern Renaissance', *Art History* 16 (1993), 554–79.

[11] Weinsberg, *Buch Weinsberg,* vol. 1, fol. 667^{v}.

[12] Hannah Amburger, 'Die Familiengeschichte der Köler: Ein Beitrag zur Autobiographie des 16. Jahrhunderts', *Mitteilungen des Vereins für Geschichte der Stadt Nürnberg* 30 (1931), 153–288, here 219.

[13] Ulinka Rublack and Maria Hayward (eds), *The First Book of Fashion: The Book of Clothes of Matthäus and Veit Konrad Schwarz of Augsburg* (London, 2015), 62.

four different outfits.[14] That Schwarz was referencing his body's shape in these images is evident when he described the paintings which depict his naked body as showing his 'true figure' (*mein rechte gstallt*).[15] With the removal of his clothes, Schwarz understood these images to provide a truer representation of his body's form than his dressed paintings, since his nakedness made visible his newly 'fat and wide' body (Figures 1.1 & 1.2).

Both Köler and Schwarz viewed clothing as fundamental to their figures. The different shapes that Köler described depending on occasion, as well as the distinction that Schwarz made between his dressed and undressed forms, suggests how clothing was viewed as a means of altering the body's form in this period, enabling a person to have multiple body shapes depending on their state of dress or undress. Clothing thus enabled the wearer to enact body size in different ways and in different contexts. Within the contemporary understanding of natural versus unnatural body size, therefore, clothing was one of the numerous external influences which could contribute towards the unnatural shaping of the body.[16] These three early modern men used clothing to construct alternative figures which departed from the bodies they possessed beneath their clothes. Schwarz's clothed portraits show that he used clothing to cinch in his expanding body and define his waist. Meanwhile Hermann von Weinsberg made clothing choices based on the thinness of his body. Weinsberg suffered with a hernia for most of his life and he used a tight-fitting girdle to support and hide the lump. The girdle, Weinsberg believed, had caused him to become 'slender (*smal*) in my lower body as though I were totally thin (*ganß mager*)'. Thus he stated, 'for this reason, I have rarely gone around in a doublet and hose', and 'for the past thirty years I have worn *sammarien* like tunics (*karsack*) instead of shorter styles or the *paltrock*'.[17] Weinsberg described a *Samarie* as fitting 'like a wide sack around the body', and this loose style contrasted with a *Paltrock*, which was cut and fitted to the body with a clearly defined waist.[18] In choosing to wear a *Samarie* instead of a *Paltrock*, Weinsberg thus indicated a desire to conceal his figure, as he preferred to wear clothing which was longer and looser and which would skim over his frame. Weinsberg used clothing to construct a figure which extended beyond the shape of his naked body, which had itself been formed through the imposition of the girdle. Weinsberg's example thus indicates the difficulty of distinguishing between natural and unnatural body size in relation to clothing, since the undressed body could nevertheless be marked by practices of dress.

14 Ibid. 91. 15 Ibid. 129. 16 See Chapter 2, 36–42.

17 Weinsberg, *Buch Weinsberg*, vol. 1, fol. 723^r.

18 Ibid., vol. 2, fol. 37^r. See also Karen Stolleis, 'Kölner Patrizier- und Bürgerkleidung in der frühen Neuzeit', in Johannes Pietsch and Karen Stolleis (eds), *Kölner Patrizier- und Bürgerkleidung des 17. Jahrhunderts: Die Kostümsammlung Hüpsch im Hessischen Landesmuseum Darmstadt* (Riggisberg, 2008), 19–57, here 26–7.

Despite widespread practices of modifying the body through dress, the use of clothing for constructing alternative figures was concerning for contemporary moralizers who insisted that dress should not be used to create the illusion of something real.[19] The manipulation of the body's form through clothing could be viewed as a deformation of one's God-given body.[20] Just as recipes for altering body size could be morally questionable, therefore, shaping the body through dress was problematic. Clothing had been created following the Fall when the disobedience of Adam and Eve resulted in shame at their nakedness. Thus Lutheran pastor Johannes Strauß of Elsterberg wrote in 1580 that wearing clothes should act as a reminder of the Fall 'out of innocence and into misery and danger'. He continued by stating that 'God dressed this depraved human nature, and so we are dressed in a new body'.[21] Strauß echoed the words of Erasmus who wrote of clothing as 'the body's body' and as such stated that it should 'harmonize with the lines of the body'.[22] The need for clothing to follow the natural contours of the body was of central importance for religious commentators. The connection between dress and morality was widely evoked throughout early modern Europe including across confessional divides.[23] In sixteenth-century Germany, the criticism of immoderate dress practices was particularly taken up by Lutheran commentators, as exemplified in the 'devil books' (*Teufelsbücher*) from 1555 onwards which took aim at elaborate dress displays, such as the wearing of baggy and expansive hose known as *Pluderhosen*.[24] While individuals of different confessional beliefs, such as Weinsberg, Schwarz, and Köler, used clothing to construct new figures for themselves, for moralizers the creation of fashionable bodily ideals for women and men was instead viewed as a vain disfigurement of the body.

Women's Bodies

With the rise of fitted clothing from the fourteenth century onwards, tailored garments increasingly accentuated sexual difference, constructing new understandings of the masculine and feminine body.[25] The fashioning of women's bodies in particular was marked by concerns surrounding honour and decency. From 1490, sumptuary legislation in the German speaking regions made clear that women

[19] Rublack, *Dressing Up*, 25–6.

[20] Dennis Bruna, 'Medieval Fashions, Bodies and Transformations', in Denis Bruna (ed.), *Fashioning the Body: An Intimate History of the Silhouette* (New York, 2015), 31–6, here 34.

[21] Johannes Strauß, *Wider den Kleyder, Pluder, Pauß und Krauß Teuffel* (Leipzig, 1581), fol. A6^{v}–A8^{r}.

[22] Rummel, *Erasmus Reader*, 109.

[23] On the moral significance of dress see Aileen Ribeiro, *Dress and Morality* (London, 1986). On the widespread application of sumptuary legislation as the enforcement of morality see Giorgio Riello and Ulinka Rublack, 'Introduction', in Giorgio Riello and Ulinka Rublack (eds), *The Right to Dress: Sumptuary Laws in a Global Perspective, c.1200–1800* (Cambridge, 2019), 1–34.

[24] Rublack, *Dressing Up*, 109–12.

[25] Ibid. 18.

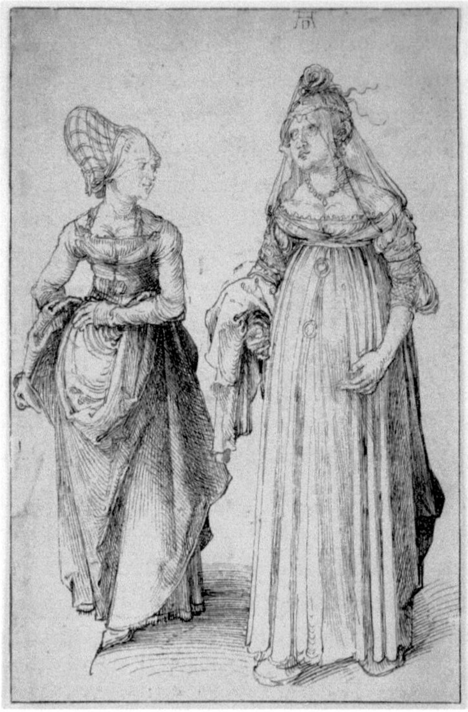

Figure 5.1 Albrecht Dürer, Nuremberg and Venetian Woman, 1495. Ink on paper, 24.5 × 15.9 cm. Städel Museum, Frankfurt am Main, public domain. The Nuremberg woman on the left is shown with a fitted bodice and narrow upper body, reflecting the neatness and control of German women's dress in contrast to the voluminous clothing of the Venetian.

should completely cover their upper bodies to ensure modesty, and such coverage became characteristic of German women's dress in contrast to other European regions such as Italy, France, and England.[26] The praise of modesty in German women's dress was connected to a growing German proto-nationalist ideology which, in combination with the Lutheran Reformation, frequently associated extravagance in dress with Catholic Italy and Spain. The honour and decency of German women was presented through the idealized slenderness of their upper bodies, which were not only completely covered by their clothing but also tightly compressed. Albrecht Dürer observed this ideal in his drawing of a Nuremberg woman and a Venetian woman from 1495 (Figure 5.1). Giving little definition to their facial features, Dürer focused on the shape of their bodies created through clothing. The wide, voluminous skirt of the Venetian woman, beginning just

[26] Ibid. 246. See also Ulinka Rublack, 'The Right to Dress: Sartorial Politics in Germany, c.1300–1750', in *The Right to Dress*, 37–73.

below her bust, is juxtaposed with the tight upper body of the German, whose dress is closely fitted to her waist, chest, and arms. With this image, Dürer celebrated the neatness and control of German dress in which modesty was enforced through sumptuary regulations.[27] Moreover, this slender ideal for German women reflected an ideal of controlled consumption and bodily comportment, suggesting that such women were not eating or drinking to excess, or indulging in luxury and extravagance. Contemporary artists repeatedly used the image of fleshy, voluptuous nude women to present uncontrolled and seductive female power.[28] Such images appear as the obverse of the dressed German women who appear in contemporary costume books and portraiture, whose slim bodies thus connoted controlled sexuality.

While the head-covering worn by Dürer's Nuremberg woman shows her to be married, given its connotations of modesty and chaste femininity, this slender ideal was particularly prominent in depictions of young, unmarried women.[29] Hans Weigel's *Habitus praecipuorum populorum* from 1577, for example, presents young women of a variety of social ranks with such narrow torsos (Figures 5.2–5.4). Like Dürer, Weigel contrasted these images with those of Italian women, whose dress he showed as more elaborate and expansive. In connection with their more extravagant fashions, the Italian women's body shapes also differ from the German women's. A woman from Naples (Figure 5.5) is shown wearing a particularly low-slung girdle, creating the image of a large and rounded belly which is accentuated through the high waistline of her gown which sits just below the bust.

Jost Amman constructed similar contrasts in his costume book from 1586. The German women presented are again characterized by their modesty. Amman depicted a young woman from Thuringia (Figure 5.6), for example, where, the accompanying text suggests, there are 'many virtuous maidens'.[30] Such virtue appears reflected in the Thuringian woman's modest dress and narrow waist. By contrast, Amman presented an 'unchaste woman of Rome' (Figure 5.7), and the text informs us that in Rome 'women without reserve / live unchaste and shameful / they give their bodies to shame / for the want of ephemeral money / and to quiet their lasciviousness'.[31] The Roman woman's bodice is shown to extend below her belly making it appear rounded and expansive. The description of her loose morals is reflected in the loosely draped fabric of her dress, in contrast to the neatly pleated skirt of the woman from Thuringia (see also Figures 5.3 and 5.4). Pleats were considered a specifically German form of dress in this period, likely

[27] Rublack, *Dressing Up*, 125–7 and 139. [28] See Chapter 3.

[29] Katherine Bond, '"Fashioned with Marvellous Skill": Veils and the Costume Books of Sixteenth-Century Europe', in Susanna Burghartz, Lucas Burkart, Christine Göttler, and Ulinka Rublack (eds), *Materialized Identities in Early Modern Culture, 1450–1750* (Amsterdam, 2021), 325–68, here 327.

[30] Jost Amman, *Frauen-Trachtenbuch.* Facsimile reprint of *Im Frauwenzimmer wirt vermeldt von allerley schöen Kleidungen* (1586) (Munich, 1880), 21.

[31] Ibid. 101.

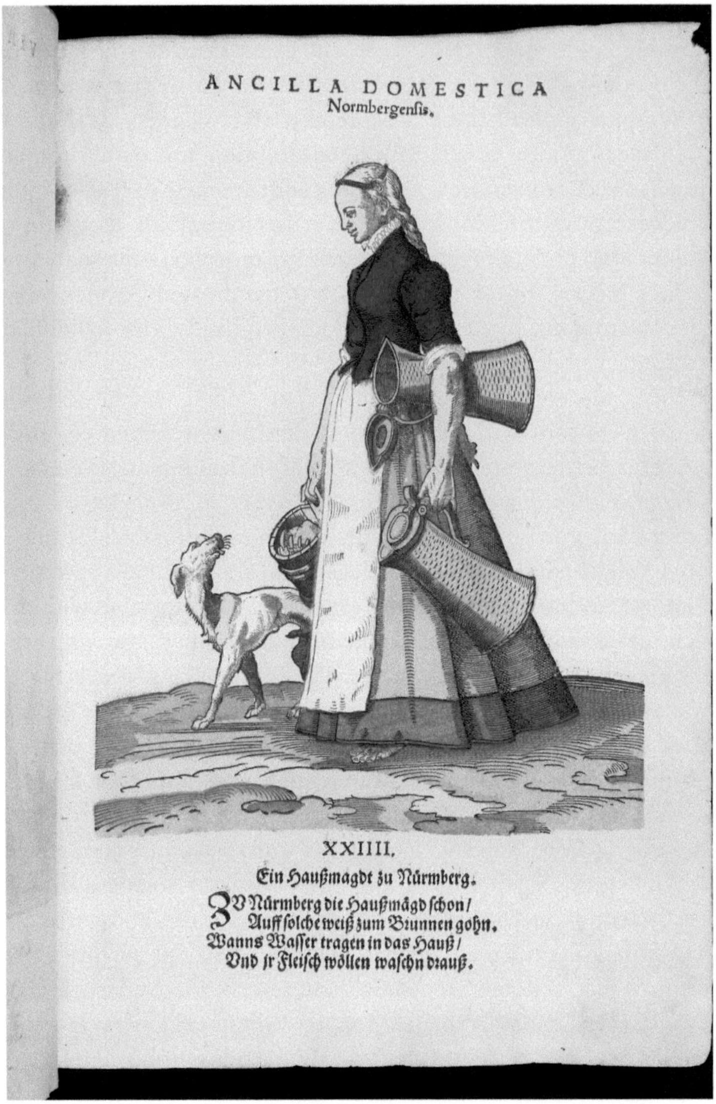
ANCILLA DOMESTICA
Normbergensis.
XXIIII.
Ein Haußmagdt zu Nürmberg.
ZV Nürmberg die Haußmägd schon/
Auff solche weiß zum Brunnen gohn.
Wanns Wasser tragen in das Hauß/
Vnd jr Fleisch wöllen waschn drauß.

Figure 5.2 'A Housemaid from Nuremberg', in Hans Weigel, *Habitus praecipuorum populorum*, (Nuremberg, 1577), fol. Fiv[r], plate 024 © The Master and Fellows of Trinity College, Cambridge. The Nuremberg housemaid, shown collecting water, wears a tight-fitting bodice and completely covers her upper body.

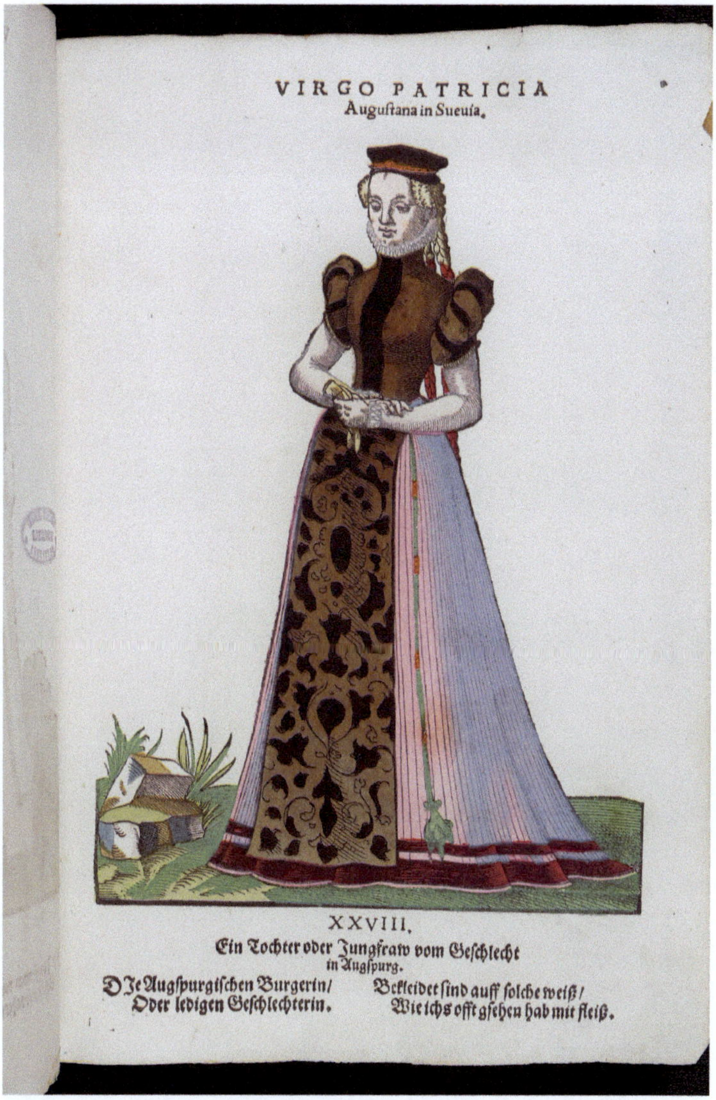
VIRGO PATRICIA
Augustana in Sueuia.
XXVIII.
Ein Tochter oder Jungfraw vom Geschlecht
in Augspurg.
DJe Augspurgischen Burgerin/
Oder ledigen Geschlechterin.
Bekleidet sind auff solche weiß/
Wie ichs offt gsehen hab mit fleiß.

Figure 5.3 'Patrician Daughter or Maid from Augsburg', in Hans Weigel, *Habitus praecipuorum populorum*, (Nuremberg, 1577), fol. Giv^r, plate 028 © The Master and Fellows of Trinity College, Cambridge. The unmarried daughters of Augsburg patricians are shown to wear garments which modestly conceal their upper bodies while tightly containing them.

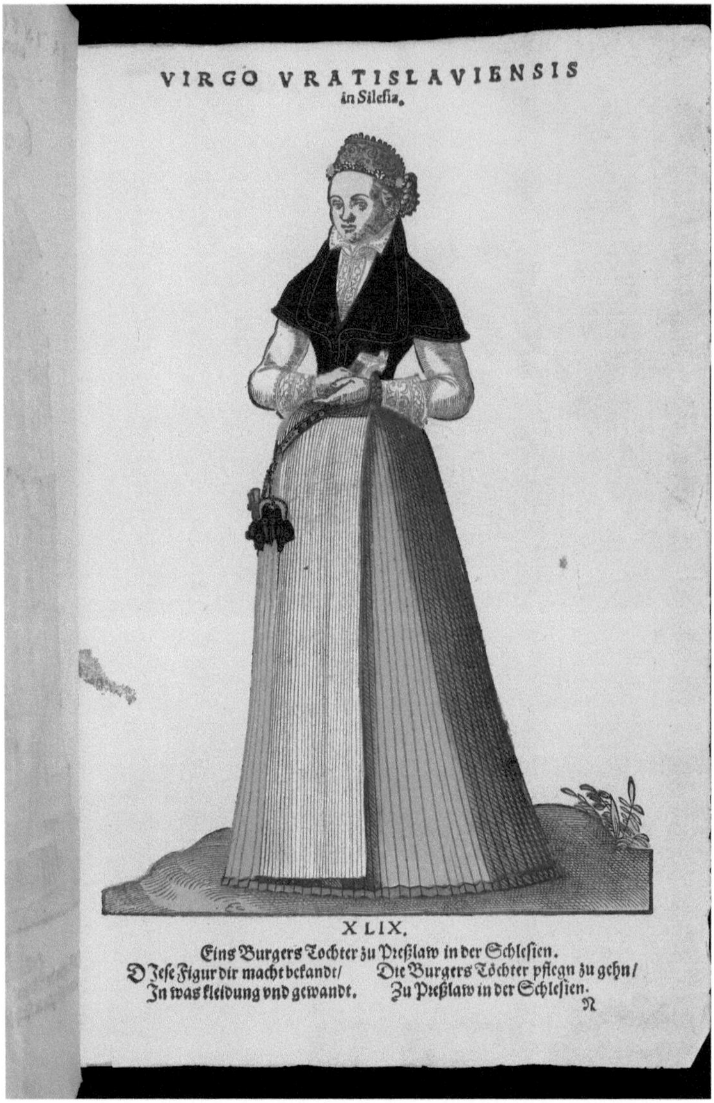
VIRGO VRATISLAVIENSIS
in Silesia.
XLIX.
Eins Burgers Tochter zu Preßlaw in der Schlesien.
DIese Figur dir macht bekandt/
In was kleidung vnd gewandt.
Die Burgers Töchter pflegn zu gehn/
Zu Preßlaw in der Schlesien.
N

Figure 5.4 'Citizen's Daughter from Breslau', in Hans Weigel, *Habitus praecipuorum populorum*, (Nuremberg, 1577), fol. Ni^{r}, plate 049 © The Master and Fellows of Trinity College, Cambridge. The young woman from Breslau is shown with a very narrow waist while her upper body is completely covered by a high-necked blouse.

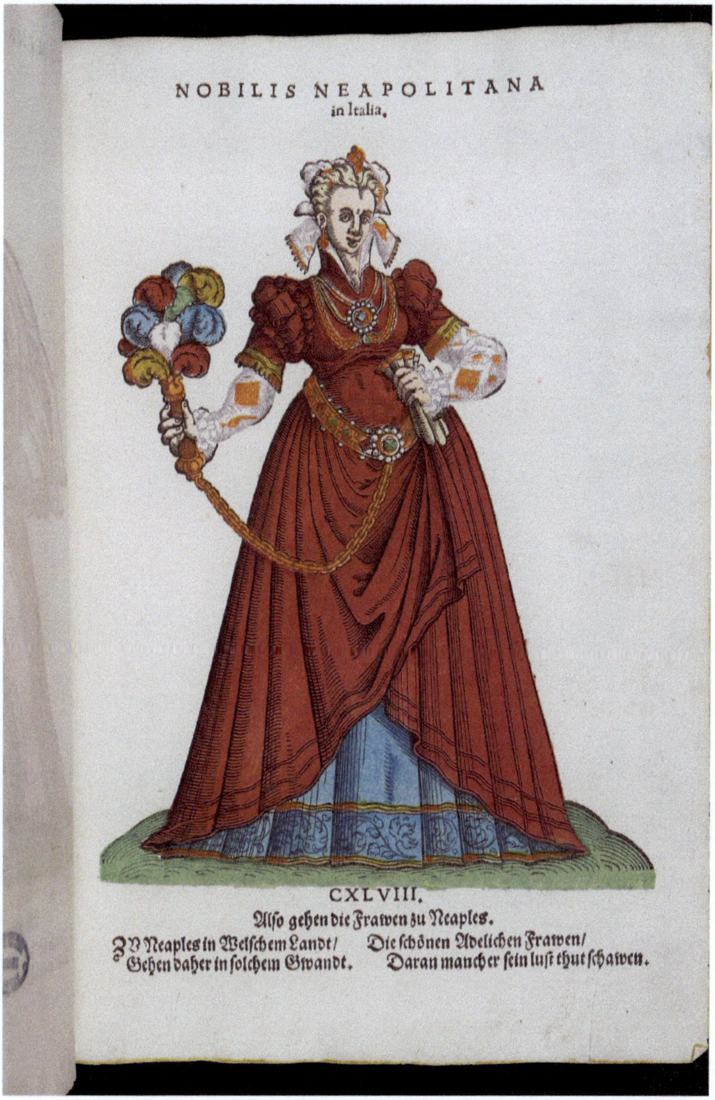
NOBILIS NEAPOLITANA
in Italia.
CXLVIII.
Alſo gehen die Frawen zu Neaples.
ZV Neaples in Welſchem Landt/
Gehen daher in ſolchem Gwandt.
Die ſchönen Adelichen Frawen/
Daran mancher ſein luſt thut ſchawen.

Figure 5.5 'Woman from Naples', in Hans Weigel, *Habitus praecipuorum populorum*, (Nuremberg, 1577), fol. Ooiv[r], plate 148 © The Master and Fellows of Trinity College, Cambridge. The Neapolitan woman is shown with a low-slung girdle beneath a rounded belly. Her dress is notably more extravagant and voluminous than that of German women.

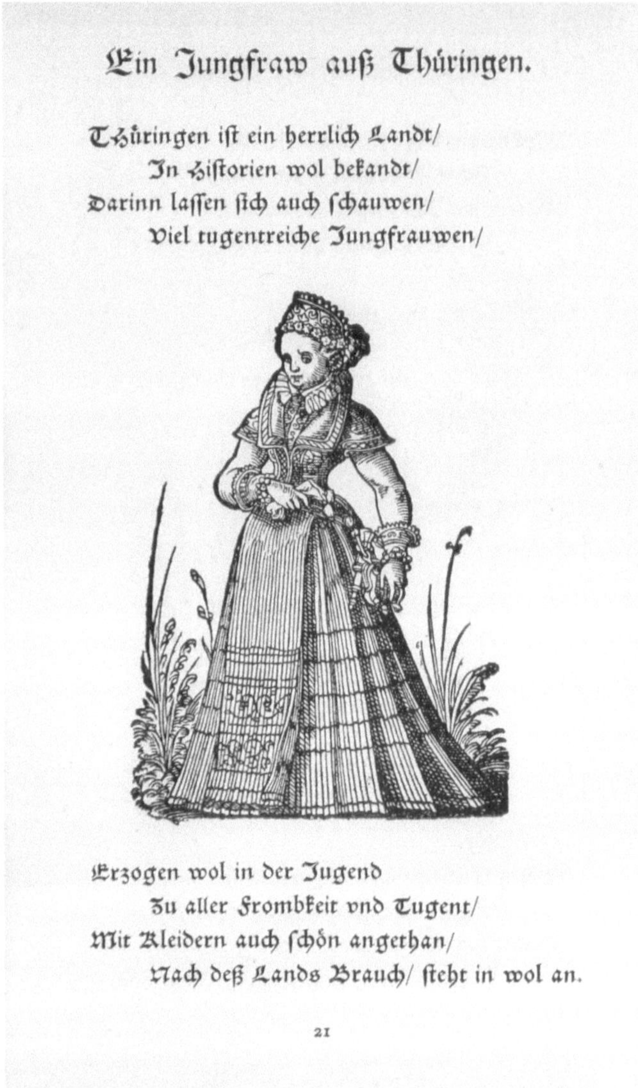

Ein Jungfraw auß Thüringen.

Thüringen iſt ein herrlich Landt/
In Hiſtorien wol bekandt/
Darinn laſſen ſich auch ſchauwen/
Viel tugentreiche Jungfrauwen/

Erzogen wol in der Jugend
Zu aller Frombkeit vnd Tugent/
Mit Kleidern auch ſchön angethan/
Nach deß Lands Brauch/ ſteht in wol an.

21

Figure 5.6 'Maiden from Thuringia', in Jost Amman, *Frauen-Trachtenbuch*, 1586. Facsimile reprint with title: *Im Frauwenzimmer wirt vermeldt von allerley schöen Kleidungen* (Munich, 1880), 21. Wellcome Collection, London, public domain. The unmarried woman from Thuringia is shown with a narrow waist and modest dress. The accompanying text describes how the region's young women are brought up to be devout and virtuous.

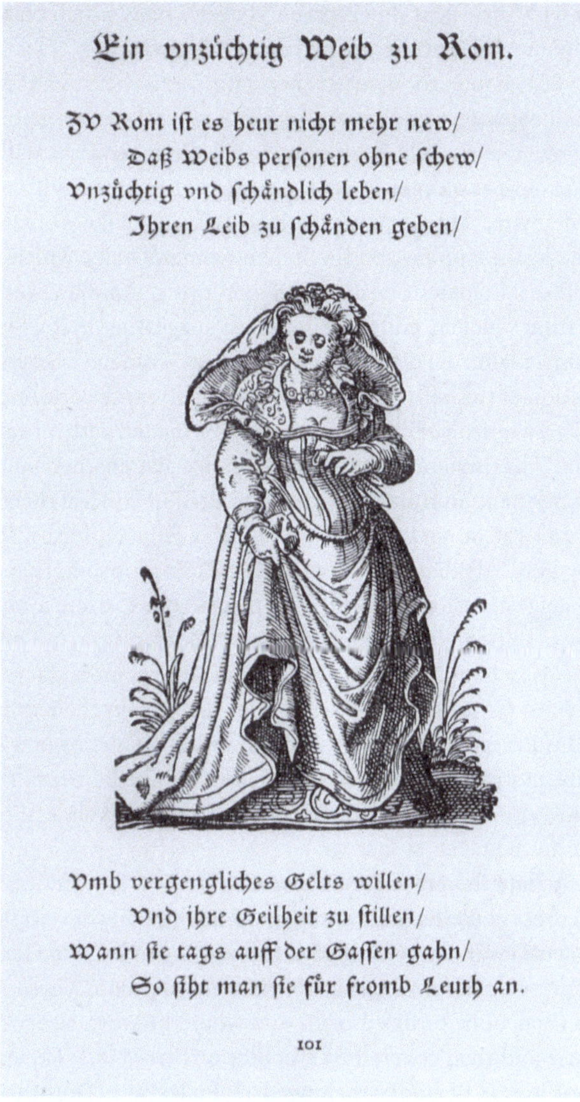

Ein vnzüchtig Weib zu Rom.

ZV Rom ist es heur nicht mehr new/
Daß Weibs personen ohne schew/
Vnzüchtig vnd schändlich leben/
Ihren Leib zu schänden geben/

Vmb vergengliches Gelts willen/
Vnd jhre Geilheit zu stillen/
Wann sie tags auff der Gassen gahn/
So siht man sie für fromb Leuth an.

101

Figure 5.7 'An Unchaste Woman from Rome', in Jost Amman, *Frauen-Trachtenbuch*, 1586. Facsimile reprint with title: *Im Frauwenzimmer wirt vermeldt von allerley schöen Kleidungen* (Munich, 1880), 101. Wellcome Collection, London, public domain. The Roman woman's bodice is shown to extend below her rounded belly, while the loose expanse of her dress reflects the text's description of her loose morals.

in connection with their neat precision and orderly lines which created a streamlined silhouette. In the run-up to her daughter's wedding, Electress Anna of Saxony (1532–85) wrote to instruct her aunt, Elisabeth von Mecklenburg-Güstrow, on appropriate wedding attire: 'Thus we ask once again in a friendly manner that you, like us, will keep your usual German dress with the pleated gowns and caps and not dress in Italian (*wälsche*) clothing with smooth skirts and un-pleated gowns.'[32] In Amman's depiction of a patrician woman from Venice (Figure 5.8), he again emphasized the Italian woman's belly, which is clearly visible through the transparent material of her dress. Amman stated that such women were from 'ancient patrician' families, suggesting that even elite Italian women lacked the controlled morality of German women.[33] Given the contemporary association of the belly with gluttony, sexuality, and worldliness, the fleshiness of the Italian women's bellies in such images is loaded with moral significance. By contrast the Thuringian woman's tight bodice flattens her belly, and she is shown resting her hand in front of her torso to further conceal the area.

Seeking to cultivate a narrow upper body to meet such ideals, some German women may have deliberately controlled their consumption. Hippolytus Guarinonius suggested that this restriction took place from a young age and would be imposed upon girls by their parents.[34] Reflecting a contemporary trope concerning the folly of mothers, he stated that some women 'starve their daughters while they are growing children…so that they retain their thin and slender bodies and do not become too large and powerful.'[35] This trope was more often used to criticize mothers and nurses who 'deformed' the bodies of young women by lacing them into tight-fitting foundation garments.[36] While such moralizing comments cannot be taken at face value, they nevertheless reflect contemporary efforts to manipulate the proportions of young bodies, as practices of both consumption and dress could be used to shape women's bodily development. Later in the sixteenth century an early form of corset was worn by elite German women, known as a pair of bodies in English or *Mieder* in German. These were typically stiffened with whalebone or dried reeds and would be worn either over or under a shirt or blouse and then covered by a bodice or *Brüstlein*.[37] The earliest surviving example of a pair of bodies belonged to Pfalzgräfin Dorothea Sabina von Neuberg and was included in her burial clothing when she died in 1598 at the age of 22 (Figure 5.9). This garment was made of a silk moiré fabric, giving it a rippled appearance, and was likely originally ivory in colour, but has now discoloured to a light brown. Lines of back stitching in a heavy silk thread indicate the

[32] Quoted in Katrin Keller, *Kurfürstin Anna von Sachsen, 1532–1585* (Regensburg, 2010), 51.
[33] Amman, *Frauen-Trachtenbuch*, 106.
[34] See Chapter 2, 41. [35] Guarinonius, *Die Grewel der Verwüstung*, 547.
[36] Sarah Bendall, *Shaping Femininity: Foundation Garments, the Body and Women in Early Modern England* (London, 2022), 156–9.
[37] Jutta Zander-Seidel, *Textiler Hausrat: Kleidung und Haustextilien in Nürnberg von 1500–1650* (Munich, 1990), 94–5. See also Janet Arnold, *Patterns of Fashion 3: The Cut and Construction of Clothes for Men and Women c.1560–1620* (London, 1985), 8, and Susan Vincent, *The Anatomy of Fashion: Dressing the Body from the Renaissance to Today* (Oxford and New York, 2009), 38–9.

Ein Geſchlechterin zu Venedig im Sommerkleid.

JM Sommer wann die Sonn warm ſcheint/
Vnd Venediſche Weiber ſeind/
Von den Vralten Geſchlechtern/
Die auß jhrem Hauß giengen gern/

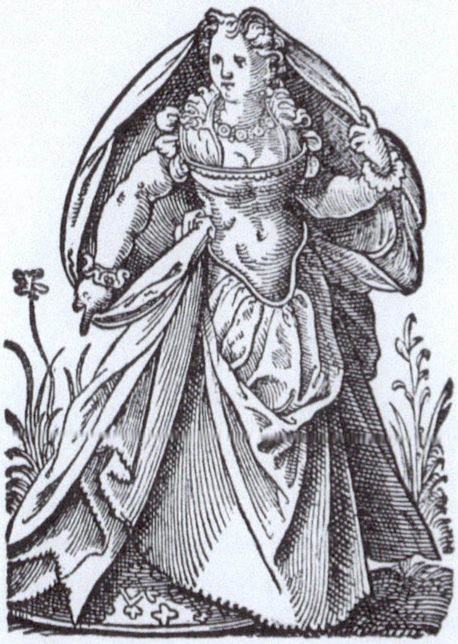

Vor eſſens ſich zu erquicken
Damit ſie nun nicht erſticken/
So legen ſie ſich lüfftig an/
Wie diſe Figur iſt gethan.

106

Figure 5.8 'Patrician Woman from Venice', in Jost Amman, *Frauen-Trachtenbuch*, 1586. Facsimile reprint with title: *Im Frauwenzimmer wirt vermeldt von allerley schöen Kleidungen* (Munich, 1880), 106. Wellcome Collection, London, public domain. The transparent material of the patrician woman's summer gown reveals the contours of her belly.

position of whale bones for stiffening and the wide casing at the centre front suggests the presence of a busk which has not survived. Both elements would have added to the rigidity of the body, flattening the torso.[38] Measurements taken from

[38] Arnold, *Patterns of Fashion 3*, 113. On this garment see also Johannes Pietsch, 'Establishing Identity: Stays from Southern Germany in the Collection of the Bayerisches Nationalmuseum', in

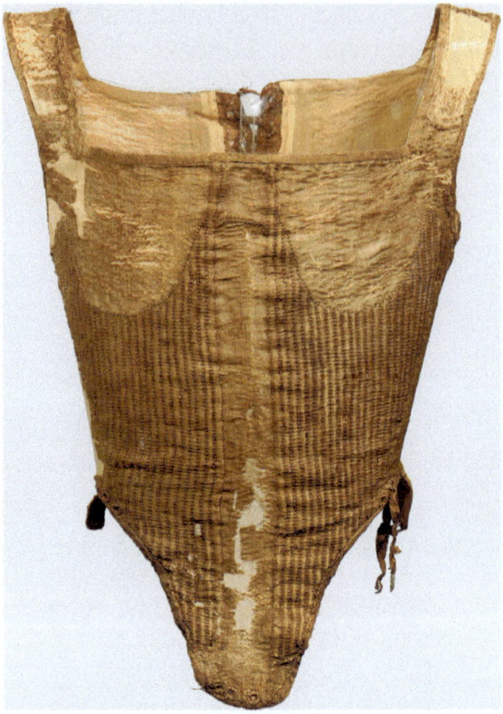

Figure 5.9 Pair of bodies belonging to Pfalzgräfin Dorothea Sabina von Neuberg, worn at her burial in 1598. Bayerisches Nationalmuseum, Munich © Bayerisches Nationalmuseum München/Photo: Bastian Krack. This is the oldest surviving example of a pair of bodies. Whalebones and a central busk, which have not survived, would have added to the rigidity and containment of the upper body in this garment.

the bodies show that Dorothea's waist while wearing the garment would have measured only 50.8 cm (20 inches) and her bust 71 cm (28 inches). Though she must have been naturally slight, to maintain such proportions it is likely that her body would have known the constraints of foundation garments throughout the course of its physiological development.[39] In contrast to nineteenth-century corsets, early bodies and stays did not significantly reduce the body's measurements upon wearing them, yet their use from an early age could inhibit the normal growth of the ribs, resulting in a narrower torso.[40] That young women's bodies

Frank Matthias Kammel and Johannes Pietsch (eds), *Structuring Fashion: Foundation Garments through History* (Munich, 2019), 73–83, esp. 74–5.

[39] Axel Moulinier and Sophie Vesin, 'Women's Undergarments and the Submission of the Body in the Sixteenth Century', in Denis Bruna (ed.), *Fashioning the Body*, 57–66, here 61. On the wearing of bodies by young girls in England see Sarah Bendall, *Shaping Femininity: Foundation Garments, the Body and Women in Early Modern England* (London, 2022), 154–7.

[40] See Bendall, *Shaping Femininity*, 153–64. Archaeological evidence shows the effects of eighteenth-century bodies on rib development, see Katherine Marie Klingerman, 'Binding Femininity: An Examination of the Effects of Tightlacing on the Female Pelvis', MA thesis, Baton Rouge, LA, 2006, 53.

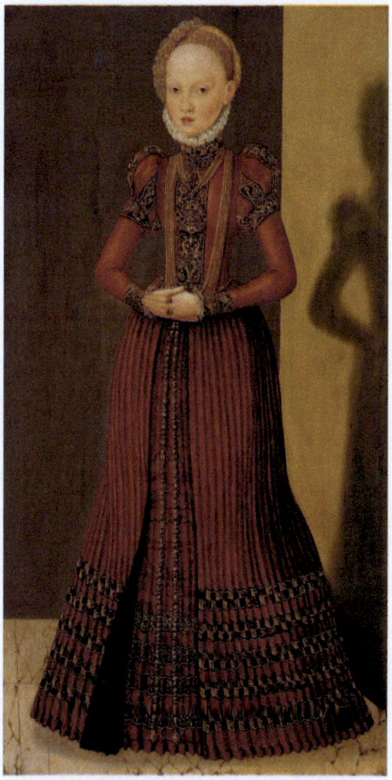

Figure 5.10 Lucas Cranach the Younger, Portrait of Elisabeth of Saxony, 1564. Oil on limewood, 166.3 × 81 cm. Staatliche Kunstsammlungen Dresden. © Rüstkammer, Staatliche Kunstsammlungen Dresden, photo: Elke Estel/Hans-Peter Klut. Elisabeth is shown at the age of 12 with an incredibly narrow torso likely indicating the manipulation of her pre-adolescent body through foundation garments.

were subject to such restrictions is suggested by portraits such as Lucas Cranach the Younger's painting of Elisabeth, Duchess of Saxony from 1564 (Figure 5.10) in which Elisabeth's pre-adolescent body is shown to be incredibly slight. While young girls were generally recognized to be naturally thinner than adult women, such practices aimed at maintaining and cultivating this slenderness as they progressed into adulthood.

The idealization of a slender upper body in this period was not a purely German phenomenon, and the structuring of this silhouette was replicated across Europe in the sixteenth century.[41] As indicated by the examples of Dürer, Weigel, and Amman, however, this figure was interpreted by contemporaries as materializing a form of German identity which played into a proto-nationalistic ideology present since the end of the fifteenth century. The modesty and decorum which German women were encouraged to display through their slenderness was

[41] Bendall, *Shaping Femininity*, 27–37.

presented as the opposite of foreign extravagance. Nevertheless, some worried that luxury was being indulged in closer to home. In 1502, the humanist and friend of Albrecht Dürer, Conrad Celtis, praised Nuremberg women for their frugality and modest appearance as well as their *cultus*. Rather than contrasting their manners with outsiders, his foil was the figure of a corrupted woman named Elsa who dressed luxuriously and erotically and who represented contemporary German decadence. Alongside the praise of German decency and honour, therefore, were concerns about the threat which decadent dress posed to the virtue and decorum of German women.[42]

This binary opposition of female virtue and vice, presented by Celtis, Dürer and others, was repeatedly framed in terms of thinness versus fatness. Yet these two models for femininity were not always so clearly opposed. In the late sixteenth and early seventeenth century, German women increasingly accentuated their narrow waists and compact upper bodies using padding around the hips and bum, in a garment known as *Weiberspeck* or 'women's lard' in German. This garment was one of a number of variations on a farthingale, an item used to add shape beneath a woman's gown which was popular across Europe.[43] The very name used for this garment in German reinforced a connection between women's bodies, food, and fatness. While intended to emphasize the slenderness of the upper body, in keeping with the widespread bodily ideal, this garment was meant to give the impression of fatness and expanse around the bottom and hips, areas associated with female fertility as well as sexual attractiveness. A Flemish satirical print from 1600 shows women being outfitted with such rolls in a tailor's shop. A caption above reads, 'Come beautiful women with skinny buttocks, quickly we shall make them round and merry' (Figure 5.11).[44]

In his critique of contemporary fashions from 1644, Johann Michael Moscherosch took aim at this deformation of the female body, building on moral criticism of dress styles which created the illusion of something real beneath one's clothing. He stated,

> What kind of misfortune do your wives and daughters engage with now with the great, cushioned, and padded holes (*grossen gepulsterten, gefuterten Löchern*)? As if they want to make a better figure and fatness (*eine bessere Leibesgestalt und Feiste*) through such a bulge; hence not unreasonably they care to call such sausages and stuffing lard, which is almost twenty-five pounds in weight and they wear it on their bodies. Those must be fat pigs (*feiste Säuwe*) indeed, and an honourable man would fairly recoil to touch such a dirty, ugly, louse-sack.

[42] Rublack, *Dressing Up*, 133.
[43] See Bendall, *Shaping Femininity*, 143–51.
[44] Ibid. 76.

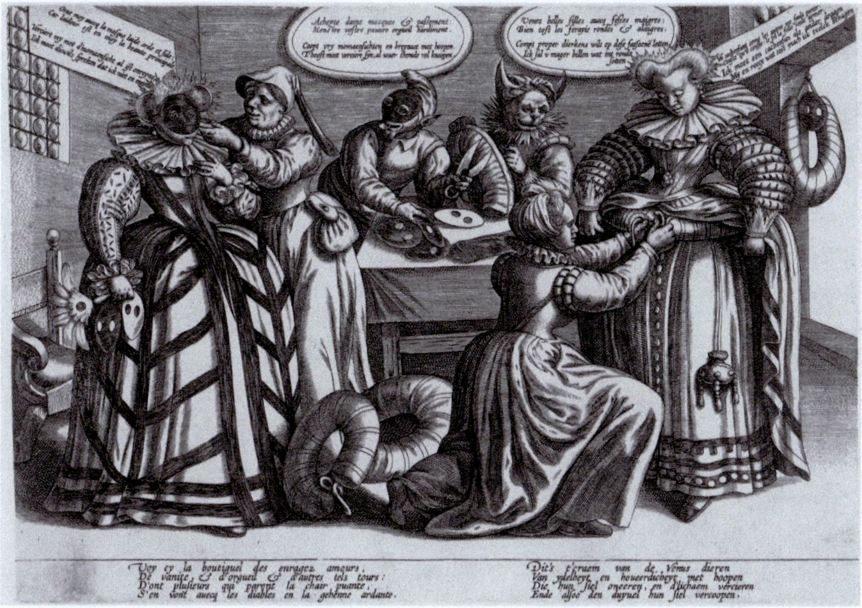

Figure 5.11 Maerten de Vos, The Vanity of Women, 1600. Engraving, dimensions not given. Metropolitan Museum of Art, New York, public domain. This Dutch print shows women dressing in bum rolls or *Weiberspeck* in German. The accompanying text describes the garments as assisting women with 'skinny buttocks'.

Just as Celtis presented the figure of Elsa as the type of woman who should not be desired by decent German men, Moscherosch depicted the dishonour of women who wore the *Weiberspeck*. He went on to relay a humorous song about the garment:

> because our women have lard (*Speck*) / now we don't need to buy any more pigs…I shall never want for lard / for a single woman can give me a centner (100 pounds) / If I have no grease (*Schmaltz*) in the house / should I crow about it? / What need have I of pigs? / Woman, hand out the lard! / Is that not a dirty life. / That the women now have lard.[45]

Moscherosch played on the term *Weiberspeck* to state that women wearing these garments were 'fat pigs', thus utilizing the tension between the dressed and undressed body, between what was visible and invisible, revealed and concealed. He criticized the deception of such women who created the illusion of fatness in their lower bodies, in turn challenging the agency which such garments enabled women to assert over their own bodies.[46]

[45] Johann Michael Moscherosch, *Anderer Theil der Gesichte Philanders von Sittewalt* (Strasbourg, 1644), 87–8.
[46] Bendall, *Shaping Femininity*, 78.

The ideal female silhouette thus consisted of a compact upper body, which was accentuated through a voluminous skirt. This figure inverted the ideal for men, whose clothing expanded the upper body, while their slender legs were displayed in tight-fitting hose. Such ideals echoed humoral understandings of the differences between women and men's 'natural' bodies. In Galenic medicine, the hot and dry nature of men developed their upper bodies, while the cool and wet complexions of women were associated with the lower body.[47] Highlighting such differences in Dürer's 1504 engraving of 'Adam and Eve' (Figure 3.5), a contemporary commentator wrote that 'the chest and shoulders of Adam [swell] with a certain manly fullness, while in contrast he has not emphasised Eve's parts except those below her belly and around her hips'.[48] Sexual difference was thus exemplified in the clothing styles of women and men which presented the complementarity of their bodily forms. This is visible in images of couples from this period. In Heinrich Aldegrever's print of wedding dancers from 1538 (Figure 5.12), for example, the folds of the woman's skirt creates volume at her lower body which is replicated in the gown which emphasizes her partner's upper body.

This ideal for women's bodies remained remarkably consistent throughout the sixteenth and early seventeenth centuries, though figures softened and broadened slightly towards the end of this period through voluminous sleeves and higher waistlines (Figure 5.13). German women of varying age and rank were consistently presented with controlled upper bodies, and while slenderness was idealized, clothing was used to mould bodies of varying size to correspond to this desired silhouette. Of the few pairs of bodies that remain from this period most, like those of Dorothea von Neuberg, are very small. Yet this is likely due to the greater potential of larger garments for repurposing or resizing for alternative wearers.[49] Larger wearers of such items did exist, however, and early modern tailors would have been trained to produce tight-fitting gowns for women of varying sizes.[50] The modesty and virtue associated with compact female bodies might thus be conveyed through larger bodies which adhered to the same idealized silhouette.[51]

Even by moulding the figure through clothing, however, people's bodies cannot always be made to conform to ideal proportions. As well as being naturally larger, women's bodies might depart from such forms with age, or through the

[47] See Susan P. Mattern, *Galen and the Rhetoric of Healing* (Baltimore, MD, 2008), 103. On the association of women with lower impulses in connection to physiology see Natalie Zemon Davis, 'Women on Top', in *Society and Culture in Early Modern France* (Stanford, CA, 1975), 124–51.

[48] Jeffrey Ashcroft, *Albrecht Dürer: Documentary Biography* (New Haven, 2017), vol. 1, 464. See also Jeffrey Chipps Smith, *Dürer* (London, 2012), 138.

[49] Bendall, *Shaping Femininity*, 173.

[50] See Jane Malcolm-Davies, Caroline Johnson, and Ninya Mikhaila, '"And her Black Satin Gown must be New-Bodied": The Twenty-First Century Body in Pursuit of the Holbein Look', *Costume* 42 (2008), 21–9.

[51] See Thessy Schoenholzer Nichols, 'It does Not Need to be Hard to Hold', in Kammel and Pietsch, *Structuring Fashion*, 29–38, esp. 30–1.

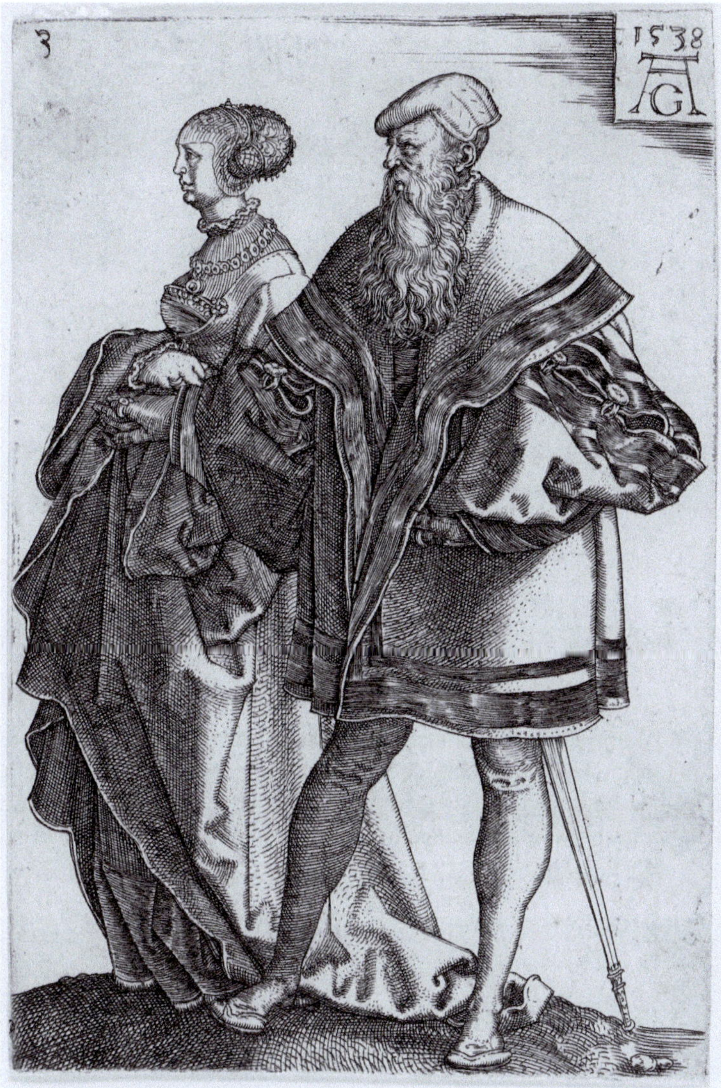

Figure 5.12 Heinrich Aldegrever, Dancing Couple, plate 3 from The Large Wedding-Dancers, 1538. Engraving, 11.7 × 7.8 cm. Art Institute of Chicago, public domain. The couple's dress emphasizes the complementarity of women and men's bodily forms, as the volume of the woman's lower body is echoed in the man's expansive gown which emphasizes his upper body.

expansion of pregnancy and longer-term bodily consequences of bearing children. While visual culture widely replicated an image of slender German femininity, therefore, the reality of women's bodies would have presented a more varied picture. The majority of Maria Jacobäa Fugger's wardrobe, for example, was made up of wide-fitting gowns known as a *weiter Rock* or *Kutte* in German which gave a

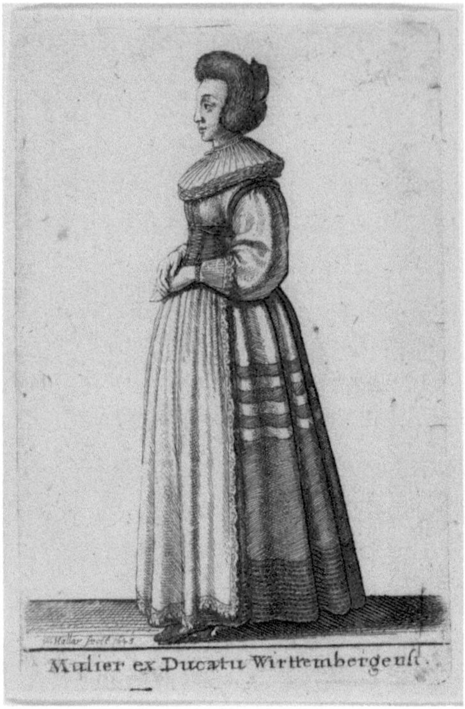

Figure 5.13 Wenceslaus Hollar, Woman from the Duchy of Württemberg, 1643. Etching, 91 × 60 mm. National Gallery of Art, Washington, DC, public domain. German women's dress in the early seventeenth century softened slightly with the addition of voluminous sleeves and higher waistlines, though a relatively close-fitting upper body remained the norm.

cone like shape to the body.[52] This shape disguised the body's contours and may have been Maria's preferred style due to the relatively large proportions of her body (as suggested by her portraits) which at her death at the age of 26 had already borne five children. Magdalena Paumgartner may have referenced a similar style of gown when she wrote to her husband in 1584 requesting that he send her four measures of damask so that she could have a loose-fitting gown made for her expanding pregnant body. She wrote that she had 'never liked to wear [this kind of garment] before, but now I have to', suggesting how changes in the body's form could dictate a person's fashion choices.[53] Moreover, in couples' portraits, married patrician women were sometimes shown wearing large gowns

[52] Karen Stolleis, 'Die Kleider der Maria Jacobäa Fugger (1562–1588)', in Mechthild Flury-Lemberg and Karen Stolleis (eds), *Documenta Textilia: Festschrift für Sigrid Müller-Christensen* (Munich, 1981), 357–70, here 361.

[53] Georg Steinhausen (ed.), *Briefwechsel Balthasar Paumgartners des Jüngeren mit seiner Gattin Magdalena, geb. Behaim (1582–1598)* (Stuttgart, 1895), 211.

(*Schauben*) which mirrored those of their husbands. This implicated the bodies of wives in conceptions of masculine honour which were embodied in these representational garments.[54] Displaying their married status, wifely restraint, and modesty, such gowns could render married women invisible as individuals by disguising their unique bodily form.[55] Yet, by wearing such gowns, women would also be able to disguise the contours of their figures and prevent the visibility of any alterations in their form over time which departed from contemporary ideals. As Grobian suggested, gowns allowed the wearer to keep the details of their body size to themselves.

Men's Bodies

While ideals for the female body remained relatively consistent across the sixteenth century, the male silhouette underwent an extreme transformation. At the end of the fifteenth century, the fashionable male figure represented in visual culture was notably slender with long, thin legs which were accentuated through high waistlines and pointed shoes. In the first half of the sixteenth century, however, men were increasingly shown with expansive upper bodies, constructing a bulky and imposing silhouette. As Aileen Ribeiro stated, therefore, with the dominance of 'German fashions' in this period, 'elegant Burgundian elongation had given way to a kind of squat solidity'.[56] While this development took place across Europe to varying degrees, this fashionably broad silhouette originated in the German context where it was especially popular. Portraits of German men, particularly those above the age of 30, consistently conform to this model of masculine bulk. Elite men in positions of power were especially likely to present themselves with large figures, and their vast size was connected to their political authority. Dürer's portrait of Emperor Maximilian I from 1519, for instance, emphasized the rounded solidity of his body.[57] Likewise, the Saxon Electors who protected Martin Luther were shown to be especially bulky in their portraits, and their large size was echoed in Luther's own presentation from the 1530s onwards.[58] Ottheinrich, Elector of the Palatinate, was presented with a particularly imposing and expansive figure (Figure 5.14). In his case, material evidence shows that this was not merely a presentational device, since a surviving garment, likely a winter

[54] See e.g. the portraits of Veronica Bimlin and Georg Herwart from the Herwart 'book of honour' in the Stadtarchiv Augsburg. Reproduced in Rublack, *Dressing Up*, 135.

[55] Susanna Burghartz makes this argument in relation to the wearing of veils by married women in Reformation Basel. Susanna Burghartz, 'Covered Women? Veiling in Early Modern Europe', tr. Jane Caplan, *History Workshop Journal* 80 (2015), 1–32, here 13.

[56] Ribeiro, *Dress and Morality*, 59.

[57] This portrait is held in the Kunsthistorisches Museum, Vienna. Inv. No. Gemäldegalerie, 825.

[58] Lyndal Roper, 'Martin Luther's Body: The "Stout Doctor" and his Biographers', *American Historical Review* 115 (2010), 351–84, here 357.

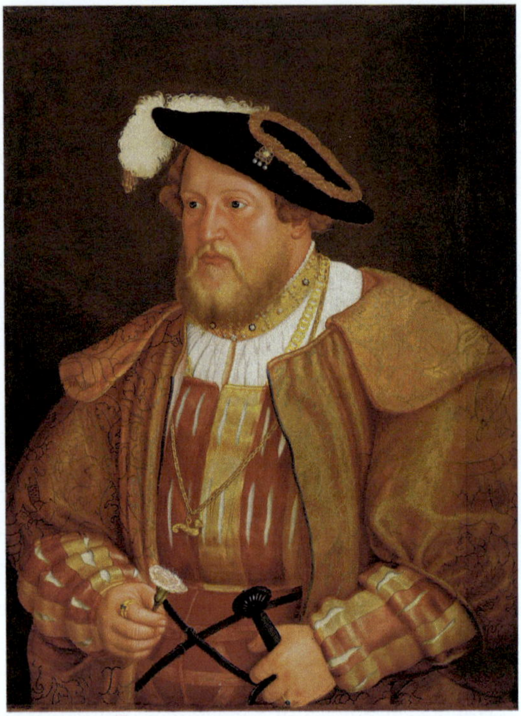

Figure 5.14 Barthel Beham, Portrait of Palatine Elector Ottheinrich, 1533. Oil on conifer wood, 97 × 71.2 cm. Bayerische Staatsgemäldesammlungen, Staatsgalerie Neuburg, licence: CC BY-SA 4.0. Ottheinrich is shown by Beham to possess a particularly expansive figure.

vest to be worn under the rest of his clothing, indicates that the circumference of the elector's chest must have measured somewhere between 200 and 235 cm (79–93 inches).[59] Ottheinrich's successor as Elector Palatine was Frederick III, a devout convert to Calvinism, whose portraits suggest that this image of bulky German masculinity transcended confessional differences.[60]

This expansive silhouette was not only reserved for elite rulers, however, but was replicated by men from both the upper and middle classes. In most cases these were married men, and since marriage was a cornerstone for male maturity, it seems that large size became associated with German manliness in this period. In 1525, Christoph Amberger created a portrait of an anonymous Augsburg man (Figure 5.15) who is shown with a large and rounded body in-keeping with the

[59] Magdalene Gärtner, 'Strickweste Ottheinrichs', in Suzanne Bäumler, Evamaria Brockhoff, and Michael Henker (eds), *Von Kaisers Gnaden. 500 Jahre Pfalz-Neuburg*, exh. cat., Schloss Neuburg (Regensburg, 2005), 300, cat. no. 7.135.

[60] See e.g. his portrait by an unknown artist sold at Sotheby's in 2015: https://www.sothebys.com/en/auctions/ecatalogue/2015/old-master-paintings-19th-century-n09303/lot.404.html?locale=en

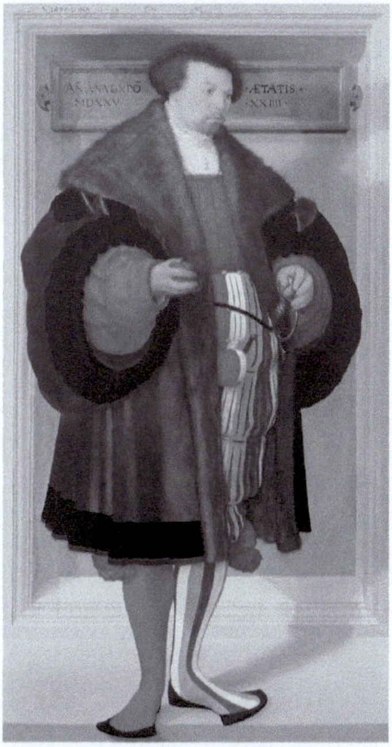

Figure 5.15 Christoph Amberger, Portrait of a Man, 1525. Oil on spruce wood, 191 × 101 cm. Kunsthistorisches Museum, Vienna. © KHM-Museumsverband. The 24-year-old man is shown with a large and rounded figure. This presentation of masculine bulk was necessitated by his marital status, particularly since his wife was seven years his senior.

contemporary ideal for mature men. The portrait states, however, that the sitter is only 24. While he may simply have possessed a larger body at a young age, his marital status would also have encouraged his bulky presentation, as his portrait is paired with that of his wife (Figure 5.16). Since her age is stated to be 31, the need for her husband to portray this image of mature masculine bulk was likely amplified due to the discrepancy in their ages.[61]

In the majority of contemporary portraits which present sitters with such imposing proportions, their bulk is accentuated through their choice of clothing. Most of these men were shown wearing expansive gowns, often referred to specifically as a *Schaube* in German, or by the more generic *Rock* (gown). Around 1500, such gowns reached to the wearer's ankles, elongating the figure. In the first half of the sixteenth century, however, shorter styles of gowns became increasingly popular, enabling men to show off shapely legs in tight-fitting hose, and giving even greater emphasis to the expanse of the upper body. *Schauben* were representational garments which created an imposing, powerful silhouette for

[61] On the importance of complementarity for married couples' bodies see Chapter 6, 214–17.

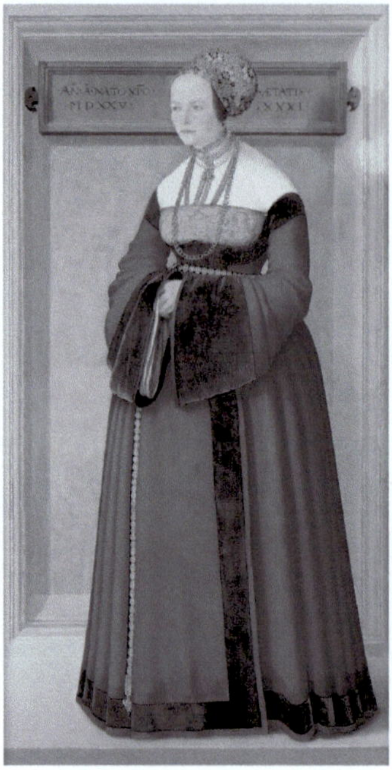

Figure 5.16 Christoph Amberger, Portrait of a Woman, 1525. Oil on spruce wood, 191 × 101 cm. Kunsthistorisches Museum Vienna. © KHM-Museumsverband.

the wearer, yet they were not the preserve of the ruling classes but were also worn by Burgher men.[62] Such gowns could take multiple forms, creating either a rounded or horizontal silhouette depending on the shape of the collar which could either slope into the waist or be cut perpendicular to the shoulders. The sixteenth century saw a development in the form of these gowns, as both the collar and shoulders became wider, reinforcing the box-like shape they created for the male body.[63] The collar of a gown would often reveal a fur lining, amplifying the role of this garment for presenting the status and authority of the wearer.[64] Sumptuary legislation dictated which furs could be worn by those of varying status, for instance imperial regulations from 1530 stated that only magistrates, patricians, and the nobility were permitted to wear gowns lined with marten fur.[65] Fur thus presented the wealth and position of its wearer, which would in turn have been related to the sensory experience of wearing such soft and luxurious materials. The

[62] Johannes Pietsch, *Zwei Schauben aus dem Bayerischen Nationalmuseum München: Ein Beitrag zur Kostümforschung* (Munich, 2004), 18.

[63] Ibid. 13.

[64] Philipp Zitzlsperger, *Dürers Pelz und das Recht im Bild: Kleiderkunde als Methode der Kunstgeschichte* (Berlin, 2012), 26–7.

[65] Rublack, 'Sartorial Politics in Germany', 51–2.

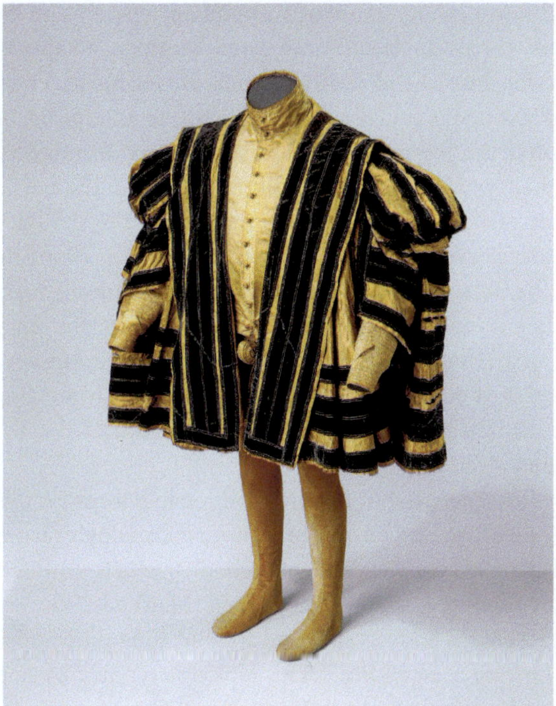

Figure 5.17 Ceremonial Dress of Elector Moritz of Saxony, 1540–5. Yellow silk damask, black silk velvet, silver cord, and gold thread, length 90 cm, hem circumference 628 cm. Staatliche Kunstsammlungen, Dresden © Abegg-Stiftung, CH-3132 Riggisberg, 2008 (Christoph von Viràg). The gown is a cross between a Spanish cape and a German *Schaube*. The gown's broad shoulders, wide lapels, and voluminous folds of heavy damask and velvet created an imposing and expansive form for the wearer.

expansion of the body and the physical space taken up by the wearer of this garment was likewise an essential part of its representational significance.

An extant garment which demonstrates this expansive, powerful silhouette, is the ceremonial gown of Elector Moritz of Saxony (Figure 5.17).[66] This garment, which is a cross between a Spanish cape and a German *Schaube*, was made of yellow silk damask and black velvet.[67] The gown has a circular cut in the style of the Spanish cape, and the circumference of this circle when laid flat is 6.38 metres. This indicates the large quantities of heavy damask and velvet that went into the

[66] See Jutta Bäumel, 'Der Kleider-Nachlaß des Kurfürsten Moritz von Sachsen: Das Inventar von 1553 und die in der Dresdener Rüstkammer überlieferten Originale', *Zeitschrift für historische Waffen- und Kostümkunde* 35 (1993), 65–106, and Bettina Niekamp and Agnieszka Woś Jucker (eds), with Jutta Charlotte von Bloh and Anna Jolly, *Das Prunkkleid des Kurfürsten Moritz von Sachsen (1521–1553) in der Dresdner Rüstkammer: Dokumentation—Restaurierung—Konservierung* (Riggisberg, 2008).

[67] Pietsch, *Zwei Schauben*, 45.

gown's creation, adding to an image of bulk and expanse.[68] With its horizontal cut at the shoulders, the gown would have given Moritz a notably wide silhouette, particularly in contrast to the relatively slim size of his surviving doublet and trunk-hose, indicating the potential for such items to enlarge the body. Moreover, the construction of the gown suggests how such garments imposed themselves on the bodies of their wearers. A strip of silk was sewn on the outside of the gown underneath the collar which went across the tops of the shoulders and was fastened within each sleeve. This was intended to evenly distribute the weight of the sleeves across the neck and shoulders while maintaining the breadth of the garment.[69] This detail suggests how the gown's great weight was recognized to impact on the wearer's comfort, posture, and movement. Moreover, the sense of added weight on the body would have contributed to an awareness of the wearer's imposing form, as well as the power and authority associated with such representational garments.

This bulky silhouette was not the only fashionable form for the male figure in this period. While broad and burly figures were increasingly favoured over previous models of Burgundian elegance, male bodies which were lean and graceful continued to be idealized among young men. Matthäus Schwarz, for instance, took pains to present his body as slim and athletic, thus cultivating a youthful and more delicate form of masculinity.[70] This look was typified by sloping shoulders, wide sleeves, and a particularly narrow waist. The increasing importance of sports such as fencing reinforced this youthful ideal for the light and flexible body and this was idealized in presentations of the hyper-fashionable Lansquenet soldiers. The height and slenderness of Lansquenets was accentuated through long peacock or ostrich feathers worn on their hats and helmets, as well as their clinging hose and flowing sleeves which were often slashed to reveal sensuous materials such as silk or velvet (Figure 5.18). The Lansquenets' slim figures thus presented a distinct form of masculinity. In an engraving from the first half of the sixteenth century, Barthel Beham deliberately inverted the popular image of the slender Lansquenet, instead showing a soldier who appears old, tired, and crucially bulky, with a fleshy belly and thighs (Figure 5.19). Beham was no stranger to utilizing body size to convey meaning in his images, and here the departure from the typical slenderness of the Lansquenet silhouette is central to the print's satirical humour.[71]

[68] Bettina Niekamp, 'Das Prunkkleid des Moritz von Sachsen', in Niekamp and Jucker (eds), *Das Prunkkleid*, 21–48, here 21.

[69] Ibid. 26.

[70] Schwarz claimed that his waist was one ell (around 60 cm). See Rublack and Hayward, *First Book of Fashion*, 94 and 260. On Schwarz's 'delicate masculinity' see Rublack, *Dressing Up*, 60. See also Karin Orchard, *Annäherungen der Geschlechter: Androgynie in der Kunst des Cinquecento* (Münster, 1992), 28–48.

[71] See Chapter 3, 106–10.

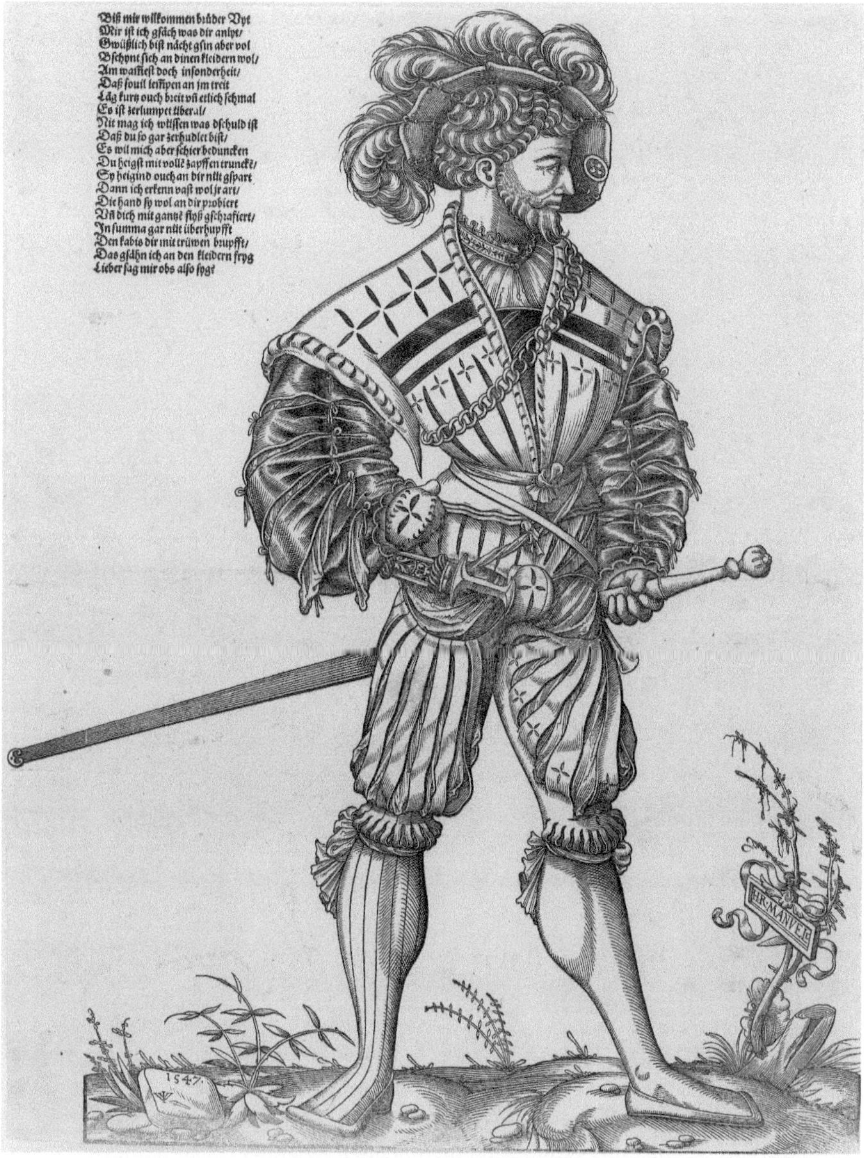
Biß mir willkommen brůder Vyt
Mir ist ich gsäch was dir anlyt/
Gwüßlich bist nächt gsin aber vol
Bschynt sich an dinen kleidern wol/
Am waffiest doch insonderheit/
Daß souil lempen an jm treit
Läg kurtz ouch breit vñ etlich schmal
Es ist zerlumpet überal/
Nit mag ich wüssen was dschuld ist
Daß du so gar zerhudlet bist/
Es wil mich aber schier bedunckẽ
Du heigst mit vollẽ zapffen trunckẽ/
Sy heigind ouch an dir nüt gspart
Dann ich erkenn vast wol jr art/
Die hand sy wol an dir probiert
Vñ dich mit gantzẽ flyß gschrafiert/
In summa gar nüt überhupfft
Den kabis dir mit trüwen brupfft/
Das gsähn ich an den kleidern fryg
Lieber sag mir obs also syg?
1547
H R MANVEL

Figure 5.18 Monogrammist IW, after Hans Rudolf Manuel Deutsch, Lansquenet, 1547. Woodcut, 39.5 × 29. 5 cm. Rijksmuseum, Amsterdam, public domain. Lansquenet soldiers were typically presented with slim, elongated bodies, often accentuated through plumes of peacock or ostrich feathers.

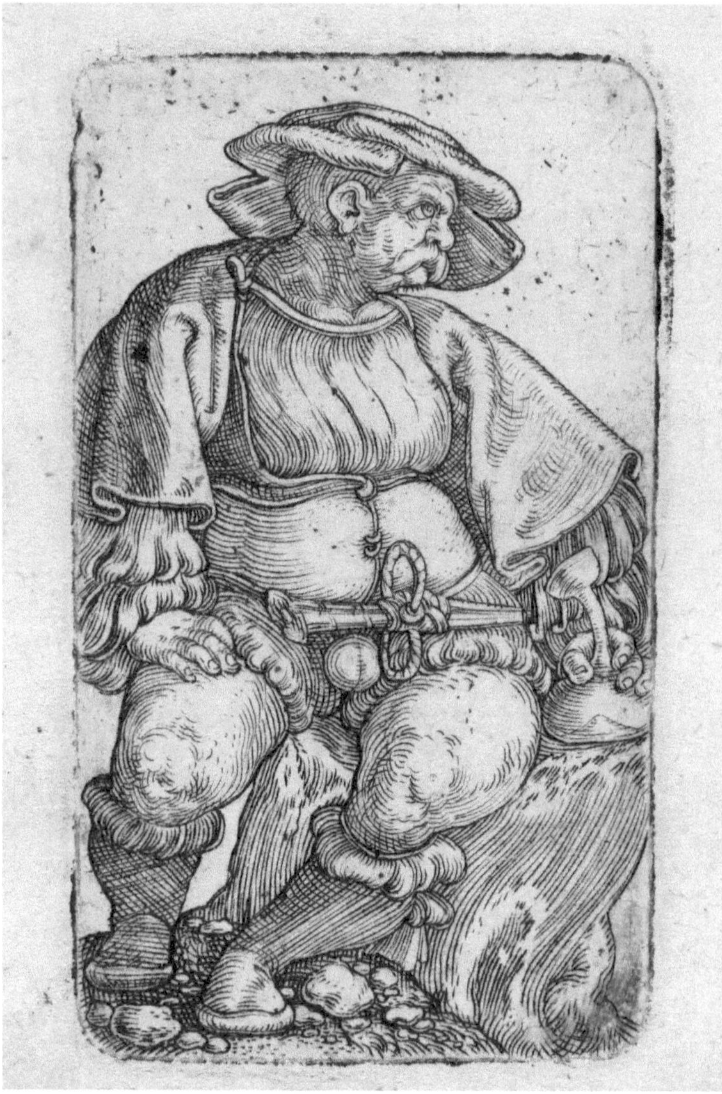

Figure 5.19 Barthel Beham, Lansquenet, 1512–40. Engraving, 4.7 × 2.7 cm. Rijksmuseum, Amsterdam, public domain. Beham deliberately inverted the popular image of the slender Lansquenet, instead presenting a satirical image of a worn-out soldier with a bulky and fleshy form.

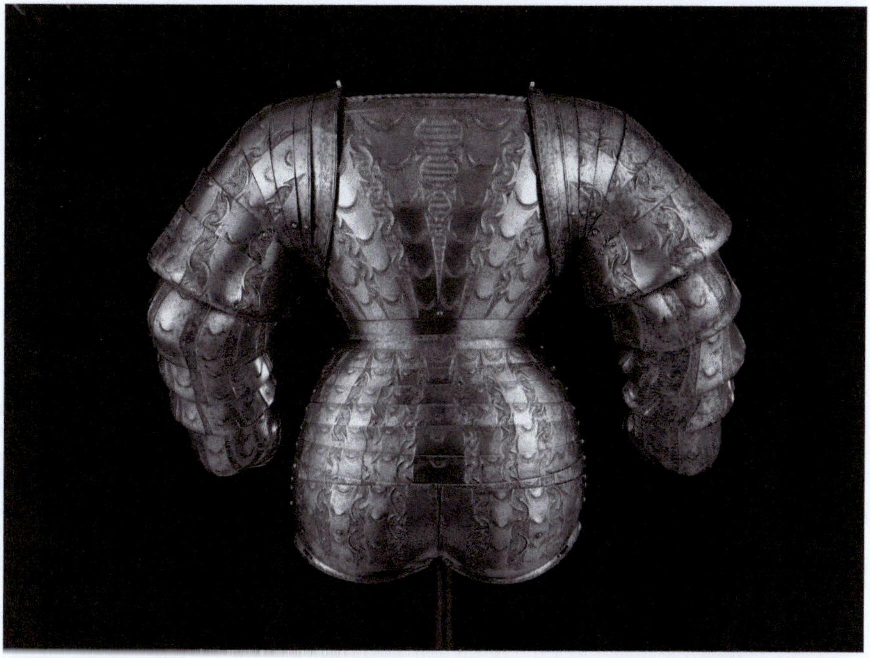

Figure 5.20 Kolman Helmschmid, Portions of a Costume Armour, 1525. Steel, copper alloy, gold, 68.6 × 45.7 cm. Metropolitan Museum, New York, public domain. Two styles of contemporary German masculinity appear combined in this armour, as the flowing sleeves and slashes of Lansquenet clothing are mixed with the breadth and solidity which characterized the presentation of mature German men.

Different categories of masculinity were associated with different bodily forms which were in turn shaped by practices of dress and adornment.[72] Yet these types were not always mutually exclusive. Costume armour created by Kolman Helmschmid in 1525 (Figure 5.20), for example, combines these two styles of contemporary masculinity. The armour appears as a facsimile of Lansquenet clothing with its flowing sleeves and slashes, yet through its breadth, as well as the solidity of its construction in steel, it also references the large and imposing form of mature German men.[73] Similarly, portraits of younger men wearing *Schauben* often showed the gown worn open at the front, enabling such men to display their narrow waists within this broad silhouette. As suggested by Köler and Schwarz, therefore, clothing allowed the wearer to take on different bodily

[72] See Ulinka Rublack, *Dürer's Coats: Renaissance Men and Material Cultures of Social Recognition*, The Natalie Zemon Davis Memorial Lectures Series (Vienna, 2025).

[73] For another of Helmschmid's creations see Stefan Krause, *Fashion in Steel: The Landsknecht Armour of Wilhelm von Rogendorf* (London, 2017).

forms depending on the kind of figure they wanted to create at a particular moment or context.[74]

In the second half of the sixteenth century, the fashionable male figure shifted again. The *Schaube* gradually fell out of fashion, eventually becoming the preserve of town councillors, scholars, and pastors, for whom the gown retained its associations with responsibility and authority.[75] German men's bodies continued to be presented as bulky, yet this volume shifted down from the shoulders to the middle of the body and the upper thighs (Figure 5.21). Ballooning, padded trunk-hose enlarged the thighs, while the contours of the lower legs remained visible in tight fitting stockings. Since the Middle Ages, shapely legs signified both beauty and rank among men, and this continued throughout the sixteenth century and into the early seventeenth century.[76] An emphasis on the middle body was reflected in the quilting and padding of men's doublets in this period, which increasingly focused on the area of the belly. A stuffed and padded belly was known as a peas-belly or peascod in English and a *Gänsbauch* ('goose belly') in German, due to the rounded shape it produced. An extant green doublet in the Germanisches Nationalmuseum in Nuremberg presents a *Gänsbauch* formed by cotton fleece padding which was sewn into the lining of the garment at the front and sides of the body (Figure 5.22).[77] A very similar though child-sized doublet is visible in a 1589 portrait of Balthasar Paumgartner, the son of Magdalena Paumgartner, whose belly is shown protruding and curving under in the classic shape of the *Gänsbauch*.[78] Like young girls, therefore, young boy's bodies were also subject to the shapes of contemporary fashion.

The fashionable form of the *Gänsbauch* was also reflected in contemporary plate armour which reconstructed these expanded bellies in steel. Breastplates were shaped into protruding, often pointed stomachs, which were intended more for display than protection.[79] Angus Patterson has written of such forms as being 'suggestive of a well-fed gentleman', and on one level these bellies played into

[74] Ulinka Rublack, 'Renaissance Dress, Cultures of Making, and the Period Eye', *West 86th: A Journal of Decorative Arts, Design History and Material Culture* 23 (2016), 6–34.

[75] Hermann von Weinsberg noted that he was already out of date by wearing his *Schaube* in 1578. Helene Dihle, 'Männerkleidung des 16. Jahrhunderts nach dem Buch Weinsberg', *Zeitschrift für historische Waffen- und Kostümkunde* (1923–25), 177–84, here 182.

[76] Rublack, *Dressing Up*, 18.

[77] Jutta Zander-Seidel, 'Grünes Wams mit "Gänsbauch"', in Jutta Zander-Seidel (ed.), *In Mode: Kleider und Bilder aus Renaissance und Frühbarock*, exh. cat., Germanisches Nationalmuseum (Nuremberg, 2015), 88–90, cat. no. 39.

[78] Nicolas Juvenal, Portrait of Balthasar IV Paumgartner, 1589. Oil on panel, 111 × 97 cm. In private collection. Reproduced in Zander-Seidel, *In Mode*, 91, cat. no. 40.

[79] See e.g. a suit of armour from late sixteenth-century Nuremberg in the Germanisches National Museum. Inv. No. W1342.

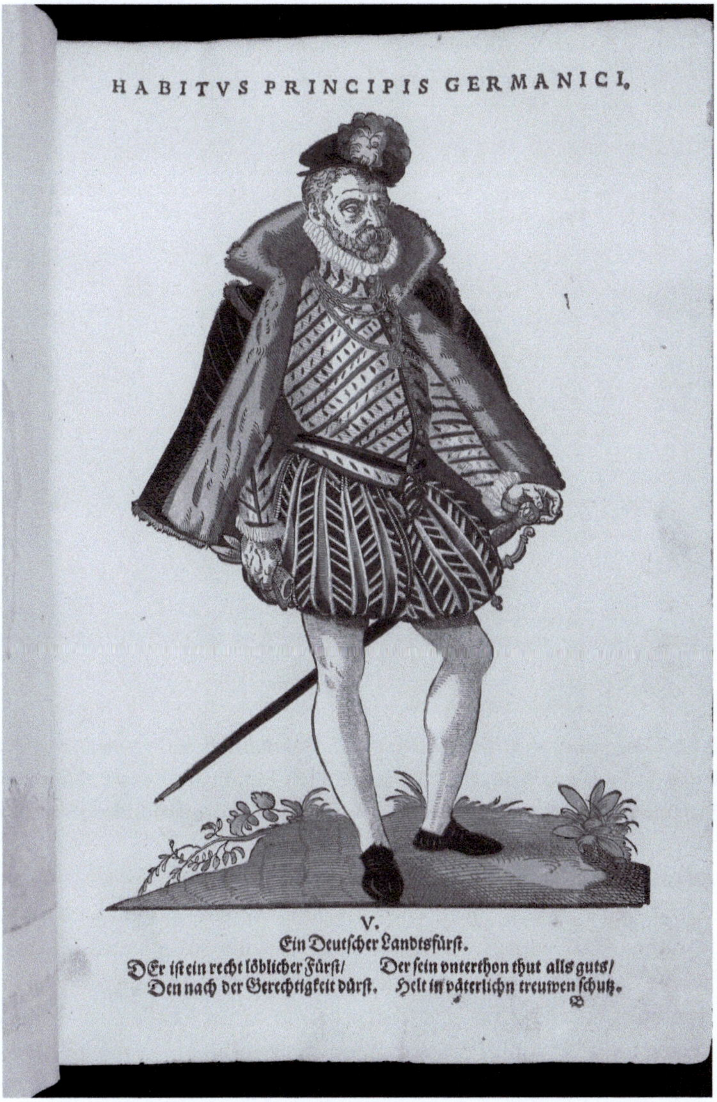
HABITVS PRINCIPIS GERMANICI.
V.
Ein Deutscher Landtsfürst.
DEr ist ein recht löblicher Fürst/ Der sein vnterthon thut alls guts/
Den nach der Gerechtigkeit dürst. Helt in väterlichn treuwen schutz.

Figure 5.21 'A German Prince', Hans Weigel, *Habitus praecipuorum populorum* (Nuremberg, 1577), fol. Bi[r], plate 005 © The Master and Fellows of Trinity College, Cambridge. The volume of the man's clothing is focused at the centre of his body through a padded doublet and trunk-hose as well as the sloping cut of his gown.

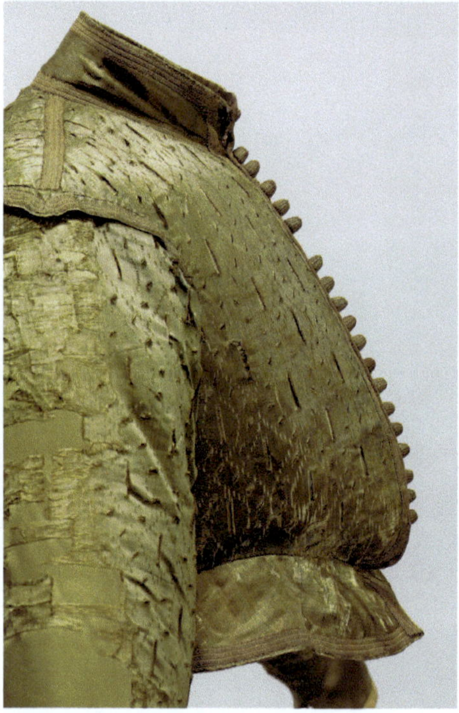

Figure 5.22 Green doublet with *Gänsbauch*, 1580–1600. Silk satin over silk taffeta, linen lining, and wadding, length 54 cm. © Germanisches Nationalmuseum, Nuremberg. Photo: G. Janssen. The doublet is padded at the belly to create a rounded shape.

contemporary associations between wealth, prestige, and large size.[80] The solidity of armoured bellies would have encouraged their association with power and strength, rather than with the fleshy, excessive bellies of gluttons or drunkards. Nevertheless, the contemporary connection between a fat belly and the vices of gluttony and drunkenness fuelled moral criticism of these expansive forms in both cloth and steel. In England, Philip Stubbes wrote in his *Anatomie of Abuses* from 1583 that 'I never saw any wear them but I have supposed him to be a man inclined to gourmandice, gluttonie and such like'.[81] In Saxony in 1593, a broadsheet by Philipp Uffenbach reported four monstrous births, including two children whose bodies replicated the shapes created by contemporary fashions. The print includes a child with an engorged and swollen stomach, intended to mimic the form of the *Gänsbauch* (Figure 5.23), and in a similar broadsheet from 1599 it was described how a child was born whose 'stomach was as big / as is now the custom with

[80] Angus Patterson, *Fashion and Armour in Renaissance Europe: Proud Lookes and Brave Attire* (London, 2009), 45.

[81] Frederick J. Furnivall (ed.), *Phillip Stubbes's Anatomy of the Abuses in England in Shakspere's youth, A.D. 1583* (London, 1877–9), 55.

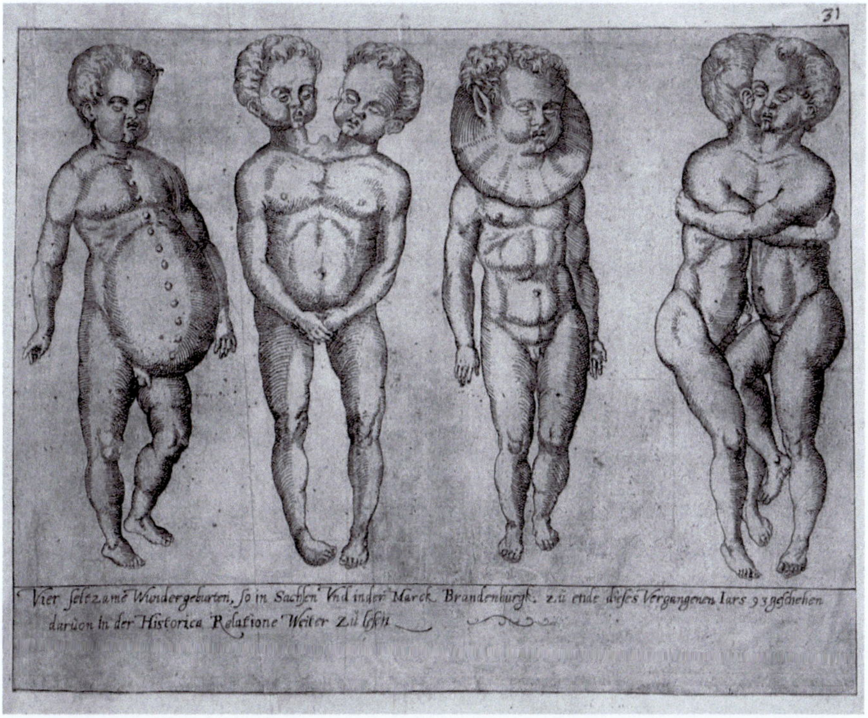

Figure 5.23 Philipp Uffenbach, Four Curious Wonder-Births Which Took Place in Saxony and the Margraviate of Brandenburg in this Past Year 1593 (*Vier seltzame Wundergeburten, so in Sachsen Vnd in der Mark Brandenburgk zu ende dieses Vergangenen Iars 93 geschehen*), 1593. Engraving, 21 × 26.7 cm. Wellcome Collection, London, public domain. Catalogued as 'Four Grotesquely Deformed Children'. On the left of the image, a child is shown with an engorged belly intended to mimic the form of a doublet with a *Gänsbauch,* as indicated by the buttons running down the centre of his chest and stomach.

doublets'.[82] These prints were part of a larger tradition of reporting monstrous births throughout the sixteenth century, in which such occurrences were frequently viewed as apocalyptic warnings.[83] Since one sign of the impending apocalypse was believed to be the proliferation of gluttony and drunkenness, and a resulting fattening of people's bodies, these images of babies born with expanded stomachs, replicating the form of the *Gänsbauch,* take on further meaning, reflecting the eschatological significance of fatness and the belly.[84] Moreover, such images present

[82] Jutta Zander-Seidel, '"Vier seltzame Wundergeburten, so in Sachsen Vnd in der Mark Brandenburgk zu ende dieses Vergangenen Iars 93 geschehen daruon in der Historica Relatione Weiter zu lesen"', in Zander-Seidel, *In Mode,* 155, cat. no. 74. Similar broadsheets were produced elsewhere in Europe, see Bendall, *Shaping Femininity,* 78.

[83] See Jennifer Spinks, *Monstrous Births and Visual Culture in Sixteenth-Century Germany* (London, 2009).

[84] See Chapter 4.

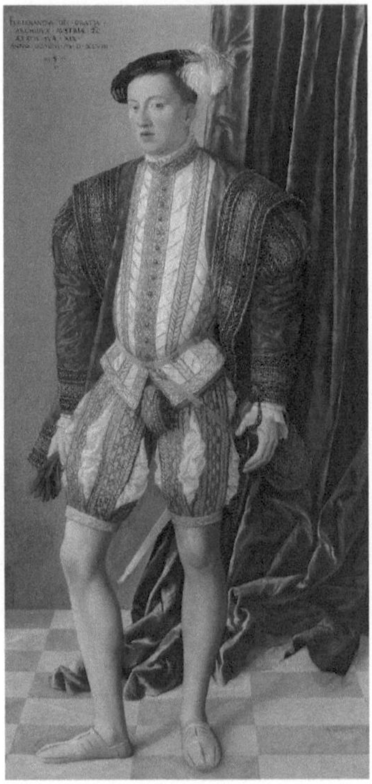

Figure 5.24 Jacob Seisenegger, Duke Ferdinand II of Tirol, 1548. Oil on canvas, 184.5 × 89 cm. Kunsthistorisches Museum, Vienna. © KHM-Museumsverband. The slenderness of Ferdinand's young body enables the *Gänsbauch* to stand out from his figure.

the tension between the dressed and the undressed body, as contemporaries questioned how far dressed forms reflected the shape of bodies beneath their clothing.

Lutheran pastor Lucas Osiander (1534–1604) drew upon this tension in his criticism of the excessive *Gänsbauch* from 1586. He began by writing: 'one completely marvellous ornament, however, are the ugly, long, puffed up *Gänsbäuch* / that begin above at the neck and hang right under the girdle (like a bay-widow hangs out from a house)' and he stated that one 'could not distort or disfigure (*verstellen vnd deformiern*) himself in any uglier way'. Osiander continued by stating,

> If one, who wears one such fabricated belly / gained one such belly in reality (*in der Wahrheit ein solchen Bauch vberkeme*) / as that with which he wants to fill out his clothes / so he would plead at several pulpits for God to remove this burden and cross from him. [Yet] when we form this belly ourselves with clothing, it is supposed to be a special prosperity (*ein sonderer Wolstand*).[85]

[85] Lucas Osiander, *Ein Predig, Von hoffertiger vngestalter Kleidung der Weibs vnd Manns Personen* (Tübingen, 1586), 14.

While wearers might indicate their prosperity through these padded stomachs, therefore, Osiander suggests that this was not intended to reflect the body beneath.

The acceptability of the *Gänsbauch* for its wearers thus appears to have rested on an acknowledged disconnection with the form of the naked body, complicating the idea that such men wished to appear 'well-fed'. Indeed, in many portraits which depict men wearing such false bellies, the pointed form of the *Gänsbauch* accentuates a narrow waist. Such images show slim young men wearing the garment, and it is their thinness that enables the *Gänsbauch* to stand out from their slender figures (Figure 5.24). The green doublet mentioned above indicates that larger men did wear these items, yet even in portraits where the sitter appears to have a relatively large body, the *Gänsbauch* acts to narrow it (Figure 5.25). Were a man to have an actual fat belly, this would make such cinching in difficult, creating an expanse around the waist which would not fit with the fashionable silhouette intended. Wearing the *Gänsbauch* may even have been meant, therefore, to suggest that the body beneath the garment was slim enough to achieve this look, just as Osiander suggests that such men would not want fat bellies 'in reality'. Masculine German

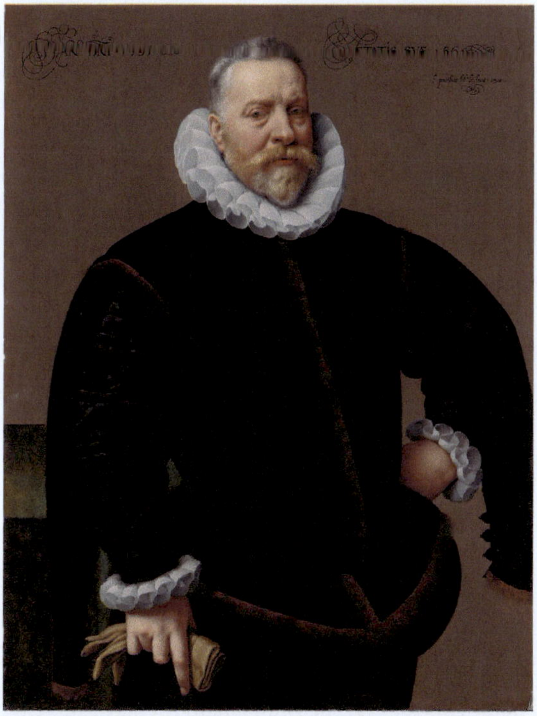

Figure 5.25 Frans Pourbus the Younger, An Unknown Man Aged 56, 1591. Oil on panel, 196 × 96.5 cm. © Private collection, image courtesy of The Weiss Gallery, London. This unknown man appears to have a relatively large body, yet the addition of the *Gänsbauch* narrows the appearance of his waist while padding the lower stomach.

bulk was not necessarily about creating an image of fatness, therefore, and a distinction between the dressed and undressed body was acknowledged.

By the early seventeenth century such structured, padded bellies were no longer in style, though emphasis continued to be placed on the middle body which increasingly took on a softer, looser form. Doublets flared out from high waistlines, while hose lengthened below the knees (Figure 5.26). Men continued to use clothing to present themselves in alternative figures, yet this softer, less structured silhouette meant that the role of dress in actively moulding the body into fashionable forms was reduced. This would also have lessened the awareness of body size and shape which the tighter, more structured fashions of the previous century had encouraged. Throughout the sixteenth century, therefore, body size was of particular significance for German men whose experience of the world was mediated through clothing items which imposed fashionable shapes on the

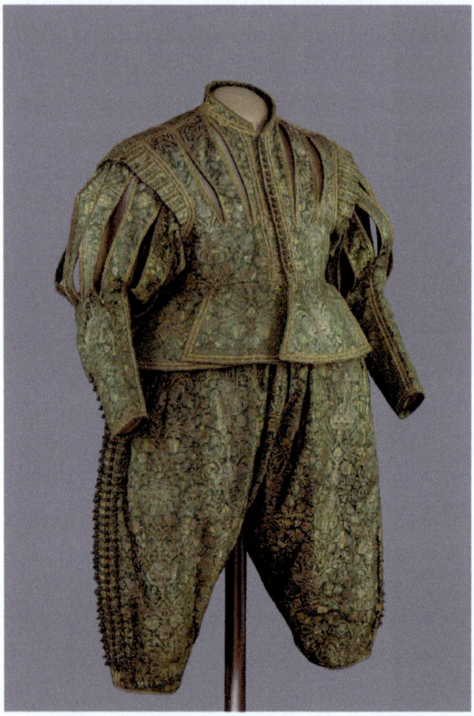

Figure 5.26 Doublet and hose from the ceremonial dress of Elector Johann Georg I. of Saxony, 1620–5. Green silk with gold thread, lined with green silk satin, green taffeta, and linen, waist circumference, 106 cm, front length (to flap), 28.2 cm. Staatliche Kunstsammlungen, Dresden. © Rüstkammer, Staatliche Kunstsammlungen Dresden, Photo: Jürgen Lösel. The Elector's doublet and hose present a typical fashionable silhouette from the early seventeenth century. The doublet's high waistline and the loose fit of the hose create a soft bulk at the centre of the body.

body. During this period, the relationship between the clothed and the naked figure was of the utmost importance for conceptions of body size, and this relationship was managed through practices of dressing, as well as making and altering clothing.

Clothing the Body

Contemporary fashions for German women and men involved shaping the body and constructing the figure through clothing that was padded, tailored, and boned. Dress items could be tightly fitted or could extend beyond the contours of the body, exaggerating particular areas of the figure. They could also be remarkably heavy, with items like the *Schaube* or *Weiberspeck* weighing down the shoulders or hips. This close interaction between clothing and the body would have encouraged an intense awareness of the body's size, shape, and stature. Moreover, since it was highly unusual for early modern bodies to be weighed, and as relatively few people owned full-length mirrors during this period, clothing would have been a central means by which changes in body size would have been sensed.[86] Magdalena Paumgartner, for example, described sensing her expanding pregnant body in relation to her dress, writing to her husband 'when I go out, I can never do up my bodice, and I have let it out as far as I can (*habs herausgelasen, so weit ich kind*)'.[87] In this case, the ability to let out the garment gave Magdalena a physical measure of how much larger her body had become.

Since the majority of garments could not be let out so easily, the proliferation of made-to-measure clothing in this period encouraged a greater production of dress items, as close-fitting garments needed to be replaced more often as people's body size altered over time.[88] This was especially the case for growing children and teenagers. In the late sixteenth century, 16-year-old Friedrich Behaim wrote to his mother to complain about the ill-fitting clothes she had sent to him at school. He stated, 'the stockings are so tight that I cannot get them on at all…the doublet is a complete misfit. Would you have it let out and lengthened for me?'[89] Trying on these garments and feeling their tightness against his flesh, Friedrich was confronted with the size of his body. In sourcing these items for her son, it's likely that Friedrich's mother had based her purchases on previous measurements

[86] Sabine Melchior-Bonnet, *The Mirror: A History* (London, 2002), esp. 14–28. On the significance of full-length mirrors for the perception of one's appearance see Jill Burke, *How to be a Renaissance Woman: The Untold History of Beauty and Female Creativity* (London, 2023), 42.

[87] Steinhausen, *Briefwechsel Balthasar Paumgartners,* 211. These letters are also discussed in Steven Ozment, *Magdalena and Balthasar: An Intimate Portrait of Life in Sixteenth-Century Europe Revealed in the Letters of a Nuremberg Husband and Wife* (New Haven, 1989), for this letter see 82.

[88] Rublack, *Dressing Up,* 18.

[89] Ibid. 214–15. See also Steven Ozment, *Three Behaim Boys: Growing Up in Early Modern Germany* (New Haven, 1990), 121–2.

of his figure. Through the act of dressing, therefore, Friedrich would also have gained an awareness of how his body had grown and developed in the intervening period.

Making alterations to existing clothing was a major part of a tailor's work in the early modern period. Bills from the tailor Karl Busenreuth of Nuremberg for Anna Maria Schmidmayr in 1592, for example, describe a 'bodice in silk made tighter' and 'the arms and body' of a female gown 'made wider'.[90] Such alterations could be intended to tailor a garment to a new owner (if it had been inherited or bought second-hand), to change the style of the item in line with new fashions, or to accommodate changes in the wearer's body size.[91] The green doublet with *Gänsbauch* shows signs of having been altered at the back seams, where satin of a slightly different shade has been added to expand the fit. Such alterations would typically be made at the back of a garment such as a doublet, to ensure that it was invisible when covered by a gown. Making such changes would entail the measurement and evaluation of the size and shape of the wearer's body by a tailor, a process which would have heightened the individual's awareness of their own corporeality.

This was also the case for the production of new clothing items. The vast majority of new garments were made-to-measure. Indeed, following a council decree from 1525, it was forbidden for Nuremberg tailors to make clothing intended for speculative sale, rather than for a designated client.[92] To commission an item of clothing, a buyer would first visit a tailor to have their measurements taken, where they would enquire about the amount of material required for the garment. They would then source this material elsewhere before returning to the tailor who would cut the pattern. The acts of measurement and pattern-cutting were so important in this process that only a master, rather than his apprentices or journeymen, was permitted to perform them.[93] Rather than measuring tape, tailors used strips of parchment into which they would cut notches for the various measurements of their customer's body.[94] These strips would be kept as a record of that client's measurements, meaning that tailors were able to compare later measurements against earlier ones, allowing for the observation of changes in the body. It is not known exactly which measurements would have been taken, but based on one of the earliest texts on tailoring, Juan de Alcega's *Libro de Geometria* (1580), these appear to have been fairly basic.[95] Alcega did not include instructions

[90] Zander-Seidel, *Textiler Hausrat,* 61.

[91] For a discussion of the difficulties in deciphering such alterations see Linda Baumgarten, 'Altered Historical Clothing', *Dress* 25 (1998), 42–57.

[92] Zander-Seidel, *Textiler Hausrat,* 377.

[93] Johannes Pietsch, 'Das Schneiderhandwerk im 17. Jahrhundert', in Pietsch and Stolleis, *Kölner Patrizier,* 59–125, here 59–60. See also Herbert Germar, *Das Schneiderhandwerk in Leipzig bis zum Ausgange des 17. Jahrhunderts,* PhD thesis, Leipzig, 1918, 96–101.

[94] Arnold, *Patterns of Fashion 3,* 4.

[95] Ibid. 3.

on how to measure the body and the patterns include little detail on this point. This suggests that much of the fitting and shaping of a garment would have been done on the client themselves. Often a mock-up or test piece for a garment would be constructed in linen which would then be incorporated into the lining or padding of the finished item.[96] That little of this process is recorded in works such as Alcega's reflects the extent to which this understanding of how to tailor a garment to the body was based on the learned, embodied knowledge of the tailor.

Such knowledge was built up over the course of a tailor's training. Tailors would first complete an apprenticeship before working as a journeyman and eventually taking the examination to become a master. To achieve this position, tailors needed to demonstrate knowledge of various kinds of fabrics, including the widths in which they were sold, their shrinkage, as well as whether their grain or nap would influence how they could be cut.[97] A pattern book from Enns in Austria from 1590 for instance states: 'a young master should know all these widths and also the shrinkage and how much he needs for the current piece as one will question him'.[98] Such information was needed in order to cut and tailor different kinds of fabric for different sized bodies. Intrinsic to the work of creating and altering clothing, therefore, was an understanding of the body and its proportions (Figure 5.27)

Tailored clothing acted to control the body and mould it into particular forms. Through clothing, bodies became socially acceptable, and questions of body size were deeply implicated within this acceptability. Dedekind's Grobian instructed readers that 'your trousers should be torn…it's a delight to have a bottom full of holes, your doublet should be holey at the breast, and your trousers split at the knees'.[99] Grobian's advice for uncouth behaviour thus involved wearing ripped and ill-fitting clothing, which failed to contain, control and conceal the body. Not only were torn clothes deemed untidy and a sign of poverty (as one did not have the means to repair or replace clothing), but they also blurred the boundary between the dressed and undressed body, coming to represent a sense of disorder and a lack of control over the body and its form.[100] The shape of the body in tailored clothing contributed to the ways in which early modern people made sense of the world around them, and this held consequences for the presentation of bodies which were not characterized by the shape of their clothing but were marked by its absence.

[96] Pietsch, 'Das Schneiderhandwerk im 17. Jahrhundert', 67.

[97] See Ingeborg Petrascheck-Heim, 'Die Meisterstückbücher des Schneiderhandwerks in Innsbruck', *Veröffentlichungen des Tiroler Landesmuseums Ferdinandeum* 50 (1970), 159–218.

[98] *Schneidermusterbuch: Käysserliche Freyhaitten d schneyder…Musterbuch des Handwerks der Schneider von Enns* (Enns, 1590), fol. 9ᵛ. Berlin, Staatliche Museen, Stiftung Preußischer Kulturbesitz, Kunstbibliothek. Ident. Nr. 14136895. See also Katherine Barich and Marion McNealy, *Drei Schnittbücher: Three Austrian Master Tailor Books of the 16th Century* (Kennewick, WA, 2015).

[99] Dedekind, *Grobianus*, fol. 45ᵛ.

[100] Rublack, *Dressing Up*, 31.

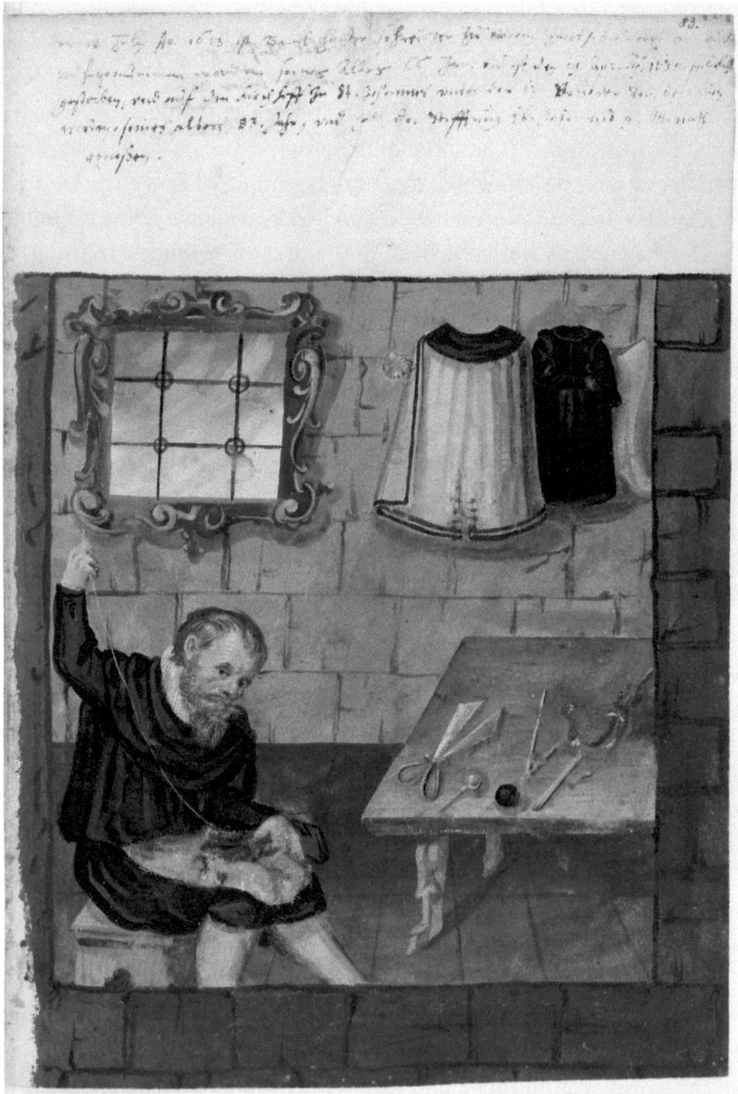

Figure 5.27 Portrait of tailor Bartl Harder, from the *Hausbücher der Nürnberger Zwölfbrüderstiftung*, Landauer I, Amb. 279.2°, fol. 83r, 1613, public domain. A Nuremberg tailor is shown at work with the tools of his trade, including a measuring stick, on the table before him.

Naked Bodies

Being naked, and therefore free of the figures which clothing could construct, made visible the size and shape of a person's body. Contexts in which bodies appeared naked in public, therefore, encouraged reflections on the differences between individual bodily forms. The bathhouse was a key site for public nudity and this setting became a crucial backdrop for artistic representations of the varying body shapes of Europeans. Like in Dürer's 'Women's Bath' (Figure 3.12) and 'Men's Bath' (Figure 3.13), Hans Bock the Elder used the context of the bathhouse to explore bodily difference in his 1580 painting (Figure 5.28). The bathers' bodies are distinguished from one another on the basis of their body shape and skin tone. A pale-skinned, rotund woman at the front of the scene, for example, is shown beside a warmer-toned, slender man with a pipe. These differences would be understood to reflect each individual's humoral balance, and in this case the fleshy woman and wiry man evoke contemporary conceptions of the embodied humoral differences between the sexes. The setting of the bathhouse, where bathers sought to rebalance the humours and could attempt to alter their body size, encourages the view that these bodies represent individuals of varying complexion in the tradition of Galenic medicine. Moreover, there is a sense in such

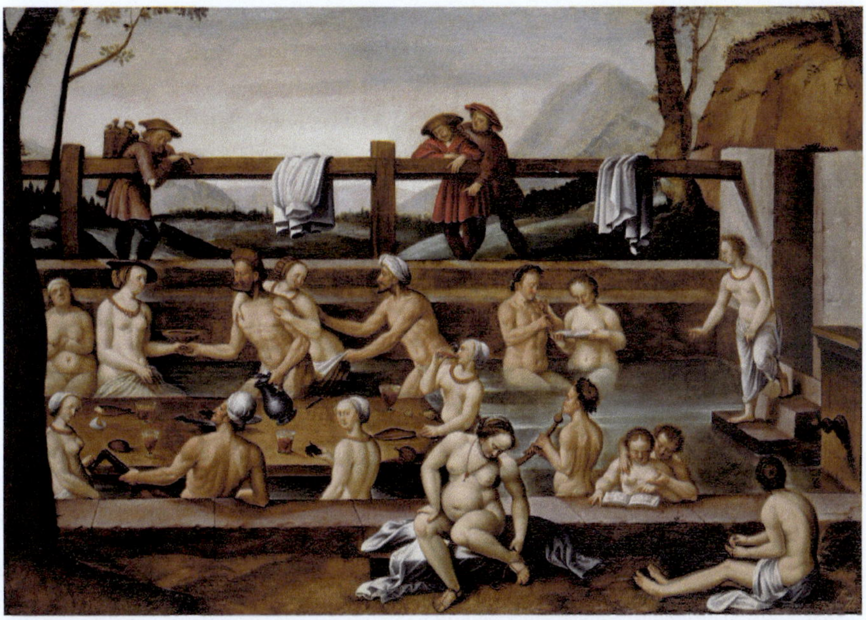

Figure 5.28 Hans Bock the Elder, the Baths at Leuk, 1580. Oil on canvas, 78.4 × 109.6 cm. Kunstmuseum, Basel, public domain. Bock used the context of the bathhouse to present the diverse figures of undressed women and men.

bathhouse scenes, which display a range of different body types, that this variety is what lies beneath the clothing which would normally mould and conceal the body into more uniform and acceptable figures.

We might also expect to see such variety, therefore, in accounts of people from the so-called 'New World', whose nakedness was repeatedly emphasized.[101] The early modern period was a time of increased global contact, connection, and exchange as European colonial projects, oceanic exploration, and large-scale international trade were intensified and consolidated.[102] Early modern Germans played an active role in the widening of European horizons.[103] The most successful German travel narrative from this period was Hans Staden's 1557 account of his time as a captive of the Tupinambá people in Brazil. Staden's text described 'what figure the people have', and he wrote that they were 'a fine people / of body and figure (*von leib vnd gestalt*) / both women and men…only that they are brown from the sun / because they all go naked / young and old / and have nothing to cover their shame'.[104] Though often based on a misinterpretation of Indigenous practices of adornment, the association of people from the Americas with nakedness was deeply entrenched and repeated by numerous European authors.[105] Describing his journey in present-day Argentina, Lansquenet soldier Ulrich Schmidel likewise described a community named 'Zemias Salvaisco' as 'mother-naked…they do not wear a single thread or anything else upon their bodies, or to cover their shame'.[106] This emphasis on nakedness encouraged a connection between Indigenous people and the biblical figures of Adam and Eve, who before the Fall had lived without clothes and had not experienced shame.[107] There was a sense, therefore, in which these communities were imagined to live

[101] See David Abulafia, *The Discovery of Mankind: Atlantic Encounters in the Age of Columbus* (New Haven and London, 2008), 54–8; Rachel Winchcombe, *Encountering Early America* (Manchester, 2021), 112–54 and Scott Manning Stevens, 'New World Contacts and the Trope of the "Naked Savage"', in Elizabeth D. Harvey (ed.), *Sensible Flesh: On Touch in Early Modern Culture* (Philadelphia, 2003), 125–40.

[102] For the consequences of early globalization for material culture and consumption practices see Beverly Lemire, *Global Trade and the Transformation of Consumer Cultures: The Material World Remade, c.1500–1820* (Cambridge, 2018).

[103] Renate Dürr et al., 'Forum: Globalizing Early Modern German History', *German History* 31 (2013), 366–82; Christine Johnson, *The German Discovery of the World: Renaissance Encounters with the Strange and Marvelous* (Charlottesville, VA, 2008). On German encounters with Indigenous people see also Stephanie Leitch, *Mapping Ethnography in Early Modern Germany* (New York, 2010).

[104] Hans Staden, *Warhaftige Historia und beschreibung eyner Landtschafft der Wilden, Nacketen, Grimmigen Menschfresser-Leuthen, in der Newenwelt America gelegen* (Marburg, 1557), fol. qi^{r}.

[105] On the longevity of this association see Philippa Levine, 'Naked Natives and Noble Savages: The Cultural Work of Nakedness in Imperial Britain', in Barry Crosbie and Mark Hampton (eds), *The Cultural Construction of the British World* (Manchester, 2015), 17–38.

[106] Ulrich Schmidel, *Vierte Schiffart. Warhafftige Historien. Einer Wunderbaren Schiffart, welche Ulrich Schmidel von Straubing, von Anno 1534. biß Anno 1554 in Americam oder Newenwelt, bey Brasilia und Rio della Plata gethan* (Nuremberg, 1599), 20.

[107] A Low German translation of Amerigo Vespucci's *Mundus Novus* from 1506 contained images drawn directly from prints of Adam and Eve's expulsion from Eden. Carina L. Johnson, *Cultural Hierarchy in Sixteenth-Century Europe: The Ottomans and Mexicans* (Cambridge, 2011), 12–13. See also Leitch, *Mapping Ethnography*, 55.

in a form of prelapsarian paradise, where their nakedness reflected their innocence and freedom from worldliness and cultural trappings. Nakedness was a key element in romanticized conceptions of the 'Noble Savage' who personified natural goodness uncorrupted by civilization.[108] The figure of the Noble Savage was one of particular fascination among Germans, for whom it connected to the nostalgic view of an ancient German past of rustic simplicity, as evoked by Tacitus.[109] On the other hand, however, the shameless nakedness of Indigenous Americans could also be interpreted as displaying a lack of civility and decorum, playing into a perception of these communities as wild or barbaric.

On encountering non-European bodies in this context, German authors regularly commented on their size and shape. These commentators' discussions of body size reflected contemporary ethno-geographical frameworks in which bodies were understood to be shaped by environments, meaning inhabitants of the Americas were expected to be physically different from Europeans.[110] In contrast to discussions of European bodies, however, these non-European bodies were described in markedly homogeneous terms, seeming to deny individuality in body size and shape. Schmidel, for example, described the people of 'Zemias Salvaisco' as being 'short and fat' (*kurze vnd dicke*), the 'Tiembus' as 'big people, and upright of body' (*grosse Leuth vnd gerad von Leib*), while the 'Parana' were 'upright and well-formed of body' (*gerad vnd wolgeschickt von Leib*).[111] While Schmidel repeatedly praised the bodies of Indigenous people as well proportioned, his descriptions remained cursory and generalizing.

The bodies of enslaved Africans were described in similar terms. By the sixteenth century, a sizeable proportion of Black Africans were present in Europe, particularly in cities such as Lisbon, Antwerp, and Venice which were key ports in the expanding slave trade.[112] In 1555 Swiss naturalist Leonhard Thurneysser travelled to Lisbon, where he commented on the bodies of enslaved Africans he encountered. He wrote 'as for their size or proportion of their bodies, they are

[108] See Levine, 'Naked Natives and Noble Savages'; Ter Ellingson, *The Myth of the Noble Savage* (Berkeley, CA, 2001); Stelio Cro, *The Noble Savage: Allegory of Freedom* (Waterloo, 1990).

[109] The idea of the 'Noble Savage', and Germans as noble savages, particularly took hold in the eighteenth century but had been present from the late Middle Ages and had its roots in antiquity. Johann J. K. Reusch, 'Germans as Noble Savages and Castaways: Alter Egos and Alterity in German Collective Consciousness during the Long Eighteenth Century', *Eighteenth-Century Studies* 42 (2008), 91–129.

[110] See Surekha Davies, *Renaissance Ethnography and the Invention of the Human: New Worlds, Maps and Monsters* (Cambridge, 2016), esp. 23–46.

[111] Schmidel, *Vierte Schiffart*, here 20, 15, and 19. See 'wohlgeschickt', *Deutsches Wörterbuch von Jacob Grimm und Wilhelm Grimm* (DWB), digital edition: www.woerterbuchnetz.de/DWB/

[112] See Thomas F. Earle and Kate J. P. Lowe (eds), *Black Africans in Renaissance Europe* (Cambridge, 2005); Kate Lowe, 'Visible Lives: Black Gondoliers and Other Black Africans in Renaissance Venice', *Renaissance Quarterly* 66 (2013), 412–52; Olivette Otele, *African Europeans: An Untold History* (London, 2020), esp. 39–66.

middling' (*An* Statur *aber oder Leibes* Proportion, *seindt sie mittelmessig*).[113] Thurneysser offered slightly more detail and allowed for some variation between bodies when he wrote that 'some among them have a longish head and high foreheads, narrow and drawn in (*ennge vnnd eingezogene*) shoulders, a hollow or pushed in (*gedempten oder nieder getruckhten*) belly, a very flat and even (*ebene vnnd gleiche*) chest'.[114] In general, Thurneysser described Black Africans as if they were a botanical or zoological species, with their bodies conforming to one identifiable type. Albrecht Dürer made similarly sweeping categorizations in his 'Discourse on Aesthetics' when he wrote that people belonged to 'two races, white and black'. He stated that the faces of Black people were 'seldom handsome', yet he continued 'I have seen a number of them who otherwise are so well-made and comely (*wolgeschickt vnnd ertig*) in their whole bodies as I have never seen better formed nor can imagine, with very good kinds of arms and all things'.[115] In an earlier draft he stated, 'their legs are knotted and usually scrawny (*dür*)'.[116] While Dürer's wider text on proportion embraced the diversity of beauty in nature, with such comments he glossed over the potential for diverse proportions in Black bodies.

Images of non-European bodies reinforced this sense of uniformity. Hans Burgkmair's woodcuts of 'People of Africa and India' (Figure 5.29), for example, have been described by Stephanie Leitch as inviting 'a prescient use' of the term 'ethnography', due to Burgkmair's care in distinguishing one group from another 'by virtue of their variance in geography, appearance, and customs'.[117] Despite this sensitivity, however, Burgkmair depicted very little variation in the forms of the bodies on show, either between or within the groups he presented. Perhaps stylistic considerations encouraged such uniformity. Yet in a period in which European bathing scenes capitalized on the visibility of variations between individual bodies, it is particularly striking that images of naked or partly covered non-European bodies would neglect to include such bodily variation.

Race has been identified as a crucial factor in the development of modern fatphobia and for informing perceptions of body size since the Renaissance.[118] Sixteenth-century German writers were certainly interested in the bodily forms of Black Africans they encountered in Europe, as well as the Indigenous people of

[113] Bernardo Jerosch Herold, 'The Diary of the Swiss Leonhard Thurneysser and Black Africans in Renaissance Lisbon', *Renaissance Studies* 32 (2018), 463–88, here 478. The article includes a transcription of the original manuscript on 475–82, and an English translation on 482–8. I have based my translations on Jerosch Herold's.

[114] Ibid. 477.

[115] Hans Rupprich, *Dürer: Schriftlicher Nachlass* (Berlin, 1956), vol. 3, 295. Translation from Jeffrey Ashcroft, *Albrecht Dürer: Documentary Biography* (New Haven, 2017), vol. 2, 878. Sabrina Strings discusses this passage in *Fearing the Black Body: The Racial Origins of Fat Phobia* (New York, 2019), 19.

[116] Rupprich, *Schriftlicher Nachlass*, vol. 3, 286. Ashcroft, *Documentary Biography*, vol. 1, 525.

[117] Stephanie Leitch, 'Burgkmair's *Peoples of Africa and India* (1508) and the Origins of Ethnography in Print', *Art Bulletin* 91 (2009), 134–59, here 135.

[118] Strings, *Fearing the Black Body*, esp. 15–64.

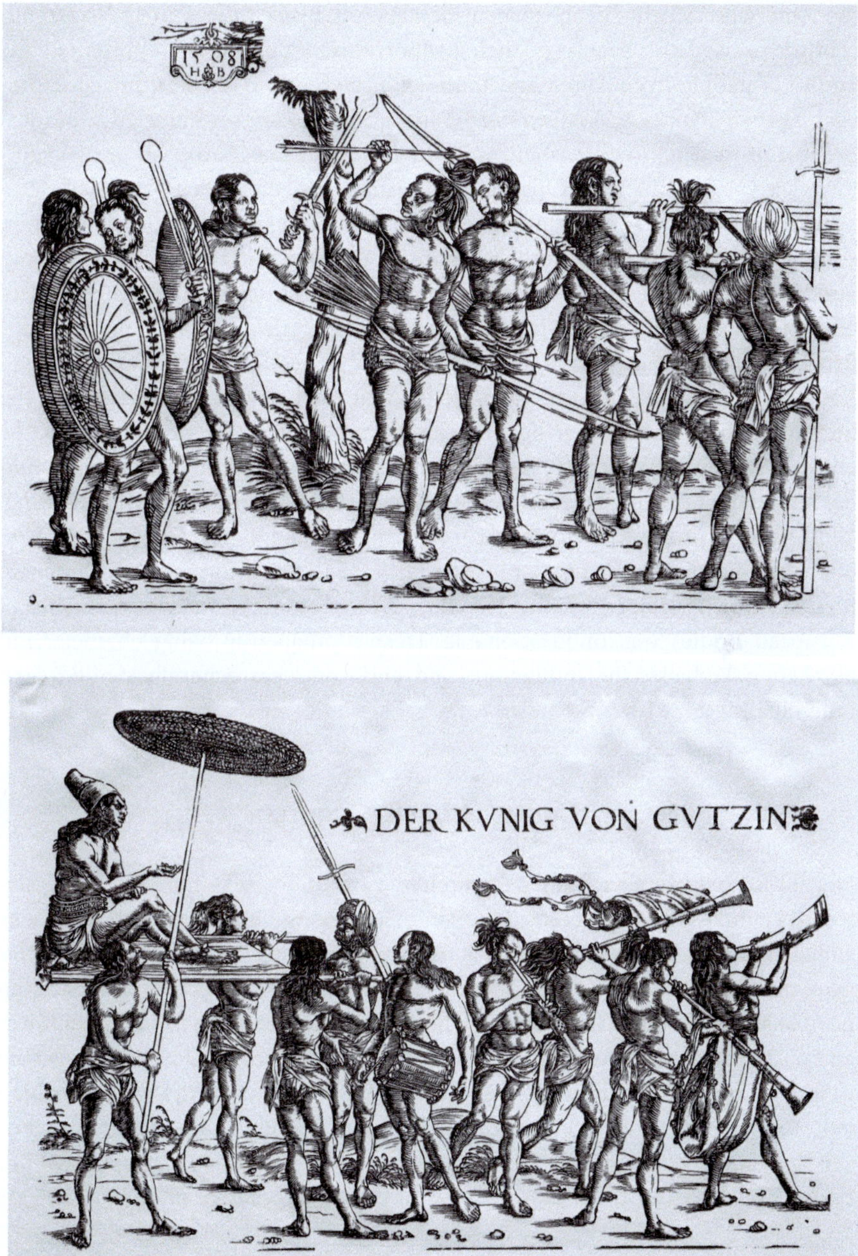

Figure 5.29 Hans Burgkmair, The King of Cochin, part of series 'People of Africa and India', 1508. Woodcut in two parts, dimensions not given. The Cleveland Museum of Art, public domain. Despite the exposure of their bodies, Burgkmair presents little variation in the bodily forms of women and men.

the Americas. Much European commentary on Black bodies in the sixteenth century praised the beauty of their proportions.[119] Burgkmair represented the bodies of people from Africa and India with reference to classical imagery, presenting their figures in contrapposto poses and applying his knowledge of ideal proportion.[120] Such representations of the beauty of non-European bodies reinforced a view of the Noble Savage, suggesting that their unadorned, physical beauty reflected inner purity and goodness. Whether praise or critique, however, commentary from German authors regarding the undressed bodies of those from outside Europe had a universalizing tendency which shows how questions of body size were implicated in processes of othering in this period, ultimately contributing towards early forms of race-making.[121] Beneath their clothes, European bodies were recognized to be individual, composed of a unique balance of the humours which meant that health regimens and dietary advice needed to be tailored to their own personal needs. Such bodies had a natural form which could be remodelled through practices of eating, bathing, and crucially dressing. Clothes were understood to construct alternative figures for European bodies, often causing them to become more uniform as they conformed to fashionable ideals or norms of acceptability. When undressed, however, the individuality of European bodies was unquestionable. Despite frequently being characterized by their nakedness, the Indigenous and enslaved were generally denied such individuality.

Constructing the Figure

Not all extra-European bodies were characterized by nakedness, and the sixteenth century witnessed the production of a growing number of costume books which reported on dress practices across the globe, including several examples from the German lands.[122] This interest in global fashions reflected the expanding horizons of early modern Germans who became fascinated by different cultures and customs. Such costume studies, like those of Europeans, glossed over bodily difference or individuality, but they nevertheless recognized the ways in which cultures outside Europe used clothing to construct different silhouettes. A manuscript costume book produced in Augsburg in the last quarter of the sixteenth century reflected on the dress practices of people in a range of global contexts

[119] Ibid. 15–41. [120] Leitch, *Mapping Ethnography*, 89.

[121] On early modern race-making see Hannah Murphy, 'Re-writing Race in Early Modern European Medicine', *History Compass* 19 (2021), https://doi.org/10.1111/hic3.12692 Christine Johnson discusses German commentators' processes of 'othering' in *The German Discovery*, esp. 3–8.

[122] On such costume books see Giorgio Riello, 'The World in a Book: The Creation of the Global in Sixteenth-Century European Costume Books', *Past and Present* 242 (2019), 281–317; Katherine Bond, 'Mapping Culture in the Habsburg Empire: Fashioning a Costume Book in the Court of Charles V', *Renaissance Quarterly* 71 (2018), 530–79; Rublack, *Dressing Up*, 180–209.

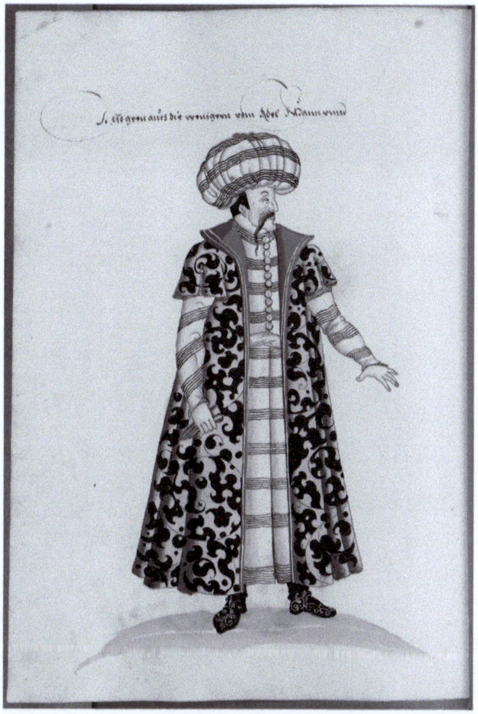

Figure 5.30 'A Noble Man from Palestine', in *Kostüme der Männer und Frauen in Augsburg und Nürnberg, Deutschland, Europa, Orient und Afrika*, fol. 146^{v}. Bayerische Staatsbibliothek, Munich, Cod.icon. 341, public domain.

including in Palestine, Syria, Egypt, and Ethiopia.[123] Its unknown creator appears intrigued, for instance, by the different silhouettes of noble Palestinian men and women which were created through gowns, either tailored or draped, and different forms of headwear, either rounded or elongated (Figures 5.30 and 5.31). The clothing of 'others' closer to home also merited scrutiny. Christoph Weiditz's earlier costume book from the 1530s contained numerous images of Muslim 'Morisco' women in Spain, and he was particularly preoccupied by the rounded shapes created through their loose-fitting and voluminous dress (Figure 5.32). The recording of different cultures of dress by early modern Germans still frequently presented a sense of generalized otherness; costume books regularly contained numerous images with various styles of clothing worn in Germany, differentiated by region, age, occasion and social status, while other cultures were represented

[123] *Kostüme der Männer und Frauen in Augsburg und Nürnberg, Deutschland, Europa, Orient und Afrika*—BSB Cod.icon. 341. Last quarter of the sixteenth century. Bayerische Staatsbibliothek, Munich. Digital reproduction: https://www.digitale-sammlungen.de/en/view/bsb00011752?page=,1

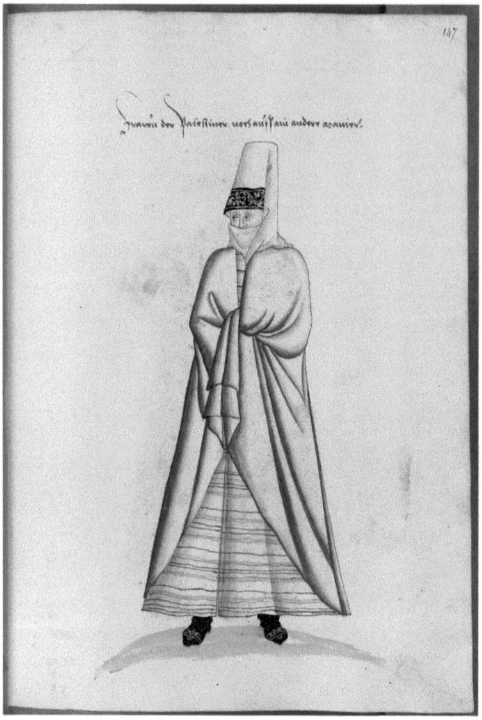

Figure 5.31 'A Noble Woman from Palestine', in *Kostüme der Männer und Frauen in Augsburg und Nürnberg, Deutschland, Europa, Orient und Afrika*, fol. 147r. Bayerische Staatsbibliothek, Munich, Cod.icon. 341, public domain. The anonymous compiler of this costume book reflected on the different bodily forms created by dress in global contexts, including in these images of a noble Palestinian man and woman whose differing figures are created through different styles of gown and headwear.

by a more limited number of studies.[124] Nonetheless, these images point to a contemporary curiosity about the creation of different body shapes through clothing, including in diverse global contexts.

Dress was recognized by early modern Germans as an essential part of a person's figure. Clothing enabled German women and men to construct alternative forms for their bodies which aligned with fashionable ideals as well as moral requirements for the gendered body. Dress thus extended embodied experiences which could in turn become associated with a sense of German identity, as women and men presented German values of honour and good government, robustness and strength, through the clothes they wore and the shapes these created for their bodies. While distinctions between the dressed and undressed body

[124] E.g. of the 506 pages of Sigmund Heldt's costume book created between 1560 and 1580 in Nuremberg 100 pages focused on the city of Nuremberg alone. See Rublack, *Dressing Up*, 199–206.

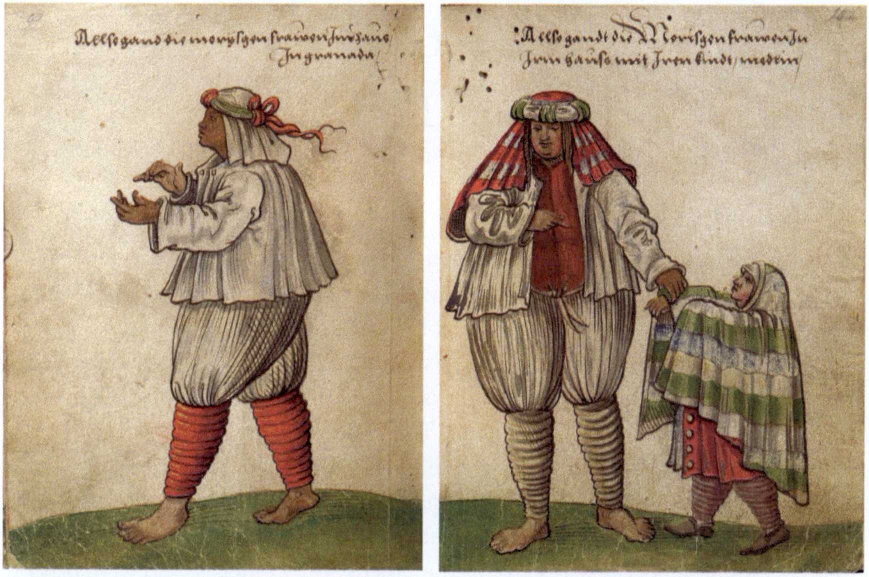

Figure 5.32 'House-clothes of Morisco Women and Children in Granada', in Christoph Weiditz, *Trachtenbuch* (1530s), 99–100. Germanisches Nationalmuseum, Nuremberg, Hs. 22474, public domain. The artist was particularly interested in the rounded body shapes created by Morisco women's voluminous dress.

were important, the ability of clothes to impose on the body and mould it into particular forms meant it was not always easy to distinguish between the two. The blurred line between dress and undress was then used by German moralizers to critique what they considered the deformation of the body through clothes. For those who revelled in contemporary fashions, as well as those who railed against them, the manipulation of body size and proportions through clothing was of critical significance.

This period witnessed a proliferation in clothing items with which to fashion the body and, combined with the increasing prevalence of tailored clothing, the sixteenth century was thus a particularly important moment for the intimate relationship between body size and dress. In following centuries, it would become more common for bodies to be weighed to measure changes in size and shape, and the role of dress as a means of sensing such alterations was reduced. Together with the increased medical, artistic, and spiritual interest in bodily form, this heightened relationship between dress and the body contributed towards the elevated significance of body size within German culture.

Body Size in Early Modern Germany. Holly Fletcher, Oxford University Press.
DOI: 10.1093/9780198972983.003.0005

6
Personal Body Size

In 1480s Florence, the Italian mathematician and architect Antonio Manetti wrote a tale about a trick of deception in which a fat woodworker called Manetto, 'the fat one' (*Il Grasso*), was convinced by a group of his acquaintances that he had become someone else. The group was made up of gentlemen from ruling Florentine families, as well as painters, goldsmiths, and sculptors, including Filippo Brunelleschi and Donatello. Their deceit involved locking 'simple-minded' Manetto out of his house while one of the group imitated his voice, addressed him as Matteo (another acquaintance) and instructed him to leave. Later, others from the group passed him in the street and addressed him as Matteo, and he was even arrested for Matteo's debts by officials who were privy to the joke. At first, Manetto insisted he was the fat woodworker, yet when no one believed him, he eventually became convinced that he really had become Matteo.[1]

In his study of early modern identity and surveillance, Valentin Groebner used this story to argue that in this period 'people had only the appearance that others perceived in them', and therefore identity depended upon external evaluation.[2] Yet this interpretation overlooks the significance of body size for this story and its humour. While the tale comes from fifteenth-century Italy, where the layers of meaning which made up ideas about fatness and thinness differed from those in the German context, it reveals much about how body size was perceived by early modern people. The fatness of Manetto is crucial to the story, not just as a sign of his simple nature, but because part of the tale's humour lies in the fact that Manetto could be persuaded he had become somebody else, despite continuing to experience the world through his fat body. In a period in which mind and body were deeply connected, and personhood was embedded within the matter of the body as much as the soul, it would have been especially laughable that Manetto could believe he had become Matteo while his clothes still fitted his form, he still took up the same amount of space, and his body still moved in, and felt, the same way.[3] The fact that Manetto was a craftsman, whose occupation required him to

[1] Antonio Manetti, *The Fat Woodworker*, tr. Robert L. Martone and Valerie Martone (New York, 1991).

[2] Valentin Groebner, *Who are You? Identification, Deception, and Surveillance in Early Modern Europe*, tr. Mark Kyburz and John Peck (New York, 2007), quotation 29. Groebner summarizes Manetti's tale on 18–21.

[3] On the person as both soul and body in medieval spiritual belief, in contrast to modern 'body-hopping' films, see Caroline Walker Bynum, 'Why All the Fuss about the Body? A Medievalist's Perspective', *Critical Inquiry* 22 (1995), 1–33, esp. 19.

be especially attuned to his bodily capabilities and sensory perceptions, pushed the joke even further.[4] The tale thus presents a contemporary expectation that one would and should have an awareness of one's own body, including its size and shape.

Individual body size informs a person's physical experience of the world, an experience which is likewise moulded by cultural beliefs and expectations. So far, this book has focused on the cultural meanings that body size took on in early modern Germany, yet it has also highlighted how personal experiences of body size related to these wider perceptions. We have seen how Hieronymus Bock advised readers to eat crushed ash leaves to slim down, while noting that his own thin body did not require such measures. Albrecht Dürer's personal embodied experiences were crucial to his study of human proportion and aesthetic beauty, while individuals such as Matthäus Schwarz, Hieronymus Köler, Hermann von Weinsberg, and Magdalena Paumgartner used garments to construct fashionable silhouettes and to reveal or conceal their body size. This chapter builds on these glimpses into personal embodied experience by focusing on personal testimonies in 'self-narrative' sources, such as letters and diaries, where early modern Germans gave accounts of their own and others' bodies. These sources enable a closer examination of how early modern people perceived their material bodies in dialogue with the cultural meanings ascribed to fatness and thinness from the late fifteenth to the early seventeenth century.

Body size was personal, yet this did not mean that the individual body was understood in isolation. As a composite and fluid entity, the body was constructed in relation to a complex array of social, religious, and political influences and was in constant material exchange with its surroundings.[5] Moreover, bodies were conceived of as belonging within a network of relations which included the other human bodies with which a person interacted. There was, therefore, an embodied dimension to the social configuration of personhood in this period.[6] Rather than conceiving of themselves primarily as individuals, early modern people thought and acted through social networks; self-narrative sources from early modern Germany show that body size was embedded within such networks in both social and material terms.[7] Body size held a crucial role within contemporary practices

[4] See Pamela H. Smith, *The Body of the Artisan: Art and Experience in the Scientific Revolution* (Chicago, 2004).

[5] On the fluid early modern body see Ulinka Rublack, 'Fluxes: The Early Modern Body and the Emotions', *History Workshop Journal* 53 (2002), 1–16.

[6] On the social configuration of personhood see David Sabean, *Power in the Blood: Popular Culture and Village Discourse in Early Modern Germany* (Cambridge, 1984); Thomas Robisheaux, *The Last Witch of Langenburg: Murder in a German Village* (New York, 2009).

[7] Gabriele Jancke and Claudia Ulbrich, 'From the Individual to the Person: Challenging Autobiography Theory', in Claudia Ulbrich et al. (eds), *Mapping the 'I': Research on Self-Narratives in Germany and Switzerland* (Leiden, 2015), 13–33. See also Mary Fulbrook and Ulinka Rublack, 'In Relation: The "Social Self" and Ego-Documents', *German History* 28 (2010), 263–72. Historians such as Gudrun Piller and Maren Lorenz have challenged the view that self-narratives may be used to

of care as conveyed through these texts. Early modern people expressed deep concern for the bodies of their family and friends, offered practical advice for their well-being, and even described the materialization of such concern through alterations in their own bodily form. The bodies of one's connections mattered to early modern people, and this was especially true for the relationship between wives and husbands. Body size was a central issue for marital compatibility and the composite body was nowhere more apparent than in marriage, where women and men co-produced one another's bodies through acts of care and shared responsibility. The relationship between body size and care meant that bodily form had immense affective potential, something which Dürer seized upon in his artworks.[8] Changes in the body of a person's loved ones could thus be expressed in deeply emotional terms. Moreover, the role of body size within these social, emotional, and material networks encouraged an association between body size and belonging, or unbelonging, which could be expressed at the level of household, family, and nation. In self-narratives, therefore, we see how early modern people 'did' body size, as the authors of these texts used and performed fatness and thinness to convey meaning and emotion and to situate themselves within networks of care and belonging. Body size thus materialized both individual personhood and collective belonging.[9]

Anna and Albrecht

Body size began to take on increasing cultural significance in Germany from the late fifteenth century. It was not until the beginning of the sixteenth century that this new culture of body size truly gathered momentum, as embodied ideals for German masculinity shifted, medical advice regarding fatness and thinness proliferated, and the Reformation heightened the spiritual significance of body size. Yet late medieval Germans were nevertheless beginning to take greater notice of the fatness or thinness of their bodies. This is evident in letters shared between Albrecht III (1414–1486), margrave and elector of Brandenburg, and his second wife Anna, daughter of Frederick II of Saxony. In his youth, Albrecht had distinguished himself for his skill and courage in battle, becoming known as Albrecht

access contemporary bodily experiences but this chapter understands them to be fruitful sources for exploring early modern bodies so long as they are not seen to simply translate experience into language. See Gudrun Piller 'Private Body: What do Self-Narratives Bring to the History of the Body?', in Ulbrich et al., *Mapping the 'I'*, 76–94; Maren Lorenz, 'Tiefe Wunden. Gewalterfahrung in den Kriegen der Frühen Neuzeit', in Ulrich Bielefeld et al. (eds), *Gesellschaft—Gewalt -Vertrauen: Jan Philipp Reemtsma zum 60. Geburtstag* (Hamburg, 2012), 332–54.

[8] See Chapter 3.

[9] On the diverse ways in which early modern Germans constructed a sense of self, qualifying the arguments of Sabean and Robisheaux, see Laura Kounine, *Imagining the Witch: Emotions, Gender, and Selfhood in Early Modern Germany* (Oxford, 2018).

Achilles due to his knightly virtues. In fifteenth-century tournament records he was celebrated as the bravest, strongest, and most skilled knight.[10] The couple were married in 1458, and sixteen years into their marriage they exchanged a series of letters while Albrecht was fighting in the Burgundian Wars. At this point Albrecht was 60 and Anna was 37. These letters offer fascinating insights into the emotional significance of body size for this couple, as Anna and Albrecht repeatedly wrote to one another with news of their bodily states, including changes in size and shape.

Writing to Anna from a military campaign in Koblenz on 26 December 1474, Albrecht reported that his body was decreasing in size. He suggested the great strength of his troops meant that rations were running short, and he noted that he was 'becoming very thin' (*ser klein*), despite the provisions that his wife had sent to sustain him.[11] Anna dutifully replied shortly afterwards, providing advice on how he could replenish his body. She sent him a hat and some 'water' (a form of tonic) and wrote 'Master Nicholas says that the water is very healthy for Your Dearness, and that you should use it. You also wrote to me that you have become much smaller (*ser abnemt*), he says it is very good for that, and that one will gain size again and become strong [from it] (*wider zunem und brestig werd*).'[12] Anna connected Albrecht's decreasing size with a weakening of his body, something that would have been concerning to both parties. Albrecht's strength was necessary for the immediate exertions of war, as well as for his embodiment of the role of male ruler. Anna expressed her worry for Albrecht, bidding him to 'I ask that you should let me know properly how you are and how things stand with you, because I know that you have become ill and weak (*blod und schwach*), and you have to undergo a great deal of travail and labour. That brings me no small worry.'[13] Anna took care over her husband's body, seeking out practical advice on his behalf, sending him provisions, as well as requesting regular updates on his health. For Anna, the maintenance of Albrecht's body, including its size, was an essential part of her role as wife and caregiver, yet it became a far more difficult task during his absence. A month later, Albrecht reassured Anna that he was feeling well despite his reduced body. He stated 'I, by God's mercy, am well, healthy, and stronger, as well as slimmer (*frisch und gesunt und stercker, auch geringer*), than I have been in ten years.'[14] Having regained his strength, Albrecht viewed his smaller body with positivity, perhaps appreciating the agility and spryness it granted him on the battlefield, as well as his return to a more youthful form.

[10] Clifford J. Rogers, *The Oxford Encyclopedia of Medieval Warfare and Military Technology*, vol. 1 (Oxford, 2010), 19–20. See also Willi Böhm, 'Albrecht, Kurfürst von Brandenburg', in *Allgemeine deutsche Biographie*, vol. 1 (Leipzig, 1875), 243–52, and Ernst Schubert, 'Albrecht Achilles, Markgraf und Kurfürst von Brandenburg 1414–1486', *Fränkische Lebensbilder* 4 (1971), 130–72.

[11] Georg Steinhausen (ed.), *Deutsche Privatbriefe des Mittelalters*, vol. 1. *Fürsten und Magnaten, Edle und Ritter* (Berlin, 1899), 128. I am grateful to Stephen Mossman for his assistance with these translations.

[12] Ibid. 139. [13] Ibid. 137–8. [14] Ibid. 143.

It was not merely Albrecht's body size that concerned the pair. In the same exchange, Albrecht wrote to Anna saying 'I want to know if your arse has become bigger or smaller (*ob dir der arß grosser oder kleiner*) than when I left you'.[15] The size of Anna's body was central to the erotic communication Albrecht shared with his wife. He wrote to her, 'we want to spare the beating (*pfeffer*) for you when we are home. If your backside has become big (*wirt dir der hinter groß*), you will suffer it all the better, and we will enjoy it as it is beautiful; if it has become thin (*türr*) we'll still keep at it'.[16] *Pfeffer* here refers to the central and south German custom of beating loved ones and acquaintances with switches or twigs to bring them good luck, often at New Year or on Holy Innocents Day on 28 December. Those who received such beatings would be rewarded with gingerbread (*Pfefferkuchen*), and thus the performance of this custom was referred to using the verb *pfeffern*.[17] Writing on 26 December, Albrecht was clearly referencing this custom, yet throughout his letters *pfeffern* also takes on erotic significance, and is perhaps better understood as a form of spanking.[18] When Albrecht writes to Anna, 'Should God grant that we return home, we want to *pfeffern* you with the young Albrecht and your ladies in waiting with the switches', it seems that he also uses the verb as a reference to intercourse, with the 'young Albrecht' referring to his penis.[19] While it was with Anna alone that Albrecht's sexual desires would be realized through coitus, he repeatedly made sexual jokes about spanking the ladies in waiting, thus including them and their bodies within his erotic fantasies.[20] The fatness of the women's bodies and specifically their arses was the focus of Albrecht's sexual attention. In his following letter Albrecht writes, 'It is a burden to me, that I have not recently beaten (*gepfeffert*) you and the ladies in waiting, and I am worried that your backsides will shrink. Therefore eat often and treat yourself well so that your undercarriage remains fat (*dir der unterleger dick bleib*)!'[21]

A fat bottom was clearly associated with eroticism for Albrecht, who teased his wife with the promise of intercourse which depended on the size of her 'backside'. Albrecht thus found a way to remain intimate with his wife's body despite being far apart. He also imposed upon her his own sexual desires, surely influencing the way in which Anna viewed her own body in response to what she knew her husband to find attractive. She responded to him with reports of her body, writing for instance, 'in relation to size (*der groß halben*) I would like to say, I have not yet

[15] Ibid. 144. [16] Ibid. 128.

[17] See for instance Hanns Bächtold-Stäubli and Eduard Hoffmann-Krayer (eds), *Handwörterbuch des deutschen Aberglaubens*, vol. 6 (Berlin, 1987), 1573–4.

[18] Cordula Nolte, 'Verbalerotische Kommunikation, *gut schwenck* oder: Worüber lachte man bei Hofe? Einige Thesen zum Briefwechsel des Kurfürstenpaares Albrecht und Anna von Brandenburg-Ansbach 1474/75', in Jan Hirschbiegel and Werner Paravicini (eds), *Das Frauenzimmer: Die Frau bei Hofe in Spätmittelalter und früher Neuzeit* (Sigmaringen, 2000), 449–61, here 455. On spanking, Nolte references Henry Kratz, *Über den Wortschatz der Erotik im Spätmittelhochdeutschen und Frühneuhochdeutschen*, PhD thesis, Ohio, 1949, 143.

[19] Steinhausen, *Deutsche Privatbriefe*, 128–9.

[20] See Nolte, 'Verbalerotische Kommunikation', 455.

[21] Steinhausen, *Deutsche Privatbriefe*, 129.

become smaller (*cleiner*), unless Lent chastises me so that I get a bit slimmer (*ein wenig geringer*)'.[22] She thus anticipated the approaching period of fasting, warning Albrecht of the material consequences it might have for her body size. This was not just an intimate conversation between two partners, however, as these letters appear to have been read aloud and discussed among the women of the *Frauenzimmer,* several of whom intervene in the exchange.[23] One of the women, for instance, was derided by Albrecht for having blonde pubic hair, prompting Anna to write 'she does not like to hear that you write from the Rhein about her [being] blonde' and so 'she has learnt an art by which she can become brown'.[24] While much of the conversation was intended to be humorous, even if Albrecht's teasing was not taken seriously, his comments about the women had the potential to influence the ways in which they viewed and maintained their bodies, taking effect in their practices of bodily care and nourishment.

In March 1475, Anna wrote to her husband saying,

> My ladies in waiting are complaining loudly that they have to get up so early and spend so much time in the church praying, at your behest, so that God helps you to return home, that they have become misshapen (*ungeschafen*) and small around the backside (*um die hindern klein*); and they want to put the responsibility for it on me, because I wake them up every morning so early. I say [to them] that I do not find that my size is vanishing (*mein grosen dafon ferge*) or that I am becoming smaller (*abnem*) on that account... If they had my constitution (*wern sie geschlacht als ich*), then the fasting and praying would do them no harm.[25]

Anna's comments reflect understandings of body size in relation to food and sleep which were repeated in medical texts throughout the following century; that restricted consumption and a lack of sleep would encourage thinness. She also suggests that spending time in church praying would likewise encourage this reduction in size, hinting at a connection between spirituality and bodily form that went beyond purely fasting. This may have reflected the late medieval association of female piety with asceticism and bodily mortification. Suggesting that she was able to sustain these activities without becoming 'misshapen', Anna teasingly presents her body as superior to those of her ladies in waiting. Moreover, by stating that she is better able to maintain a large bottom than they are, Anna shows herself to be the most attractive of the women, drawing on her knowledge of Albrecht's sexual ideal. Despite the humour therefore, there is a slightly more serious undertone to this passage, reflecting the need for Anna to be at the forefront of Albrecht's erotic fantasies.[26]

22 Ibid. 133. 23 See Nolte, 'Verbalerotische Kommunikation', 455.
24 Steinhausen, *Deutsche Privatbriefe*, 139–40. 25 Ibid. 139.
26 See Nolte, 'Verbalerotische Kommunikation', 451.

In this long-running exchange, body size is shown to play an important role in Anna and Albrecht's marriage. The couple wrote to one another requesting news of the other's bodily form, notably focusing on the strength of Albrecht's body and the sexual attractiveness of Anna's, thus mirroring gendered ideals in both the fifteenth and sixteenth centuries in which men were expected to act as the strong head of a household, while women's bodies were valued for their fecundity. Nevertheless, body size appears part of a shared language of care for the couple, who used these discussions to remain intimate with one another's bodies during their separation. Anna and Albrecht 'did' body size, therefore, as they performed thinness and fatness as symbols of weakness and vulnerability, pleasure, eroticism, and attraction to convey messages to one another in their letters.

Caring for the Body

Body size as a subject of care and concern is often present in self-narratives from early modern Germany. Changes in the body's form could be indicative of changes in health, causing worry for those who observed such alterations in the bodies of their loved ones. In the early seventeenth century, Elisabeth Starhemberg wrote to her sister-in-law, expressing her concern that her daughter Margareta was in great pain and had become much thinner.[27] A year later, Judith Starhemberg wrote to her mother-in-law with worries about her son who was unwell and had become 'emaciated, skinny and pale (*abzördt mager vnd pleih*)' as a result.[28] An unnatural and unintended reduction in body size was a particular cause for concern since such thinness was a recognized sign of bodily deterioration. Some diseases wasted the body to such an extent that they were said to gorge themselves on a person's flesh. Albrecht Dürer wrote of the French pox (syphilis) as 'devouring (*fressen*) away many people until they die', while Balthasar Sibenhar, a parson in Beyerberg, wrote in his autobiography around 1590 of suffering from an illness which had 'eaten (*gefressen*) him fully to death'.[29] In both cases the verb *fressen*, used to denote animal eating habits or gluttonous human consumption, suggests an aggressive devouring of the body. Remembering an illness he suffered aged 24,

[27] Einzelbrief 19, 25 Briefe der Elisabeth geb. Ungnad (1578–1631), am 2.2.1598 mit Erasmus II. von Starhemberg (1575–1648) verheiratet, an ihre Schwägerin Juliana Starhemberg geb. Roggendorf (1574–1633). Briefkonvolut Starhemberg, Bestand Riedegg 43, Oberösterreichisches Landesarchiv, Linz. www.univie.ac.at/Geschichte/Frauenbriefe/briefliste1.htm

[28] Einzelbrief 10, 18 Briefe der Judith Sabina geb. Jörger (1604–1630), am 4.6.1624 mit Erasmus den jüngeren von Starhemberg (1595–1664) verheiratet, an ihre Schwiegermutter Juliana Starhemberg geb. Roggendorf (1574–1633) und ihren Schwager Kasper (1598–1646) und Heinrich Wilhelm Starhemberg (1593–1675). Briefkonvolut Starhemberg, Bestand Riedegg 47, Oberösterreichisches Landesarchiv, Linz. www.univie.ac.at/Geschichte/Frauenbriefe/briefliste1.htm

[29] Hans Rupprich, *Dürer: Schriftlicher Nachlass* (Berlin, 1956), vol. 1, 53; J. Bickel, 'Die Selbstbiographie des Balthasar Sibenhar, Pfarrers in Beyerberg 1572–1601', *Beiträge zur bayerischen Kirchengeschichte* 7 (1901), 256–74, here 268.

Hermann von Weinsberg similarly noted that 'so much flesh disappeared from my legs that I saw the bone through the flesh.'[30] Dramatic changes in body size prompted by sickness were frightening, memorable, and worthy of note.

Infancy and childhood were the most dangerous stages of life in this period, and young bodies were known to be particularly vulnerable to disease. Changes in a child's body size would thus be alarming for their parents. In 1590, Magdalena Paumgartner wrote to her husband expressing concern for their son 'little Balthasar' who was suffering from dropsy, now known as edema, in which fluid retention causes the body to swell. While Balthasar appeared to have recovered, Magdalena worried about his future health, stating 'I hope that a fever will not come out of it, although his size has reduced (*abgenumen*) so much.'[31] Two years later, young Balthasar's dropsy returned more aggressively, and his body took on the illness's characteristic bloated stomach. Magdalena wrote to her husband 'eternal God grace us, that he will become smaller again (*abnem*) before you return home!'[32] In both cases, little Balthasar's body size took on great significance for Magdalena as a representation of her son's health, for which she expressed her care through letters to his father.[33]

When children grew up and left home, early modern parents continued to care for the size of their children's bodies through letters containing dietary and health advice. Indeed, such concern was heightened since the separation made it more difficult for parents to actively intervene in their children's health. Wolfgang Reichart frequently wrote to his son Zeno while he was away studying, instructing him on the kinds of things, as well as the amount of food, he should be eating. While his son was in Tübingen in 1522, Wolfgang wrote that due to the weakness of Zeno's stomach he should avoid fresh fruits such as strawberries, cherries, apples, pears, and grapes, informing his son that it was not only books that were important for students but also bodily health.[34] A month later, he told Zeno to eat and drink everything necessary for his body but to avoid excess; when he was hungry he should eat supplementary foods, but he must not give into the temptations of excessive drinking. Wolfgang thus followed contemporary medical advice regarding the maintenance of a person's body, including their size, which required them to eat just as much as their bodies required to be satiated. He also reflected the humoral understanding of younger people as hot and dry and thus requiring a greater amount of food than older people. He stated that he understood Zeno would need to consume a lot to grow and develop, and thus he should eat and drink as much as he needed to become full, but he forbade

[30] Hermann Weinsberg, *Buch Weinsberg*, transcribed by Abteilung für Rheinische Landesgeschichte, Universität Bonn. Digital Edition: www.weinsberg.uni-bonn.de, vol. 1, fol. 128^{v}.

[31] Georg Steinhausen (ed.), *Briefwechsel Balthasar Paumgartners des Jüngeren mit seiner Gattin Magdalena, geb. Behaim (1582–1598)* (Stuttgart, 1895), 105.

[32] Ibid. 166.

[33] Sadly, little Balthasar died during this second period of illness. Ibid. 168–9.

[34] Walther Ludwig (ed.), *Vater und Sohn im 16. Jahrhundert Der Briefwechsel des Wolfgang Reichart genannt Rychardus mit seinem Sohn Zeno (1520–1543)* (Hildesheim, 1999), 89–90.

Zeno from participating in drinking sprees where one was neither hungry nor thirsty.[35] While not explicitly mentioning body size, Wolfgang's advice followed dietary understandings of how to prevent either an unnatural fattening or slimming of the body, which was understood to occur if one ate more or less than their body needed. Similarly, while studying at the Altdorf academy as a teenager, Friedrich Behaim informed his mother, 'your letter scolding me for my excessive table has been delivered'. She was clearly concerned about Friedrich's excessive consumption, yet he rejected her view that he did 'nothing but eat and drink to excess and lead the life of a dissolute youth', instead reassuring her 'I do remain over my books which are my dearest possession'.[36]

Parental concern during separation might also be materialized through changes in a parent's own body size. The passions or emotions were known to cause alterations in body size, and feelings of worry or anxiety were believed to encourage thinness.[37] When Swiss physician Felix Platter returned home to Basel after studying in Montpellier, he observed how his mother's body had changed in his absence. He wrote, 'my mother was at the neighbours, but she came running, cried and received me, she was so scrawny and thin (*gar thir und mager*)'.[38] In noting his mother's thinness, Platter seemed concerned by the ageing and deterioration of her body, yet his comment was also connected to her outpouring of emotion at their reunion and points to the worry their separation had caused her. Body size thus encoded the concern that both parties had for each other.

As well as parents and children, married couples expressed care for one another's bodies through self-narratives like the letters of Anna and Albrecht. In correspondence between Magdalena Paumgartner and her husband Balthasar, the couple frequently reported on the condition of their bodies, anticipating a caring response from their partner. Balthasar, a merchant, frequently reported changes in his body size to his wife while he was travelling abroad. In 1582, for example, he wrote to Magdalena, 'thanks to God's love my health is good, I have somewhat recovered from my boring journey, from which I arrived wasted and thin (*dürr unnd mager*)'.[39] Bodies were understood to be particularly vulnerable and unstable while travelling, as they passed through unfamiliar landscapes and climates.[40] Balthasar specifically blamed the heat for the thinness of his body when he arrived at the thermal baths in Lucca in 1584. He sent two separate letters, five days apart, in which he reported this change in his body size to

[35] Ibid. 96.

[36] Steven Ozment, *Three Behaim Boys: Growing Up in Early Modern Germany* (New Haven, 1990), 143–4.

[37] See Chapter 2, 46–8.

[38] Heinrich Boos (ed.), *Thomas und Felix Platter, zur Sittengeschichte des XVI. Jahrhunderts* (Hirzel, 1878), 297.

[39] Steinhausen (ed.), *Briefwechsel Balthasar Paumgartners*, 8. See Steven Ozment, *Magdalena and Balthasar: An Intimate Portrait of Life in Sixteenth-Century Europe Revealed in the Letters of a Nuremberg Husband and Wife* (New Haven, 1989), 125.

[40] On the instability of the body and travel see Rublack, 'Fluxes', 1.

Magdalena. In the first he wrote that he had become 'very thin (*sehr mager*)' due to the 'outstanding heat' on his journey, and in the second he stated 'from the great heat which was present until Bologna, my size has reduced a lot (*sehr abgenohmmen hab*), and now I will take time to fatten (*mesten*) myself again'.[41] The reduction of his body size was clearly a concern for Balthasar and he urgently wanted Magdalena to be aware of it. Using the verb *mästen* which indicates deliberate fattening, Balthasar noted an intention to prioritize the replenishment of his body. To do this he would likely have increased his food consumption and focused on consuming food and drink which were known to be fattening such as red wine, honey, eggs, various kinds of milk and plenty of meat.[42] When Balthasar wrote to Magdalena later that month that at the baths he had 'until now no other complaint, other than that I am not getting enough to eat', this grievance was almost certainly connected to his desire to fatten his body.[43] Balthasar suggested to his wife that other visitors at the baths were just there 'for the sake of pleasure, taking the waters now so that thereafter they can eat and drink all the more exuberantly'.[44] Numerous types of thermal waters were understood to assist with slimming the body, and Balthasar thus presented the baths as a site for bodily restriction and reduction in advance of future excess.[45] Yet he recognized that this was not what his own body required, writing that, for the sake of his bodily health, 'I must have the good life totally against my will'.[46]

In her response, Magdalena expressed concern for her husband's body and offered him advice for his recovery. She stated, 'since you have not been able to eat or sleep enough, you want to replenish yourself again in Lucca, stay [there] until you are well and do not spare yourself anything'.[47] Magdalena's comments indicate an awareness of factors that were recognized to contribute to changes in body size, namely those of food and rest, and she too prioritized Balthasar's bodily replenishment. Her advice on this occasion echoed her repeated instructions for her husband's health as she worried about Balthasar going to bed on an empty stomach and forgetting to eat meals.[48] Such habits were associated with the wasting away of the body which required regular sustenance, which would be distributed throughout the body during sleep.[49] If one had not eaten within a reasonable time of going to bed there would be too little food to refuel and replenish the body. Balthasar's body size was thus implicated in the practice of care which Magdalena's letters fulfilled. In this medium, the concern she expressed for Balthasar held particular significance since their separation limited her ability to actively look after his body.

[41] Steinhausen, *Briefwechsel Balthasar Paumgartners*, 43–4. [42] See Chapter 2, 32–4.
[43] Steinhausen, *Briefwechsel Balthasar Paumgartners*, 46.
[44] Ibid. 44–45. Translation from Ozment, *Magdalena and Balthasar*, 125–6.
[45] See Chapter 2, 49. [46] Steinhausen, *Briefwechsel Balthasar Paumgartners*, 45.
[47] Ibid. 50. [48] See e.g. ibid. 107; Ozment, *Magdalena and Balthasar*, 119.
[49] Ken Albala, *Eating Right in the Renaissance* (Berkeley, CA, 2002), 136.

Body size was implicated within the familial relationships and networks of care through which parents nurtured the bodies of their children and wives intervened in the maintenance of their husband's figures. A greater degree of reciprocity in such care was expected for relations between wives and husbands than parents and children, however, as in marriage, women and men were required to sustain one another's bodies, sharing responsibility for the health and fortunes of the household. This integrates a consideration of embodiment within the reciprocity which characterized early modern marriage, in which women and men gained and preserved their social independence jointly through integration within the shared household.[50] The co-production of the household took on particular importance with the Reformation, as reformers placed marriage 'at the heart of the new reformed order' and Lutheran marriage tracts emphasized the significance of the body within marital relationships.[51] In his text on marital order from 1545, for example, Johann Spangenberg wrote that, 'in marriage, each has power over the other's body'.[52] As the letters of Magdalena and Balthasar suggest, the successful fulfilment of wives' and husbands' marital roles was materialized through their partner's bodily form. While acts of care and provision were required from both wives and husbands, the attention paid to a wife's body size by her husband was more often framed in terms of sexual attractiveness and compatibility, as well as fertility and pregnancy, all of which were closely intertwined. Since childbearing inevitably involved alterations in a woman's figure, body size was thus intrinsically linked to the fulfilment of women's roles as wives and mothers in ways that were specific to their sex.

Wives and Mothers

When seeking a wife, men and their families took note of the body size of a potential bride. Marital compatibility mattered to ensure a happy and fertile marriage, and since marriage formed the 'very basis of all social order', unsuitable matches had consequences which reached beyond the confines of the household.[53] As well as emotional, humoral, social, financial, and religious compatibility, bodily form needed to be taken into account to ensure a good match.[54] In some cases,

[50] Heide Wunder, *He is the Sun, She is the Moon: Women in Early Modern Germany*, tr. Thomas Dunlap (Cambridge, 1998), 37–8.

[51] Lyndal Roper, *The Holy Household: Women and Morals in Reformation Augsburg*, Oxford Studies in Social History (Oxford, 1989), 165.

[52] Johann Spangenberg, *Des Ehelichen Ordens Spiegel vnd Regel* (Magdeburg, 1544), fol. Jvi^{v}.

[53] Joel Harrington, *Reordering Marriage and Society in Reformation Germany* (Cambridge, 1995), 3.

[54] On the importance of marital compatibility see Leah Astbury, 'When a Woman Hates her Husband: Love, Sex and Fruitful Marriages in Early Modern England', *Gender and History* 32 (2020), 523–41. On humoral compatibility in relation to body size see Jill Burke, *How to be a Renaissance Woman: The Untold History of Beauty and Female Creativity* (London, 2023), 46–7.

this meant that a woman's body needed to provide a counterbalance to her husband's. As we have seen, bodily ideals for women inverted those for men in this period, as an ideal of controlled consumption meant women were presented with slender upper bodies, in contrast to the bulk which characterized German men. If a man was naturally slender, however, to ensure their bodies were complementary, he might require a wife whose robustness made up for his own svelte form.[55] Magdalena Paumgartner's letters suggest this may have been the case for her brother Paul. She requested Balthasar's assistance in smoothing negotiations for Paul's marriage to Hieronymus Paumgartner's daughter Rosina, writing 'she is right for him, big and strong (*fein gros und starck*), just as he needs'.[56] Rosina's bodily size and strength was a crucial factor in Magdalena's endorsement of the match, which likewise hinged on her opinion of her brother's body which she viewed as necessitating a 'big and strong' wife.

Rather than countering his slenderness, it is also possible that Paul required a large and robust wife to match his own strong and vigorous body. Bodily affinity was a central factor for ensuring a fruitful marriage, and early modern people expressed (often humorous) concerns about the feasibility of positive sexual outcomes where an extreme imbalance characterized the bodies of wives and husbands.[57] Martin Luther marvelled, for instance, at the vast size of Elector Johann Friedrich's body: 'were he given to venery, it would not be a wonder if he worked his young woman to death'.[58] Similarly the chronicle of the counts of Zimmern, believed to have been written by Count Froben Christoph von Zimmern (1519–66), contains an account of the sexual practices of Count Christoph von Tengen whose extremely large body required mechanical assistance to engage in sex with his wife. The author recounted how Christoph travelled to Augsburg for the Reichstag of 1530, where the size of his body was admired by Emperor Charles V. The emperor wondered at the fact that Christoph had recently married a young countess and asked how the count, who was 'so very big and fat and unwieldy (*so gar groß, faist und ungefüeg*)', was able to have sex with his new wife and 'with so great inconvenience, accomplish something with her'. The chronicle then described the special contraption which Christoph had devised for this purpose, by which he was hoisted up on a taut sheet above the bed, with his wife lying beneath him. He would then 'fall into her, as one says of peasants in the land of Cockaigne who grow on trees, and when they're ready, fall down with their feet

55 Susanne Helene Betz, 'Verhandeln über Ehe: Die Suche nach der idealen Braut für Cosimo (II.) de' Medici', *Der diplomatische Körper: Frühneuzeitliche Diplomatie als Körperpolitik. Frühneuzeit Info* 29 (2018), 39–56.

56 Steinhausen, *Briefwechsel Balthasar Paumgartners*, 135.

57 On bodily affinity see Astbury, 'When a Woman Hates', 529.

58 'A. Lauterbachs und H. Wellers Nachschriften', Martin Luther, *D. Martin Luthers Werke: Kritische Gesamtausgabe. Tischreden*, 6 vols (Weimar, 1912–21), vol. 3, 338, no. 3468. Translation from Martin Luther, *Luther's Works*, 55 vols (St Louis, 1955–86), vol. 54, 206. Luther's comments on the Elector's body are discussed in Chapter 4, 148.

entering directly into boots which fit them perfectly and which have grown from under the trees'.[59] While the tone of this tale is comedic, it nevertheless reflects the requirement for marriage to involve sexual union with the expectation of fruitfulness, which the emperor referenced through the question of how the count could 'accomplish' something with his wife. This extreme example indicates the role of body size within such expectations, and while in this case the count's body required modification, more often it was a wife's form that needed moulding to meet a husband's requirements.

Another tale from the Zimmern Chronicle described how Count Alwig von Sulz had 'set for his wife, the countess of Helfenstain, a limit for her fatness (*ein zil irer faiste halb*); where, if she out-grew (*überwachsen*) it, she should not come to his sides any more (*ime an die seiten nit mehr kommen*)'.[60] The chronicler suggests that Alwig imposed his expectations for attractiveness onto his wife's body, insisting that she did not become any fatter than the limit he had set. His comment that she could no longer 'come to his sides' is ambiguous. It might refer to her appearing beside him in public, yet it also contains sexual connotations, suggesting she could not lie beside, or straddle him. Since marriage necessitated sexual fulfilment, her body size is shown as potentially endangering the marriage's success, echoing (though inverting) Albrecht's concerns regarding the size of Anna's bottom. It is stated that Alwig revealed this facet of their relationship at the court of the Margrave and Marchioness of Brandenburg, and since the Marchioness was 'equally so fat and big (*faist und groß*)', the chronicler suggests this caused much gossip at court, displeasing Alwig's hosts. This anecdote also reveals, therefore, how talking about body size held social cues, which when disregarded, could undermine social and political relationships.

Wives' bodies were repeatedly discussed in terms of their compatibility with their husbands' desires and physical requirements. Sexual affinity was so important because it was essential to fulfil the key purpose of marriage: generation. Here too women's bodies took centre stage. Changes in body size for women of childbearing age took on particular significance in connection with pregnancy and childbirth. It has been estimated that married women in early modern Europe were pregnant on average every other year, and this cyclical alteration in the size and shape of women's bodies would have profoundly shaped their experience of bodily form.[61] Magdalena Paumgartner wrote of the discomfort she experienced in relation to her expanding pregnant body, asking Balthasar to send four measures of damask for a new, looser-fitting garment. This was necessary, she stated, since 'when I go out, I can't do up my bodice, and I have let it out as far as I can.

[59] Froben Christof Graf von Zimmern, *Die Chronik der Grafen von Zimmern: Handschriften 580 und 581 der Fürstlich Fürstenbergischen Hofbibliothek Donaueschingen*, ed. Hansmartin Decker-Hauff and Rudolf Seigel, 3 vols (Konstanz, 1964–72), vol. 3, 35–6.

[60] Ibid., vol. 3, 214–15.

[61] Lyndal Roper, *Witch Craze: Terror and Fantasy in Baroque Germany* (New Haven, 2006), 145.

If I were even just a little fatter (*ein weniger dicker*), I'd suffocate from it, which I do not want to do.' She expressed her intention to avoid becoming pregnant again writing, 'another time I will get away from you, dearest love, so that what's happening to me now will not happen again.'[62] Magdalena was adamant that her body would never be so large and uncomfortable as in her pregnancy with little Balthasar, and indeed she never fell pregnant again.

The anticipation of pregnancy, in combination with expectations for a wife's fertility, granted women a particular vigilance when it came to experiencing changes in body size. In 1527, Elisabeth of Saxony wrote to her cousin Johann Friedrich of Saxony telling him 'write to me with news and how you are, whether your wife becomes fatter around the stomach (*ab e[uer] l[ieben] gemalt auch decker wertt umb dein bouch*) etc. I am well but my stomach still does not grow (*der bucht wesck mir nochtt nichtt*).'[63] Later that year, Johann Friedrich wrote to Elisabeth having heard that she was pregnant. She replied,

> And as Your Dearness, among other things, suggests that I am pregnant, about that I could not write anything certain. I am wary...one says that it is certain, but another says that I am getting dropsy. Therefore, I do not know for sure, whether it is true or not. But I let Your Dearness know that I am wholly healthy...I am also not swollen, either in my hands or feet, my stomach alone is a little fatter (*mir der buch ein winck decker ist*) and I let myself think that I have felt the child, if it is a child.[64]

Elisabeth longed for a child and as a result was intensely aware of the changes that took place in her body. Moreover, Johann Friedrich's questions about Elisabeth's reported pregnancy, and similarly her enquiries about the size of his wife's belly, indicate that the attention paid to a woman's body size extended to the wider family circle. The mistaking of dropsy for pregnancy, which Elisabeth feared, appears to have been somewhat common. One handbook for midwives gave advice on how to tell the difference between the two stating, 'with dropsy the limbs will generally swell, but with pregnancy they will reduce in size (*nemmen sie ab*).'[65] Elisabeth's statement that only her stomach had swollen, while her hands and feet remained the same, suggests she may have received similar advice. The description of her swollen belly reveals the emotional significance which changes in body shape could hold for women like Elisabeth. The expansion of her belly is

[62] Steinhausen, *Briefwechsel Balthasar Paumgartners*, 211. See Ozment, *Magdalena and Balthasar*, 82.

[63] André Thieme (ed.), *Die Korrespondenz der Herzogin Elisabeth von Sachsen und ergänzende Quellen* (Leipzig, 2010), 211. Elisabeth was later known as Elisabeth of Rochlitz. She is not the same Elisabeth of Saxony who was painted by Cranach the Younger in 1564.

[64] Ibid. 225–6.

[65] Jacob Rueff, *Hebammen Buch, daraus man alle Heimligkeit desz weiblichen Geschlechts erlehrnen, welcherley gestalt der Mensch in Mutter Leib empfangen, zunimpt vnnd geboren wirdt* (Frankfurt, 1588), 98.

tinged both with the excitement of a possible pregnancy as well as the anxiety that it may be a false alarm. Sadly, Elisabeth's following letter to her cousin reveals that she was not pregnant, and her marriage to Johann of Saxony was ultimately childless.[66]

Whether pregnant or not, and whether able or not to bear children, women's experiences of body size were fundamentally connected to conceptions of female fertility, pregnancy, and childbirth. Since the successful fulfilment of a wife's role depended on producing children, early modern women were conscious of alterations in their bodily form in ways that did not apply to their husbands. The composite married body, co-produced together with one's partner, remained markedly gendered, with care for women's body size focusing on the fruitfulness of sexual union in marriage.

Belonging

Since concern for body size was deeply embedded within practices of care among early modern people, it was also tied to conceptions of belonging. To possess a well-looked-after body, particularly one which was not extremely thin or undernourished, indicated that a person was cared for and thus belonged within a network of care. The travel account of Johannes Butzbach (1477–1516), a prior and monastic author who wrote about his travels in Bohemia as a young boy, presents the obverse of such belonging as he reflected on his own foreignness and disconnection in terms of body size. Johannes travelled to Bohemia with the son of his family's neighbour whom he described as a *Beanus*, a term used for an older student who had not yet gone to university, often denoting incivility or uncouthness. This boy had persuaded Johannes's family that he should accompany the *Beanus* to school, promising Johannes a life of plenty since 'elsewhere the Saturdays are fatter than our Sundays'.[67] This was not the case, however, and the *Beanus* soon squandered the allowance they had been given, forcing Johannes to beg for food. He wrote,

> When we neared a village, he [the *Beanus*] sent me in to beg and he waited for me in front of another door. Once when I returned with empty hands he hit me…when I had got something good, however, he ate it all by himself and only gave me his leftovers. So it remained during the whole time that I was with him.[68]

[66] Thieme, *Die Korrespondenz*, 227–30.

[67] Andreas Beriger (ed. and tr.), *Johannes Butzbach, Odeporicon: Eine Autobiographie aus dem Jahre 1506. Zweisprachige Ausgabe* (Weinheim, 1991), 151. This volume contains a German translation of Butzbach's text from the original Latin. I have not worked with the original Latin and therefore I have not highlighted original language in the quotations above.

[68] Ibid. 177.

Johannes was away from home between the ages of 7 and 12, a time when contemporary medical understanding described a need for increased nourishment to fuel the strong inner heat of youth.[69] Johannes later stated that the *Beanus* made him start stealing food as well as begging, because 'with begging I could not get enough for his sustenance'.[70] As Johannes was only eating the *Beanus*'s leftovers he too would have been unable to sustain his body on what he was consuming, resulting in him becoming thin and weak.

It is noteworthy, therefore, that when Johannes described his perception of Bohemians at this time, he characterized them in terms of their fatness. Johannes wrote of rich Bohemians who were 'so fat like the Epicureans, that they have to support their bellies, which hang in front of them, with a sling that they wear around their necks'. In general he stated, among the Bohemians, 'the men are burly, bulky, and muscular and the women are also solid and corpulent'.[71] Even the peasants, he wrote, 'like to eat well...when they come to town they fill up their cheeks and stuff their stomachs full'.[72] Writing in 1505, almost twenty years after he had set out on his journey with the *Beanus,* Johannes presented an image of being surrounded by large, gluttonous, and corpulent bodies, a view which was influenced by his own contemporary experience of hunger, deprivation, and emptiness. The contrast that Johannes presented between the excessive bodies of the Bohemians and his own privation thus shows how his embodied experience materialized his lack of belonging during this period. Not only was Johannes a foreigner who did not belong among the Bohemians, but he was also at the mercy of the *Beanus*, being deprived of parental or familial care. This lack of belonging continued when he finally returned home, where he appeared 'not as a German, as I had gone away, but as a Bohemian, as a Barbarian and, as it were, a Heathen in my clothes, my manners and my long blonde hair'. This meant that Johannes was 'unrecognized' and 'regarded with shyness by all'.[73] After six years away, Johannes' body, appearance, and habits had changed to such an extent that he was no longer recognized as part of the family, showing how the body could symbolize belonging at the level of both household and nation, since he was also no longer 'a German'.

Within the context of the family, body size was also connected to a sense of embodied belonging in discussions of the similarities between the bodies of family members, as well as inherited bodily traits. In this way, body size was embedded in discussions of lineage, the recording and preservation of which was a central motivating factor for several self-narrative authors. The author of the Zimmern Chronicle, for example, repeatedly described the bodily beauty of his ancestors, positioning himself as their worthy descendant. His thirteenth-century relative Wörnher von Zimmern was stated to have been an 'upright, well-formed

[69] Albala, *Eating Right*, 105. [70] Beriger, *Odeporicon*, 181. [71] Ibid. 219.
[72] Ibid. 223. [73] Ibid. 245.

and beautiful (*gerade, lidtmeßige und schöne*) person'.[74] Meanwhile Froben Christoph's great-grandfather Werner the Younger (1423–83), was considered 'the most upright and well-built (*gredest, lidmeßigest*) man by all'.[75] He continues by writing that, 'just as his brother, Herr Werner, was a strong, upright, tall (*starker, grader, langer*) man, so Herr Gottfried was a small (*claine*) person', making clear which family line he considered superior.[76]

Cologne townsman, Hermann von Weinsberg was similarly obsessed with his lineage. His memory book, written over a period of more than fifty years, was intended to preserve the history of the Weinsberg family as Hermann wished it to be portrayed. Hermann and his father claimed that their family was descended from a line of Weinsbergs which reached back to a twelfth-century baron, and Hermann and his cousin Christian even painted a fabricated family tree in their home to present their supposedly noble origins.[77] In light of this obsession, Hermann's detailed descriptions of the bodies of his relatives appear to be part of this effort to present his lineage and his position within a well-bred family. He stated, for instance, that his mother 'was of middling height (*mittelmeissiger lengden*), not too slender (*small*)... moderate of figure (*zimlicher gestalt*)'. His father's mother 'was all middling in height and width (*dickten*), not heavy of body (*nit swar van leibe*)'. His mother's mother 'was of middling height, and not fat or wide (*nit fett oder dick*)' and his father's sister was 'of middling height like her mother... not thick or thin (*nit dick noch mager*)'.[78] As contemporary health advice warned against both extremes of fatness and thinness, praising the middling body as the ideal form, Hermann thus presented his superior embodied lineage. Crucially, he focused his attention on the bodies of his female relatives, especially his mother and grandmothers, reflecting the significance of women's body size in relation to childbearing and thus for inherited bodily traits.

On another occasion Hermann described the bodies of his siblings and in this case he related their figures and features directly to his own and to one another's. He wrote, 'my brother Gotschalk is half a head shorter than me, a bit fuller of face and body (*etwaß volliger von angesicht und leib*) than I', and 'my brother Christian is certainly a bit taller than him [Gotschalk], but not much, also a little bit thinner (*ein kleinß smaler*)'. Hermann described his sisters Maria and Catharin as 'shorter than me', and his sister Sibilla was taller than both of them, but 'a hand's-width shorter than me'.[79] Hermann thus situated their bodies in relation to each other, reflecting their position within the same family group, as well as their shared lineage. While the body was composite, being constructed, supported,

[74] Froben Christof, *Die Chronik der Grafen von Zimmern*, vol. 1, 106.

[75] Ibid. 173. [76] Ibid. 209.

[77] Matthew Lundin, *Paper Memory: A Sixteenth-Century Townsman Writes his World* (Cambridge, 2012), 62.

[78] Hermann Weinsberg, *Buch Weinsberg*, vol. 2, fol. 266^{v}. [79] Ibid., vol. 2, fol. 89^{r}.

and maintained through networks of care and external interactions, in this example Hermann also recognized the individuality of bodily form. Despite everything they shared, the siblings' bodies were different and personal, and throughout his memory book Hermann was intensely aware of the characteristics that made his own body unique.

Personal Body Size in Hermann von Weinsberg's Memory Book

Hermann's memory book aimed at preserving the Weinsberg lineage, yet he was equally preoccupied with personal memory.[80] He made detailed observations of his body, habits, health, dietary regimens, and clothing practices at various stages of his life, thus recording how these interconnected elements of his identity changed over time and with age. Hermann was intensely aware of his body size, taking meticulous measurements of his head, shoulders, arms, back, stomach, hands, feet, and facial features. Beginning his 'Book of Youth' at the age of 43, Hermann retrospectively described the form of his body ten years earlier. At the age of 33 his height had been 'three Cologne ells', with an ell being a unit of measurement in Cologne equivalent to 57.5 cm. At 173 cm tall, his waist 'from navel round to navel' measured 94 cm.[81] When noting his measurements, Hermann did not offer any judgement of his body size, though he did go on to state that at this age he 'ate very covetously (*aß seir begerlich*), and quite a lot'. He noted, however, that his stomach was able to digest this amount of food at this stage in his life, suggesting he was not eating beyond the capacity of his body. Nevertheless, since his belly was often so full of food and drink, 'it could throw it back up if I had too much to drink in an evening'.[82] While suggesting that his consumption could tend towards excess, Hermann echoed contemporary health advice by which the strong inner heat of younger people meant they were able to consume and digest a greater amount of food than those who were older. At the age of 33, however, Hermann was entering a stage of life at which the inner heat was thought to cool, encouraging excess to accumulate in the body and potentially resulting in a range of illnesses as well as the expansion of the body's form.

Hermann was clearly aware of such teachings, as by the age of 60 he had reduced his food intake to two meals a day and focused on eating simple foods without too much fat.[83] As a result, he suggested he was 'just as healthy now, as I ever was in youth or in the meantime'. He reported that at this age he suffered

[80] Lundin suggests that a desire for personal memory eventually eclipsed the concerns of lineage which occupied Hermann at the beginning of his project. Lundin, *Paper Memory*, 224.

[81] Weinsberg, *Buch Weinsberg*, vol. 1, fol. 243^{v}. See also Robert Jütte, 'Aging and Body Image in the Sixteenth Century: Hermann Weinsberg's (1518–97) Perception of the Aging Body', *European History Quarterly* 18 (1988), 259–90, here 263.

[82] Weinsberg, *Buch Weinsberg*, vol. 1, fol. 244^{v}.

[83] Ibid., vol. 2, fols 34^{v}–35^{r}.

from less pain in the body than he did as a young man, 'perhaps from the reason that I am more measured and orderly and not as excessive'.[84] He described his body as 'middling in length and width, not too short or long, too slender or fat (*small oder dick*)'.[85] In his late fifties, Hermann wrote with pride of his body's form, stating that he had 'an upright figure (*uffrichtich gestalt*) with broad shoulders', that his 'stomach did not stick out (*der bauch war nit uisstunde*)', and his 'thighs are not great of flesh (*die schunken nit gross van fleischs*)'. Though Hermann was pleased with the way he had managed to maintain his body with age, curbing his excess in line with the changes in his constitution, he acknowledged that 'I used once to be fuller (*folliger*) of body and my limbs were much stronger and more upright (*starcker und gerader*)'.[86] Though he was glad to be healthy and slim, Hermann missed the robustness of his youthful body, perhaps reflecting on the contemporary presentation of German masculinity through a broad and powerful figure. Indeed, the reduction of his size was Hermann's main observation with regard to age. He wrote that 'in adolescence I was fuller of flesh and more of body (*etwaß von fleiß volliger und mehe bei leibe gewesen*)'.[87] At 60, he noted that his waist had become 'one half-quarter ell more slender, skinnier and thinner (*smaler, dorrer, und magerer*)', and at 70 he stated, 'I am a little bit skinnier and thinner (*durer und magerer*) of body and limb...but otherwise my length, thickness and width (*lengde dickte und weite*) of the body, head and limbs is as before'.[88] Growing thinner with age was to be expected according to contemporary health advice. Though the decreasing internal heat could encourage fatness in middle age if one did not reduce consumption accordingly, ultimately this internal cooling meant that the body's flesh was replenished less effectively, causing it to shrink and dry out over time.[89]

Even when he was younger and more robust, however, Hermann had long felt that his body did not meet contemporary ideals. From the age of 9 he had suffered from a hernia which made standing, riding, and walking difficult.[90] To hide and support the hernia, Hermann wore a tight-fitting girdle around his hips which he claimed had caused him to 'become slender (*smal*) in my lower body as though I were totally thin (*ganß mager*)'.[91] This encouraged Hermann to wear loose-fitting garments which disguised his figure, rather than the fashionable doublet and hose.[92] While his waist measurement at the age of 33 suggests that he was not particularly thin around his middle, it seems that Hermann was self-conscious about the difference between the size of his waist and the size of his hips. At the age of 60, he wrote 'the thickness of my body is around one and a half ells [86 cm]'.[93] Beneath his girdle, however, his hips measured 'one ell and one

84 Ibid., vol. 2, fol. 32^{v}.
85 Ibid., vol. 2, fol. 30^{v}.
86 Ibid., vol. 1, fol. 666^{r}.
87 Ibid., vol. 2, fol. 30^{v}.
88 Ibid., vol. 2, fol. 30^{r}, and vol. 3, fol. 5^{v}.
89 Albala, *Eating Right*, 53.
90 Weinsberg, *Buch Weinsberg*, vol. 1, fol. 27^{r}.
91 Ibid., vol. 1, fol. 723^{r}.
92 See Chapter 5, 156.
93 Weinsberg, *Buch Weinsberg*, vol. 2, fol. 30^{r}.

and a half quarters [79 cm]'. He also wrote that previously he had been thinner 'under the girdle…because I bound myself more tightly (*ich mich steiffer bant*), than at this time'.[94] The girdle itself could thus act as a form of measurement through which Hermann could assess changes in his body's size. Through dress Hermann sought to conceal the lack of proportion in his body which he understood to have resulted from the interaction of his body with the materiality of the girdle. He recognized therefore that it was not just his age or the amount of food he ate which dictated his figure, since this also resulted from his body's material engagement with the world around him.

Like the other authors discussed in this chapter, Hermann understood himself and his own personal body to belong within a network of relations. As well as describing his siblings' bodies in relation to his own, Hermann also gave accounts of the bodies of his acquaintances. He described a distant relative called Leisgin who he said was 'as fat (*dicke*) a woman, as I have ever seen in my life'.[95] In 1583 he wrote about a papal legate, Bishop of Vercelli in Italy, as being a 'long, thin and weak man', while in 1585 he described a former acquaintance as 'a very heavy, fat, clumsy (*sware, dicke, unbeholfen*) woman, but very compassionate, understanding and good'.[96] Hermann thus revealed a negative view of fatness as he described the woman's good character as being in spite of the size of her body. Indeed, with these descriptions Hermann appears to take particular note of the bodies of women and men which diverged from contemporary ideals of feminine slenderness and masculine bulk, perhaps reflecting his own self-consciousness of his disproportionate form. At the age of 70, Hermann described the oldest men he knew. These included Johan von Delft, who he believed to be 84, who was 'tall of person and very old, though still coherent, he now struggles to walk', and Jaspar van Mulhem who was 79 and described as 'thin [and] scrawny (*mager, dur*) of person but still with good reason and character'.[97] These descriptions are from the beginning of the third volume of his memory book titled the 'Book of Very Old Age' where Hermann also noted that his own 'decrepitude' was not yet so great.[98] He thus took note of the older men in his circle, anticipating the changes which his own body and mind might undergo in the following years. It was at this point that Hermann noted his own increasing thinness, and when he commented on Jaspar's good reason and character despite his scrawny body, he was perhaps encouraged that his own ageing body would not necessarily be accompanied by incoherence or ill-temper. Hermann conceived of his body in relation to the bodies of those around him, and the minute attention he paid to his own form was reflected in his awareness of his acquaintances' figures.

When it came to his family, body size took on emotional significance for Hermann. In 1589 he worried about his sister Sibilla who was 'becoming fuller of

94 Ibid., vol. 2, fol. 31^{v}.
95 Ibid., vol. 1, fol. 62^{v}.
96 Ibid., vol. 2, fols 408^{v} and 491^{r}.
97 Ibid., vol. 3, fol. 16^{r}.
98 Ibid., vol. 3, fol. 5^{v}.

body (*folliger von Leib*) and growing bigger (*zunimpt*) than she ever has in her life'. He considered whether she should stay with him at his home, where 'a good diet keeps me so healthy, spritely and merry'. Hermann thus contemplated the material care that he could offer Sibilla to help ensure her body's health. In the same entry he noted that Sibilla's husband Johan von Woringen 'is not getting any thinner (*magerer*) either, but remains heavy (*swar*) enough', and suggested that he too might benefit from following Hermann's dietary regimen.[99] Hermann's brother-in-law was a key figure in his social circle, with whom he celebrated birthdays and New Years and for whom Hermann had considerable affection and respect. He was worried by Johan's body size, and repeatedly commented on his figure. In 1590 Hermann thought Johan looked slimmer, writing, 'I have seen that he has become thin (*mager*) because he used to be fuller and fatter (*volliger und fetter*)'.[100] By 1592 however, Johan was suffering with his size. His right leg had swollen to such an extent that he could not walk or stand, and he was anxious that this was a sign of dropsy. Hermann wrote, 'I do not know a man in Cologne who is heavier (*swarer*) than he is', referring to the bulky expanse of Johan's body.[101] Johan took to his bed, where he steadily deteriorated, being unable to eat, drink, or speak. Hermann noted that at the beginning of his illness Johan's legs had been swollen, but they had since become lean. This caused him and his family to wonder 'where the thickness (*dickte*) had come from'. Some believed it was excess water while others thought it was fat or other moist humours which had become trapped in the body, infecting the liver or lungs.[102] Hermann did not know the cause, but when Johan died shortly afterwards it was discovered that he had not been suffering from dropsy after all. Hermann stated 'for several years his body had been naturally wide, big, fat and heavy (*dick, gross, groiß und swair*)', suggesting that it was not an unnatural fatness that had caused his death.[103]

Changes of body size for Hermann's relatives often resulted in their untimely passing. In 1583 he noted that his sister Cathrin's belly had swollen, possibly from dropsy, and he wrote that 'on the fifth of October I saw her alive and spoke to her for the last time and never saw her after that morning with her swollen fat belly (*gespannen dicken bauch*)'.[104] Later that month he described how she 'died of the fat belly which grew from water or another [cause] (*deß dicken bauchs von wasser oder ander gewaxß gestorben*)'.[105] The fatness of Cathrin's stomach was thus viewed by Hermann as the reason for her death. Ten years earlier he had lost his second wife Drutgin to a similar illness, writing that 'her legs became so thick (*so dick*) that her white woollen hose had to be made wider than boots (*weiter dan lersen*), which was a great concern to us'.[106] Again clothing is shown to measure

99 Ibid., vol. 3, fol. 130v. 100 Ibid., vol. 3, fol. 165r.
101 Ibid., vol. 3, fol. 263r. 102 Ibid., vol. 3, fol. 269r.
103 Ibid., vol. 3, 270r. See Chapter 2 on the distinction between natural and unnatural body size.
104 Ibid., vol. 2, fol. 422r. 105 Ibid., vol. 2, fol. 423v. 106 Ibid., vol. 1, fol. 631v.

changes in body size as these necessitated dress alterations. When it became clear that Drutgin was dying, Hermann 'cried bitterly and kissed her on her cheeks, and she spoke but not coherently, but she understood'. He gave an emotional account of Drutgin's death, stating that as the last rites were administered, he 'had to leave to cry'.[107] Drutgin and Hermann had built a household together and cared for one another for almost twenty years. They had looked after and worried about each other's bodies, yet Hermann had been unable to prevent the swelling of Drutgin's figure which led to her death. Given Hermann's experiences with changes in his loved ones' body size, it is little wonder that he remained so vigilant about his own bodily form. For Hermann, body size could represent illness, yet it was also intertwined with notions of family, belonging, care, and personal identity.

Body Size and Personhood

For early modern Germans, body size was deeply personal. The authors of these self-narratives maintained an intimate awareness of changes in their bodily form, which they were eager to record and share with loved ones. Body size thus played a key role in maintaining social relationships and individual bodies were extended through networks of care and belonging. Spouses, family members, and friends expressed concern for one another's bodies and offered practical advice to alter their size and form. Through the production of self-narratives, therefore, early modern Germans had an outlet through which to perform body size; the authors of such texts presented their bodies in specific ways and for particular motivations, whether to encourage a response from the recipient of a letter, or as part of a wider effort of self-memorialization. Body size clearly mattered to these individuals, who used their bodies to convey meaning and emotion and to situate themselves within the broader networks of relations which made up early modern personhood.

While an individual's uniquely formed body always determines their physical perspective on the world, the personal bodily vigilance displayed by early modern Germans reflected the growing significance of body size in Germany from the late fifteenth to the early seventeenth centuries. During this period, body size became deeply implicated in conceptions of health, emotional well-being, morality, spirituality, and even Germanness itself. Individuals perceived of their bodies in relation to these contemporary expectations and ideals for bodily form, and in their letters and diaries early modern people drew on these wide-reaching cultural associations to discuss their own and others' bodies. Gender structured these discussions, as women's body size took on particular significance in relation

[107] Ibid., vol. 1, fol. 632^{v}.

to expectations surrounding marital compatibility and childbearing. Meanwhile male anxieties about body size focused on the strength and robustness of their figures which came under pressure through sickness, travel, and old age.

For German women and men, concerns about body size had become part of everyday life. Ideas about fatness and thinness informed the ways in which they experienced and made sense of their bodies, how they expressed care and support, and how they conceived of both personal and communal identity.

Body Size in Early Modern Germany. Holly Fletcher, Oxford University Press. © Holly Fletcher 2026.
DOI: 10.1093/9780198972983.003.0006

Conclusion

A Culture of Body Size

In 1644, Johann Michael Moscherosch envisaged a fictional meeting between a courtier named Philander von Sittewald and a court of old German heroes. Philander asked the heroes, who laughed at his clothing and appearance, what was the cause of the 'weak limbs and softness (*schwache Glieder vnd Weichigkeit*)' which characterized his body, in contrast to their 'great gravitas and strength (*grosse Gravität vnd Stärke*)'. In addition to foreign influences, the heroes attributed the deterioration of contemporary German bodies to the 'worry and fear of the wretched life which we are in…which suppresses the natural powers of the body'. Meanwhile, 'among the old Germans, nobody was so burdened with worry and fear, and that gave them great power, so that they became big and strong (*groß vnd starck*)'.[1] Moscherosch was writing during the period of the Thirty Years War, and his satirical texts, including the tale of Philander von Sittewald, frequently described the chaos and suffering wrought upon Germany by the conflict. With this passage, Moscherosch suggested that the affective consequences of war had reshaped a generation of Germans. War also had direct physical consequences. Contemporary reports indicate that food shortages became so extreme during the conflict that some resorted to cannibalism.[2] Both starvation and the consumption of human flesh would have been understood to hold serious ramifications for the form and matter of the body.[3] In this period of violence and devastation, in which the social, political, and cultural landscape of Germany was transformed, therefore, body size took on new meaning, coming to materialize the ravages of war.[4]

Moscherosch's use of body size in this way drew on a culture of body size which had developed across sixteenth-century Germany. From the last decades of the 1400s, body size had grown in significance throughout German culture, becoming a subject of medical, artistic, and spiritual concern, and informing the ways in which early modern Germans experienced and made sense of the world

[1] Johann Michael Moscherosch, *Anderer Theil des Gesichte Philanders von Sittewald* (Strasbourg, 1644), 63 and 109. On early modern comparisons of ancient and contemporary German bodies see Nancy Siraisi, *History, Medicine, and the Traditions of Renaissance Learning* (Ann Arbor, MI, 2007), 55–61.

[2] Geoff Mortimer, *Eyewitness Accounts of the Thirty-Years War 1618–1648* (Basingstoke, 2002), see 2, 99, 165, and 173–4; Sigrun Haude, *Coping with Life during the Thirty Years War (1618–1648)* (Leiden, 2021), 53–6.

[3] See Rachel Winchcombe, 'The Limits of Disgust: Eating the Inedible During Jamestown's "Starving Time"', *Global Food History* 11 (2023), 1–23.

[4] Hans Medick, *Der Dreißigjährige Krieg: Zeugnisse vom Leben mit Gewalt* (Göttingen, 2018).

around them. It is little wonder, therefore, that Moscherosch used body size as a frame of reference through which to convey the impact of war on German society. The notion that fear and worry could be materialized in a weak and feeble body reflected the emotional associations and affective potential attributed to body size in medical texts such as Walther Herman Ryff's and utilized in contemporary self-narratives, while the image of the great size and strength of the old Germans owed much to the proto-nationalistic rhetoric of the previous century. Moreover, the view that the state of society was mirrored in the bodies of its members connects to understandings of an extended early modern body which was constructed in relation to external forces, both material and cultural. Body size had become embedded in German culture yet, as Moscherosch's example suggests, ideas about bodily form continued to evolve as new pressures shifted cultural values, ideals, and expectations.

Rather than warfare, in sixteenth-century Germany, concerns about body size were heightened through the conjunction of several factors. A new proto-nationalist ideology established the significance of body size for conceptions of Germanness, particularly among German men who performed masculine German robustness through portraits which presented their bulky and expansive bodies. Across the sixteenth century, body size, fatness, and thinness also became the subject of growing medical scrutiny, prompting the publication of a range of recipes and instructions for how to alter the size and shape of the body which utilized the new medium of print. Following the example of Albrecht Dürer, German artists became increasingly interested in the presentation and theorization of bodies of various sizes and proportions. Informed by his own embodied experience, Dürer demonstrated the potential for body size to convey beauty, meaning, and emotion in artworks, and his study of the body dynamized the investigation of bodily form in German art across the sixteenth century. The upheaval of the Lutheran Reformation had profound consequences for German society and culture, as Luther's critique of the papacy radically transformed Christianity. Body size was embedded in beliefs concerning the coming apocalypse and the resurrection of the body and played a central role in Luther's critique of the excess and hypocrisy of the Catholic Church. Luther's language of fatness and the belly was then taken up by, and applied to, those of varying confessions, thus becoming a permanent feature of Christian theological vocabulary. Also during this period, an increasing array of fashionable garments became available to German women and men which could be used to mould the body into idealized silhouettes with the help of tailoring, padding, and boning. Women had access to a growing range of foundation garments, including the *Mieder* and *Weiberspeck*, while the *Schaube* and *Gänsbauch* granted men a new sense of body size through the expansion of the figure. Such developments both reflected and constituted a culture of body size in early modern Germany, which likewise shaped how early modern Germans perceived and experienced their bodies.

Body size thus became intertwined with gendered conceptions of personhood and belonging in this period.

Body size assumed meaning in a range of settings within the context of early modern Germany; it was 'done' by historical actors in various ways and for differing purposes. There was not one view of body size, fatness, or thinness. When German men used bulk and expanse to stage masculine power and German robustness, they did not necessarily consider their large bodies to result from the comfort, sensory pleasure, and luxury which medical authors associated with fatness. Likewise, Martin Luther understood his enlarged body in a different way from the fatness of gluttons or hypocritical monks, a distinction which he focused around the worldliness associated with a fat belly. While some parents might deliberately restrict the food intake of their daughters and use tightly laced pairs of bodies to mould their figures from childhood, medical authors and moralisers took issue with 'unnatural' thinness which was seen to deform the body. At the same time, a slender and controlled upper body for women could nevertheless represent the virtues of honour, order, and modesty. This nuanced view of body size confirms Caroline Walker Bynum's suggestion that people in the past did not have a concept of 'the body' any more than we do, that 'ideas differed according to who held them, and where and when', and thus that 'even within what we would call discourse communities, ideas about matter, body and person could conflict and contradict'.[5] This awareness of the various ways in which different forms of the body could be made to matter in alternative contexts is lost in historical approaches which only consider fatness, and which track attitudes towards fat over vast time periods stretching from antiquity to the present day. The concept of 'doing body size' thus allows us to more fully explore the significance of body size in the past.

By focusing the scope of its investigation on early modern Germany, this book has sought to approach early modern bodies on their own terms. Teleological accounts, which take modern attitudes towards fatness as their point of reference, tend to map present-day preconceptions about body size onto the past. But as historians such as Laura Gowing and Ulinka Rublack have shown, early modern bodies existed 'in a different conceptual world' and may even have behaved differently.[6] Early modern attitudes towards body size were likewise formed in relation to different cultural and conceptual forces, resulting in different embodied experiences. While questions of diet (in the modern sense of the word) and exercise dominate discussions of fatness and thinness today, for example, for early modern people these were elements of a much more holistic attitude towards

[5] Caroline Walker Bynum, 'Why All the Fuss about the Body? A Medievalist's Perspective', *Critical Inquiry* 12 (1995), 1–33, here 7 and 27.

[6] Laura Gowing, *Common Bodies: Women, Touch and Power in Seventeenth Century England* (New Haven, 2003), 6; Ulinka Rublack, 'Fluxes: The Early Modern Body and the Emotions', *History Workshop Journal* 53 (2002), 1–16.

body size as a health concern. From a medical perspective, the size of a person's body was not just determined by the amount of food they ate, since practices relating to sleep and bathing, sensory stimulation, emotions, and even the materials which came into contact with the body also had the potential to alter body size. Ideas about body size, fatness, and thinness thus entered into early modern conceptions of the body in which bodily boundaries were known to be porous and permeable, physical and mental subjectivity were closely entwined, and emotions had bodily consequences.

Building on existing understandings of the early modern body, this book has also shown body size to be implicated within a view of the extended body in this period. The understanding that body size was determined by an array of external, non-natural influences, was part of a larger conception of the body in which human bodies were understood to exist in co-dependent, material relationships with both non-human agents and their physical surroundings. An 'embodied chain of effects' meant that agricultural practices underpinning food production were recognized to materially shape the bodies of consumers. Management of body size thus extended well beyond the boundaries of the body itself. On a material level, the body was extended through practices of dress which moulded the figure into idealized forms, shaping the posture and movement of the wearer, and granting an intense awareness of body size. Yet the material experience of the body was formed in dialogue with the complex matrices of social, religious, aesthetic, and personal influences which combined to create the early modern body. Early modern bodies were thus extended through social networks, religious beliefs, and political ideologies as well as through engagement with matter, all of which shaped contemporary ideas about body size.

Body size was made to matter in everyday life, and this was not just the case for one kind of bodily form or condition. It does not make sense, therefore, to consider early modern attitudes towards fatness or thinness in isolation, since these held consequences for all early modern bodies. Medical authors taught their readers how to increase or decrease the size of the body, to become either fatter or thinner, but these lessons could be applied to bodies of all sizes. Moreover, body size held meaning for early modern people regardless of whether they considered their own bodies to be particularly fat or thin. Based on his measurements and appearance, for example, Hermann von Weinsberg viewed his body as 'middling'. In his sixties, he commented that he used to be 'fuller of flesh' and was now 'skinnier', but he never viewed himself as having a particularly fat or thin body, and yet body size still mattered immensely for his account of himself. In his theorization of the body, Dürer understood beauty to exist in the proportion of each body part to the whole, rather than how fat or thin the body was. Likewise, the reformers' teachings on moderation suggested that all bodily forms, regardless of fatness or thinness, could be deemed acceptable so long as they did not result from either gluttony or hypocritical fasting. Such bodies, which were nourished by just enough food to sustain them, displayed 'natural' body size. 'Natural' versus 'unnatural' form was arguably a more important distinction for shaping early modern attitudes towards body size than 'fat' versus 'thin'.

It was understood that all bodies possessed a 'natural' size and shape which was determined by their complexion, in turn being influenced by factors of age, gender, and environment. This natural bodily form was thought to be given by God and could also be subject to the movement of the planets at the time of one's birth. Natural body size would be maintained through the consumption of the correct amount of nourishment; excess nourishment would cause the body to become fatter, while excessive restriction would cause it to slim down. The other non-naturals could likewise act to mould the body into unnatural forms, or alternatively to return the body to its natural form following a period of unnatural fatness or thinness. As the reformers indicated, bodily forms which diverged from one's natural figure were problematic because they deformed the God-given body and indicated excessive behaviour. The notion of unnatural body size thus also drew on contemporary discourses concerning excess in which perfect balance, between the extremes of excess and deprivation, was idealized. Yet the line between natural and unnatural was blurry. If a person's body took on different sizes and shapes throughout the life course, what was their natural body size? This question underlay discussions concerning the form of the resurrected body; if one returned with the size and shape they had in life, which version of their figure would that be? The fluid dichotomy of natural versus unnatural also fed into the distinction between the dressed and undressed body. Dress was used to mould the body into various figures, causing contemporary moralizers to complain about the creation of unnatural silhouettes through garments such as the *Weiberspeck* and *Gänsbauch*. Yet body size was so intimately connected to dress in this period, with clothing physically moulding the body and embodied behaviour, that it could be difficult to determine a person's bodily form without taking clothing into account.

When Germans encountered Indigenous people from the Americas and enslaved Africans in Europe, they frequently described their bodies in terms of nakedness, yet this state of undress did not encourage a recognition of the individuality of natural bodily form. Such ethnographic descriptions were instead notably universalizing and impersonal, suggesting how body size played into processes of othering in this period. This standardizing presentation of non-European bodies was in marked opposition to understandings of European bodies which were recognized to be unique. While scholars have suggested that early modern people did not conceive of themselves as individuals but rather as part of extended networks of relations, the uniqueness of bodily form encouraged an awareness of individual personhood (for Europeans) which was nevertheless understood in relation to embodied networks of care and belonging. Personal experiences of body size were also intertwined with broader cultural understandings of fatness and thinness. In particular, personal, embodied experiences of fatness and thinness were shaped by gendered expectations and ideals for the body. Body size was connected to the fulfilment of women's roles as wives and mothers, feeding into questions of attractiveness, sexuality, and fertility, in ways which were specific to their sex and which informed their embodied experiences, as described by Magdalena Paumgartner and Elisabeth of Saxony. Among men, body size could present youthful grace and athleticism, as well as robust, masculine authority. Individuals such as Matthäus Schwarz and Albrecht of Brandenburg thus lamented changes in their bodies which prevented them from meeting these gendered ideals.

This book has uncovered a transformative phase in which body size took on increasing prominence in early modern German society and culture. As questions of fatness and thinness were integrated within discussions concerning health, food, fashion, and gendered bodily ideals, the culture of body size that emerged in sixteenth-century Germany appears, in some ways, to be remarkably familiar. The pervasiveness of ideas about body size connects their world to our own, yet ideas about fatness and thinness are historically and culturally specific and need to be approached on their own terms. There is still much more to discover about body size in the early modern world. Attitudes towards body size among poorer communities have only briefly been touched on by this book, and solely via the accounts of others. Moreover, while this study has drawn on German descriptions of bodies from beyond Europe, far more research is required to understand attitudes towards body size in non-European cultures during this period and to better understand the role that bodily form could play within cultural encounters. However future research develops, I hope it will encompass bodily forms beyond just fatness and recognize the rich diversity of ideas about, and experiences of, early modern bodies. It is inescapably clear that body size mattered to early modern people beyond the availability of food or the refinement of manners. Rather, early modern Germans 'did body size' in specific ways and in particular contexts, as part of cultural and embodied arguments about values and identities.

Body Size in Early Modern Germany. Holly Fletcher, Oxford University Press. © Holly Fletcher 2026.
DOI: 10.1093/9780198972983.003.0007

Bibliography

Manuscripts

Oberösterreichisches Landesarchiv, Linz. Briefkonvolut Starhemberg, Bestand Riedegg 43 and 47.

John Rylands Library, University of Manchester. MS 24. *Deutsches salernitanisches Arzneibuch*, late 15th century.

Bayerische Staatsbibliothek, Munich. BSB Cod.icon. 341. *Kostüme der Männer und Frauen in Augsburg und Nürnberg, Deutschland, Europa, Orient und Afrika.*

Staatliche Museen, Stiftung Preußischer Kulturbesitz, Kunstbibliothek, Berlin. Ident. Nrs. 14136879-14136985. *Schneidermusterbuch: Käysserliche Freyhaitten d schneyder [...] Musterbuch des Handwerks der Schneider von Enns* (Enns, 1590).

Published Sources

Primary

Agricola, Johannes, *Die Sprichwörtersammlungen*, ed. Sander L. Gilman (2 vols, Berlin, 1971).

Amburger, Hannah, 'Die Familiengeschichte der Köler: Ein Beitrag zur Autobiographie des 16. Jahrhunderts', *Mitteilungen des Vereins für Geschichte der Stadt Nürnberg* 30 (1931), 153–288.

Amman, Jost, *Frauen-Trachtenbuch.* Facsimile reprint of *Im Frauwenzimmer wirt vermeldt von allerley schöen Kleidungen* (1586) (Munich, 1880).

Ashcroft, Jeffrey, *Albrecht Dürer: Documentary Biography* (2 vols, New Haven, 2017).

Bauhin, Johann, *Ein New Badbuch* (Stuttgart, 1602).

Beriger, Andreas (ed. and tr.), *Johannes Butzbach, Odeporicon: Eine Autobiographie aus dem Jahre 1506. Zweisprachige Ausgabe* (Weinheim, 1991).

Bickel, J., 'Die Selbstbiographie des Balthasar Sibenhar, Pfarrers in Beyerberg 1572–1601', *Beiträge zur bayerischen Kirchengeschichte* 7 (1901), 256–74.

Birlinger, Anton (ed.), *Alemannia: Zeitschrift für Sprache, Litteratur und Volkskunde des Elsaszes, Oberrheins und Schwabens* 16 (1888).

Boccaccio, Giovanni, *Decameron*, ed. Cormac O Cuilleanain (Ware, 2004).

Bock, Hieronymus, *Kreutterbuch* (Strasbourg, 1580).

Boos, Heinrich (ed.), *Thomas und Felix Platter, zur Sittengeschichte des XVI. Jahrhunderts* (Hirzel, 1878).

Calvin, John, *Institutes of the Christian Religion*, ed. John T. McNeill, tr. Ford Lewis Battles (Louisville, 2001).

Christof, Froben, Graf von Zimmern, *Die Chronik der Grafen von Zimmern: Handschriften 580 und 581 der Fürstlich Fürstenbergischen Hofbibliothek Donaueschingen*, ed. Hansmartin Decker-Hauff and Rudolf Seigel (3 vols, Konstanz, 1964–72, and Sigmaringen, 1972).

Cochlaeus, Johannes, 'The Deeds and Writings of Martin Luther from the Year of the Lord 1517 to the Year 1546 Related Chronologically to All Posterity by Johannes Cochlaeus', in Elizabeth Vandiver and Ralph Keen (eds), *Luther's Lives: Two Contemporary Accounts of Martin Luther* (Manchester, 2003), 56–355.

Coler, Johannes, *Oeconomia oder Haußbuch* (Wittenberg, 1599).

Culpepper, Nicholas, *Pharmacopœia Londinensis* (London, 1653).

Dedekind, Friedrich, *Grobianus und Grobiana: Von unfletigen, groben, unhöflichen Sitten, und Bäwrischen Gebärde*, tr. Wendelin Helbach (Frankfurt, 1572).

Dürer, Albrecht, *Hierinn sind begriffen vier Bücher von Menschlicher Proportion* (Nuremberg, 1528).

Erb, Matthias (ed.), *Von sauffen vnd fressen: Den zweyenn greülichen Lasteren wie die durch den heiligen Chrysostomum Hieronymum vnd Basilium Magnum vnd anderen Vätteren vor tausent Jaren in jren predigen sind gestraafft worde(n)* (Mülhausen, 1559).
Erhard, Christoph, *Gründliche kurtz verfaste Historia: Von Münsterischen Widertauffern* (Munich, 1589).
Fabri, Michael, *Von der Allgemeinen Aufferstehung der Todten* (Frankfurt am Main, 1564).
Fischer, Christoph Andreas, *Vier und funfftzig Erhebliche Ursachen Warumb die Widertauffer nicht sein im Land zu leyden* (Ingolstadt, 1607).
Forster, Leonard (ed. and tr.), *Selections from Conrad Celtis, 1459–1508* (Cambridge, 1948).
Franck, Sebastian, *Von dem grewlichen laster der Trunckenheit so inn disen letzten zeytenn erst schier mit den Frantzosen auffkommen* (Augsburg, 1531).
Friderich, Matthäus, *Wider den Saufteuffel: Etliche wichtige Ursachen, warumb alle Menschen sich für dem Sauffen hüten sollen* (Leipzig, 1552).
Funck, Johann, *APOCALYPSIS: Der Offenbarung Künfftiger Geschicht Johannis, Von widerwertigkeit vnd verfolgung der waren Christlichen Kirchen sind der Apostel zeit, bis an der welt ende, Auslegung*, ed. Zacharias Engelhaubt (Wittenberg, 1560).
Furnivall, Frederick J. (ed.), *Phillip Stubbes's Anatomy of the Abuses in England in Shakspere's youth, A.D. 1583* (London, 1877–9).
Geisberg, Max (ed.), *The German Single-Leaf Woodcut 1500–1550*, vol. 4 (New York, 1974).
Gessner, Conrad, *Vogelbuch Darin[n] die art, natur und eigenschafft aller vöglen, sampt jrer waren Contrafactur, angezeigt wirt* (Zurich, 1557).
Gessner, Conrad, *Thierbuch, das ist ein kurtze beschreybung aller vierfüssigen Thieren* (Zurich, 1563).
Gregory the Great, *Pastoral Care*, tr. Henry Davis (Westminster, MD, 1950).
Guarinonius, Hippolytus, *Die Grewel der Verwüstung Menschlichen Geschlechts* (Ingolstadt, 1610).
Hermann, Nikolaus, *Ein geistliches Lied von der Auferstehung der Toten und dem ewigen Leben* (Nuremberg, 1555).
Hess, Ernst Ferdinand, *Flagellum Iudeorum, Juden Geissel, Das ist Ein Neuwe sehr nütze und gründliche Erweisung, daß Jesus Christus, Gottes und der H. Jungkfrauwen Marien Sohn, der wahre verheissene und gesandte Messias sey* (Erfurt, 1598).
Hollstein, Wilhelm, *German Engravings, Etchings, and Woodcuts, c.1400–1700*, vol. 52 (Amsterdam, 2000).
Hubner, Bartholomäus, *New Speisebüchlein: darinnen kurtzer Unterricht von Essen und Trincken, auch von allerley Speisen und Getranck* (Erfurt, 1583).
Lemnius, Levinus, *Von den wunderbarlichen Geheimnissen der Natur*, tr. Jakob Horst (Leipzig, 1572).
Ludwig, Walther (ed.), *Vater und Sohn im 16. Jahrhundert. Der Briefwechsel des Wolfgang Reichart genannt Rychardus mit seinem Sohn Zeno (1520–1543)* (Hildesheim, 1999).
Luther, Martin, *Auslegung der Episteln vnd Euangelien vom Advent an bis auff Ostern* (Wittenberg, 1528).
Luther, Martin, *D. Martin Luthers Werke: Kritische Gesamtausgabe* (120 vols, Weimar, 1883–2009).
Luther, Martin, *D. Martin Luthers Werke: Kritische Gesamtausgabe. Tischreden* (6 vols, Weimar, 1912–21).
Luther, Martin, *Luther's Works* (55 vols, St Louis, 1955–86).
Magnus, Albertus, *Dauraus man alle heimligkeit dess Weiblichen geschlechts erkennen kan.* (Frankfurt am Main, 1581).
Manetti, Antonio, *The Fat Woodworker*, tr. Robert L. Martone and Valerie Martone (New York, 1991).
Mathesius, Johannes, *Leychpredigten. Auß dem fünfftzehenden Capitel der I. Epistel S. Pauli zun Corinthiern* (Nuremberg, 1565).
Mathesius, Johannes, *Postilla. Das ist, Außlegung der Sontags vnnd fürnembsten Fest Euangelien, über das gantze Jar* (Nuremberg, 1584).
Melanchthon, Philipp, *Der BapstEsel durch M. Philippum Melanchthon gedeutet und gebessert* (Wittenberg, 1535).

Melanchthon, Philipp, 'History of the Life and Acts of Dr Martin Luther', in Elizabeth Vandiver and Ralph Keen (eds), *Luther's Lives: Two Contemporary Accounts of Martin Luther* (Manchester, 2003), 15–40.

Moscherosch, Johann Michael, *Anderer Theil der Gesichte Philanders von Sittewalt* (Strasbourg, 1644).

Müller, Gernot Michael, *Die 'Germania generalis' des Conrad Celtis: Studien mit Edition, Übersetzung und Kommentar* (Tübingen, 2001).

Müntzer, Thomas, *Auszlegung des andern vnterschyds Danielis* (Allstedt, 1524).

Müntzer, Thomas, *Hoch verursachte Schutzrede und antwort wider das Gaistloße Sanfft lebende fleysch zu Wittenberg* (Nuremberg, 1524).

Oetheus, Jakob, *Gründtlicher Bericht, Lehr unnd Instruction, von rechtem und nutzlichem brauch der Artzney* (Dillingen, 1574).

Opitz, Josua, *Eine Fastenpredigt von christlichem und antichristischem Fasten: wider den bäpstischen abgöttischen Fastenteuffel* (Regensburg, 1573).

Osiander, Lucas, *Ein Predig, Von hoffertiger vngestalter Kleidung der Weibs vnd Manns Personen* (Tübingen, 1586).

Otto, Bishop of Freising, *The Two Cities: A Chronicle of Universal History to the Year 1146 A.D.*, tr. Charles Christopher Mierow, ed. Austin P. Evans and Charles Knapp (New York, 1928).

Pegius, Martin, *Geburtsstundenbuch darinen eines jetlichen Menschens Natur und Eigenschafft sampt allerley Zufählen auß den gewissen Leuffen deren Gestirn nach rechter warhafftiger und grundtlicher Ahrt der Gestirnkunst mit geringer Müh außgereitet und derselb vor zufelligem Unfahl gewarnet* (Basel, 1570).

Pictorius, Georg, *Baderbüchlein* (Mülhausen, 1560).

Pictorius, Georg, *Leibs Artzney: Ein sehr Nutzliches Handtbüchlein vom grund und innhalt der gantzen Artzney* (Frankfurt am Main, 1566).

Rösslin, Eucharius, *Der schwangeren Frawen vnd Hebammen Rosengarten* (Augsburg, 1528).

Rublack, Ulinka, and Maria Hayward (eds), *The First Book of Fashion: The Book of Clothes of Matthäus and Veit Konrad Schwarz of Augsburg* (London, 2015).

Rueff, Jacob, *Hebammen Buch, daraus man alle Heimligkeit desz weiblichen Geschlechts erlehrnen, welcherley gestalt der Mensch in Mutter Leib empfangen, zunimpt vnnd geboren wirdt* (Frankfurt, 1588).

Rummel, Erika (ed.), *The Erasmus Reader* (Toronto, 1990).

Rupprich, Hans, *Dürer: Schriftlicher Nachlass* (3 vols, Berlin, 1956–69).

Ruscelli, Girolamo, *Weiber Zierung*, tr. Hans Jacob Wecker (Basel, 1570).

Ryff, Walther Hermann, *New Kochbuch für die Kranken* (Frankfurt am Main, 1545).

Ryff, Walther Hermann, *Spiegel der Gesundheit* (Frankfurt am Main, 1555).

Sachs, Hans, *Sämmtliche Fastnachtspiele*, ed. Edmund Goetze, (7 vols, Halle, 1880–7).

Schmidel, Ulrich, *Vierte Schiffart. Warhafftige Historien. Einer Wunderbaren Schiffart, welche Ulrich Schmidel von Straubing, von Anno 1534. biß Anno 1554 in Americam oder Newenwelt, bey Brasilia und Rio della Plata gethan* (Nuremberg, 1599).

Schön, Erhard, *Unnderweissung der Proportzion vnnd Stellung der Possen* (Nuremberg, 1540, first published 1538).

Simons, Menno, 'Foundation of Christian Doctrine', in John Christian Wenger (ed.), *The Complete Writings of Menno Simons: c.1496–1561* (Scottdale, PA, and Waterloo, 1986).

Spangenberg, Johann, *Des Ehelichen Ordens Spiegel vnd Regel* (Magdeburg, 1544).

Staden, Hans, *Warhaftige Historia und beschreibung eyner Landtschafft der Wilden, Nacketen, Grimmigen Menschfresser-Leuthen, in der Newenwelt America gelegen* (Marburg, 1557).

Steinhausen, Georg (ed.), *Briefwechsel Balthasar Paumgartners des Jüngeren mit seiner Gattin Magdalena, geb. Behaim (1582–1598)* (Stuttgart, 1895).

Steinhausen, Georg (ed.), *Deutsche Privatbriefe des Mittelalters*, vol. 1. *Fürsten und Magnaten, Edle und Ritter* (Berlin, 1899).

Strauß, Johannes, *Wider den Kleyder, Pluder, Pauß und Krauß Teuffel* (Leipzig, 1581).

Strauss, Walter L., *The Complete Drawings of Albrecht Dürer* (6 vols, New York, 1974).

Strauss, Walter (ed.), *The Illustrated Bartsch*, vol. 13 (New York, 1981).

Strigenitz, Gregor, *IEIVNIVM, Das ist: Vom Fasten/Einfeltiger vnd gruendlicher bericht* (Leipzig, 1598).

Tacitus, Publius Cornelius, *Agricola. Germania. Dialogue on Oratory,* tr. M. Hutton and W. Peterson. Loeb Classical Library 35 (Cambridge, 1970).
Tallat, Johannes, *Artzney Büchlein der Kreutter, oder Margarita medicine* (Augsburg, 1502).
Theodorus, Jacobus, *New Wasserschatz* (Frankfurt, 1581).
Thieme, André (ed.), *Die Korrespondenz der Herzogin Elisabeth von Sachsen und ergänzende Quellen* (Leipzig, 2010).
von Amsdorf, Nicolaus, *Fuenff fuernemliche vnd gewisse Zeichen aus heiliger gottlicher Schrifft/ so kurtz vor dem Juengsten tag geschehen sollen* (Jena, 1554).
von Gersdorff, Hans, *Feldbuch der Wundartzney newlich getruckt vnd gebessert* (Strasbourg, 1528).
von Hohenheim, Theophrastus (Paracelsus), 'Opus Paramirum', in Andrew Weeks (ed. and tr.), *Paracelsus (Theophrastus Bombastus von Hohenheim 1493–1541): Essential Theoretical Writings* (Leiden, 2008), 297–501.
von Matrei, Klaus, and Jeremias Martius, *Artzneybuch Deß Hochberümbten und Weyterfahrnen Herrn Nicolai de Metri* (Augsburg, 1572).
von Megenberg, Conrad, *Planctus Ecclesiae in Germaniam*, ed. Richard Scholz, *Staatsschriften des späteren Mittelalters* (Stuttgart, 1977).
von Watt, Joachim, *Das Büchlein ist genant vom alten vnd neüwen Got, Glauben und Leer* (Strasbourg, 1521).
Vredeveld, Harry (ed.), *The Poetic Works of Helius Eobanus Hessus,* vol. 3 (Leiden, 2012).
Weinsberg, Hermann, *Buch Weinsberg,* transcribed by Abteilung für Rheinische Landesgeschichte, Universität Bonn (2003). Digital edition: www.weinsberg.uni-bonn.de
Wier, Johannes, *De lamiis. Das ist: Von Teufelsgespenst Zauberern vnd GIfftbereytern/kurtzer doch gründtlicher Bericht...Samt einem angehängten kleinen Tractätlein von dem falschen vnd erdichten Fasten* (Frankfurt am Main, 1586).
Winckler, Gottfried Christian, *Wunder der Natur/Nach der Menschen Unterschiedlichen Beschaffenheit* (Frankfurt and Leipzig, 1690).
Wittich, Johannes, *Praeservator Sanitatis* (Leipzig, 1590).
Zincgref, Julius Wilhelm, *Teutsche Apophthegmata, das ist, Der Teutschen Scharfsinnige kluge Sprüche,* vol. 2 (Leiden, 1644).

Secondary

Abulafia, David, *The Discovery of Mankind: Atlantic Encounters in the Age of Columbus* (New Haven and London, 2008).
Albala, Ken, *Eating Right in the Renaissance* (Berkeley, CA, 2002).
Albala, Ken, 'Weight Loss in the Age of Reason', in Christopher E. Forth and Ana Carden-Coyne (eds), *Cultures of the Abdomen: Diet, Digestion and Fat in the Modern World* (Basingstoke, 2005), 169–83.
Andersen, Elizabeth, Henrike Lähnemann, and Anne Simon (eds), *A Companion to Mysticism and Devotion in Northern Germany in the Late Middle Ages* (Leiden, 2014).
Andersson, Christianne, 'Jungfrau, Dirne, Fortuna: Das Bild der Frau in den Zeichnungen von Urs Graf', *Kritische Berichte* 16 (1988), 26–35.
Anzelewsky, Fedja, 'Dürers "ästhetischer Exkurs" in seiner Proportionslehre', in Friedrich Mielke (ed.), *Kaleidoskop. Eine Festschrift für Fritz Baumgart zum 75. Geburtstag* (Berlin, 1977), 70–8.
Arnold, Janet, *Patterns of Fashion,* vol. 3. *The Cut and Construction of Clothes for Men and Women c.1560–1620* (London, 1985).
Arrizabalaga, Jon, 'Medical Responses to the "French Disease" in Europe at the Turn of the Sixteenth Century', in Kevin Siena (ed.), *Sins of the Flesh: Responding to Sexual Disease in Early Modern Europe* (Toronto, 2005), 33–55.
Astbury, Leah, 'When a Woman Hates her Husband: Love, Sex and Fruitful Marriages in Early Modern England', *Gender and History* 32 (2020), 523–41.
Baer, Leo, 'Vorwort', in Erhard Schön, *Unterweisung der Proportionen und Stellung der Possen, Nuremberg 1542,* ed. Leo Baer (Frankfurt am Main, 1920).
Bächtold-Stäubli, Hans (ed.), *Handwörterbuch des deutschen Aberglaubens,* vol. 2 (Berlin, 1929/30).

Bächtold-Stäubli, Hanns, and Eduard Hoffmann-Krayer (eds), *Handwörterbuch des deutschen Aberglaubens,* vol. 6 (Berlin, 1987).

Barich, Katherine, and Marion McNealy, *Drei Schnittbücher: Three Austrian Master Tailor Books of the 16th Century* (Kennewick, WA, 2015).

Barnes, Robin B., *Prophecy and Gnosis: Apocalypticism in the Wake of the Lutheran Reformation* (Stanford, CA, 1988).

Barnes, Robin B., *Astrology and Reformation* (Oxford, 2015).

Bartrum, Giulia, *German Renaissance Prints 1490–1550* (London, 1995).

Baum, Jacob, *The Reformation of the Senses: The Paradox of Religious Belief and Practice in Germany* (Urbana, IL, 2019).

Baumgarten, Linda, 'Altered Historical Clothing', *Dress* 25 (1998), 42–57.

Bäumel, Jutta, 'Der Kleider-Nachlaß des Kurfürsten Moritz von Sachsen. Das Inventar von 1553 und die in der Dresdener Rüstkammer überlieferten Originale', *Zeitschrift für historische Waffen- und Kostümkunde,* 35 (1993), 65–106.

Bäumler, Suzanne, Evamaria Brockhoff, and Michael Henker (eds), *Von Kaisers Gnaden: 500 Jahre Pfalz-Neuburg,* exh. cat., Schloss Neuburg (Regensburg, 2005).

Baxandall, Michael, *The Limewood Sculptors of Renaissance Germany* (New Haven, CT, 1980).

Bell, Rudolph, *Holy Anorexia* (Chicago, 1985).

Belozerskaya, Marina, *Rethinking the Renaissance: Burgundian Arts across Europe* (Cambridge, 2002).

Bendall, Sarah, *Shaping Femininity: Foundation Garments, the Body and Women in Early Modern England* (London, 2022).

Benesch, Otto, *The Art of the Northern Renaissance: Its Relation to the Contemporary Spiritual and Intellectual Movements* (London, 1965).

Benninga, Sara, 'The Faces of Fatness in Early Modern Europe', FKW. *Zeitschrift für Geschlechterforschung und visuelle Kultur,* 62 (2017), 24–35.

Benzing, Josef, *Walther H. Ryff und sein literarisches Werk: Eine Bibliographie* (Hamburg, 1959).

Betz, Susanne Helene, 'Verhandeln über Ehe: Die Suche nach der idealen Braut für Cosimo (II.) de' Medici', *Der diplomatische Körper: Frühneuzeitliche Diplomatie als Körperpolitik, Frühneuzeit Info* 29 (2018), 39–56.

Bischoff, Christina Johanna, 'Ultra Mensuram tendere: Zur Maßlosigkeit mönchischer Askese', in Isabelle Mandrella and Kathrin Müller (eds), *Maß und Maßlosigkeit im Mittelalter* (Berlin, 2018), 29–47.

Bitz, Matthias, *Badewesen in Südwestdeutschland 1550 bis 1840: Zum Wandel von Gesellschaft und Architektur* (Idstein, 1989).

Blanc, Odile, *Parades et Parures: L'invention du corps de mode à la fin du Moyen Age* (Paris, 1997).

Böhm, Willi, 'Albrecht, Kurfürst von Brandenburg', in *Allgemeine deutsche Biographie,* vol. 1 (Leipzig, 1875), 243–52.

Bond, Katherine, '"Fashioned with Marvellous Skill": Veils and the Costume Books of Sixteenth-Century Europe', in Susanna Burghartz, Lucas Burkart, Christine Göttler, and Ulinka Rublack (eds), *Materialized Identities in Early Modern Culture, 1450–1750* (Amsterdam, 2021), 325–68.

Bond, Katherine, 'Mapping Culture in the Habsburg Empire: Fashioning a Costume Book in the Court of Charles V', *Renaissance Quarterly* 71 (2018), 530–79.

Bonnet, Anne-Marie, *Der Akt bei Dürer und die Rezeption durch zeitgenössische Künstler.* Partially published Habilitationsschrift (Munich, 1992).

Bonnet, Anne-Marie, 'Der Akt im Werk Lucas Cranachs. Bedeutung und Spezifität der "nacketen Bilder" innerhalb der deutschen Renaissance-Malerei', in Claus Grimm, Johannes Erichsen, and Evamaria Brockhoff (eds), *Lucas Cranach: Ein Maler-Unternehmer aus Franken,* exh. cat., Haus der Bayerischen Geschichte, Augsburg (Regensburg, 1994), 139–49.

Bonnet, Anne-Marie, *'Akt' bei Dürer* (Cologne, 2001).

Bonnet, Anne-Marie, *Albrecht Dürer: Die Erfindung des Aktes* (Munich, 2014).

Borchardt, Frank L., *German Antiquity in Renaissance Myth* (Baltimore, MD, 1971).

Borggrefe, Heiner, 'Anatomie, Erotik, Dissimulation. Nackte Körper von Dürer, Baldung Grien und den Kleinmeistern', in Andreas Tacke and Stefan Heinz (eds), *Menschenbilder: Beiträge zur Altdeutschen Kunst* (Petersberg, 2011), 33–55.

Bouley, Bradford, 'A Plague of Meat: Food, Politics, and Warfare in Early Modern Italy', *Isis* 114 (2023), 631–7.

Boyarin, Daniel, 'Literary Fat Rabbis: On the Historical Origins of the Grotesque Body', *Journal of the History of Sexuality* 1 (1991), 551–84.

Brecht, Martin, *Martin Luther: Sein Weg zur Reformation, 1483–1521* (Stuttgart, 1981).

Brinkmann, Bodo, 'Die Hexe als Aktmodell: Künstlerstreit um Körperformen. The Witch as a Nude Model: The Artist's Debate on Body Forms', in Bodo Brinkmann (ed.), *Hexenlust und Sündenfall: Die seltsamen Phantasien des Hans Baldung Grien. Witches' Lust and the Fall of Man: The Strange Fantasies of Hans Baldung Grien*, exh. cat., Städel Museum, Frankfurt am Main (Petersberg, 2007), 74–96.

Brinkmann, Bodo, 'Liebe von hinten, Liebe von vorn: Dürer und Pirckheimer lesen Lukian. Love from the Back, Love from the Front: Dürer and Pirckheimer Read Lucian', in Bodo Brinkmann (ed.), *Hexenlust und Sündenfall: Die seltsamen Phantasien des Hans Baldung Grien. Witches' Lust and the Fall of Man: The Strange Fantasies of Hans Baldung Grien*, exh. cat., Städel Museum, Frankfurt am Main (Petersberg, 2007), 97–108.

Brisman, Shira, 'Sternkraut: "The Word that Unlocks" Dürer's Self-Portrait of 1493', in Daniel Hess and Thomas Eser (eds), *The Early Dürer*, exh. cat., Germanisches Nationalmuseum, Nuremberg (Nuremberg, 2012), 194–207.

Bruna, Dennis, 'Medieval Fashions, Bodies and Transformations', in Denis Bruna (ed.), *Fashioning the Body: An Intimate History of the Silhouette* (New York, 2015).

Bubenik, Andrea, *Reframing Albrecht Dürer: The Appropriation of Art, 1528–1700* (Farnham, 2013).

Buck, Lawrence, *The Roman Monster: An Icon of the Papal Antichrist in Reformation Politics* (Kirksville, MO, 2014).

Bücking, Jürgen, *Kultur und Gesellschaft in Tirol um 1600: Des Hippolytus Guarinonius' 'Grewel der Verwüstung Menschlichen Geschlechts' (1610) als kulturgeschichtliche Quelle des frühen 17. Jahrhunderts* (Lübeck and Hamburg, 1968).

Burghartz, Susanna, 'Covered Women? Veiling in Early Modern Europe', tr. Jane Caplan, *History Workshop Journal* 80 (2015), 1–32.

Burke, Jill, *How to be a Renaissance Woman: The Untold History of Beauty and Female Creativity* (London, 2023).

Burke, Jill, Thomas Kren, and Stephen J. Campbell (eds), *The Renaissance Nude*, exh. cat., J. Paul Getty Museum, Los Angeles (Los Angeles, 2018).

Burke, Peter, *The Historical Anthropology of Early Modern Italy: Essays on Perception and Communication* (Cambridge, 2005).

Buskirk, Jessica, 'Man tragt nit schwer an guter kunst. Das Goldene Zeitalter der Kunst und des Patriotismus im Nürnberg des 16. Jahrhunderts', in Jürgen Müller and Thomas Schauerte (eds), *Die gottlosen Maler von Nürnberg—Konvention und Subversion in der Druckgrafik der Beham-Brüder*, exh. cat., Albrecht-Dürer-Haus, Nuremberg (Nuremberg, 2011), 56–63.

Butler, Judith, *Gender Trouble: Feminism and the Subversion of Identity* (New York and London, 1990).

Butler, Judith, *Bodies that Matter: On the Discursive Limits of Sex* (New York, 2011, first published, 1993).

Cabré, Montserrat, 'Beautiful Bodies', in Linda Kalof (ed.), *A Cultural History of the Human Bodies in the Medieval Age* (London, 2014), 121–39.

Campbell, Caroline, 'The Artist known as Lucas Cranach', in Caroline Campbell (ed.), *Temptation in Eden: Lucas Cranach's Adam and Eve*, exh. cat., Courtauld Institute of Art, London (London, 2007), 12–17.

Cavallo, Sandra, 'Health, Air and Material Culture in the Early Modern Italian Domestic Environment', *Social History of Medicine* 29 (2016), 695–716.

Cavallo, Sandra, and Tessa Storey, *Healthy Living in Late Renaissance Italy* (Oxford, 2013).

Cavallo, Sandra, and Tessa Storey (eds), *Conserving Health in Early Modern Culture: Bodies and Environments in Italy and England* (Manchester, 2017).

Chipps Smith, Jeffrey, 'Dürer's Losses and the Dilemma of Being', in Lynne Tatlock (ed.), *Enduring Loss in Early Modern Germany: Cross Disciplinary Perspectives* (Leiden, 2010), 71–101.
Chipps Smith, Jeffrey, *Dürer* (London, 2012).
Chipps Smith, Jeffrey, *Nuremberg, a Renaissance City, 1500–1618* (Austin, TX, 2021).
Chung-Kim, Esther, *Economics of Faith: Reforming Poor Relief in Early Modern Europe* (Oxford, 2021).
Cislo, Amy Eisen, 'Paracelsus's Conception of Seeds: Rethinking Paracelsus's Ideas of Body and Matter', *Ambix* 55 (2008), 274–82.
Clark, Kenneth, *The Nude: A Study in Ideal Form* (Princeton, 1990, first published 1956).
Clementi, Siglinde, *Körper, Selbst und Melancholie: Die Selbstzeugnisse des Landadeligen Osvaldo Ercole Trapp (1634–1710)* (Cologne, 2017).
Clever, Iris, and Willemijn Ruberg, 'Beyond Cultural History? The Material Turn, Praxiography, and Body History', *Humanities* 3 (2014), 546–66.
Colbertaldo, Roberta, and Christine Ott (eds), 'Fat Worlds: Feasters and Loafers in Medieval and Early Modern Europe', Special Issue of *Food and History* 21 (2023).
Constable, Giles, *Attitudes toward Self-Inflicted Suffering in the Middle Ages* (Brookline, MA, 1982).
Constable, Giles, 'Moderation and Restraint in Ascetic Practices', in Haijo Jan Westra (ed.), *From Athens to Chartres: Neoplatonism and Medieval Thought* (Leiden, 1992), 315–27.
Coveney, John, *Food, Morals and Meaning: The Pleasure and Anxiety of Eating* (London, 2006).
Crawford, Katherine, *European Sexualities, 1400–1800* (Cambridge, 2007).
Cro, Stelio, *The Noble Savage: Allegory of Freedom* (Waterloo, 1990).
Crofts, Frederick G., 'Visualizing Germanness through Costumes in the Sixteenth Century', *Historical Journal* 64 (2021), 1198–1229.
Crowther, Kathleen, *Adam and Eve in the Protestant Reformation* (Cambridge, 2010).
Csordas, Thomas, 'Somatic Modes of Attention', *Cultural Anthropology* 8 (1993), 135–56.
Dackerman, Susan (ed.), *Prints and the Pursuit of Knowledge in Early Modern Europe*, exh. cat., Harvard Art Museums (Cambridge, MA, 2011).
Davies, Surekha, *Renaissance Ethnography and the Invention of the Human: New Worlds, Maps and Monsters* (Cambridge, 2016).
Demele, Christine, *Dürers Nacktheit: Das Weimarer Selbstbildnis* (Münster, 2012).
Deutsch, Yaacov, *Judaism in Christian Eyes: Ethnographic Descriptions of Jews and Judaism in Early Modern Europe* (Oxford, 2012).
de Waardt, Hans, 'Witchcraft, Spiritualism, and Medicine: The Religious Convictions of Johan Wier', *Sixteenth Century Journal* 42 (2011), 369–91.
Dihle, Helene, 'Männerkleidung des 16. Jahrhunderts nach dem Buch Weinsberg', *Zeitschrift für historische Waffen- und Kostümkunde* 1 (1923–5), 177–84.
Doumergue, Émile, 'Calvin: Epigone or Creator?', in William Park Armstrong (ed.), *Calvin and the Reformation* (Eugene, OR, 2004), 1–55.
Dück, Katharina, *Materia prima: Zur Semantik des Begriffs in naturkundlichen Sachschriften des 16. Jahrhunderts* (Wiesbaden, 2019).
Duden, Barbara, *The Woman Beneath the Skin: A Doctor's Patients in Eighteenth-Century Germany*, tr. Thomas Dunlap (Cambridge, 1991).
Dürr, Renate, Ronnie Hsia, Carina Johnson, Ulrike Strasser, and Merry Wiesner-Hanks, 'Forum: Globalizing Early Modern German History', *German History* 31 (2013), 366–82.
Eamon, William, *Science and the Secrets of Nature: Books of Secrets in Medieval and Early Modern Culture* (Princeton, 1996).
Earle, Rebecca, *The Body of the Conquistador: Food, Race and the Colonial Experience in Spanish America, 1492–1700* (Cambridge, 2014).
Earle, Thomas F., and Kate J. P. Lowe (eds), *Black Africans in Renaissance Europe* (Cambridge, 2005).
Eberlein, Johann Konrad, *Albrecht Dürer* (Reinbek, 2003).
Eichberger, Dagmar, and Charles Zika (eds), *Dürer and his Culture* (Cambridge, 1998).

Eknoyan, Garabed, 'A History of Obesity, or How What was Good Became Ugly and Then Bad', *Advances in Chronic Kidney Disease* 13 (2006), 421–7.
Elias, Norbert, *The Civilising Process: Sociogenetic and Psychogenetic Investigations,* ed. Eric Dunning, Johan Goudsblom, and Stephen Mennell (Oxford, 2000).
Ellingson, Ter, *The Myth of the Noble Savage* (Berkeley, CA, 2001).
Engineer, Urmi, 'Sugar Revisited: Sweetness and the Environment in the Early Modern World', in Anne Gerritsen and Giorgio Riello (eds), *The Global Lives of Things: The Material Culture of Connections in the Early Modern World* (London, 2015), 198–220.
Entwistle, Joanne, *The Fashioned Body* (Cambridge, 2015).
Entwistle, Joanne, and Emma McClendon (eds), *The Body: Fashion and Physique*, special issue of *Fashion Theory* 23 (2019).
Flavin, Susan, Marc Meltonville, Charlie Taverner, Joshua Reid, Stephen Lawrence, Carlos Belloch-Molina, and John Morrissey, 'Understanding Early Modern Beer: An Interdisciplinary Case-Study', *Historical Journal* 66 (2023), 516–49.
Fletcher, Holly, 'Age, Gender and the Body in the Bronze and Pearwood Statuettes of 1520s' Germany', *Gender and History* 32 (2020), 341–372.
Fletcher, Holly, '"Belly-Worshippers and Greed-Paunches": Fatness and the Belly in the Lutheran Reformation', *German History* 39 (2021), 173–200.
Fletcher, Holly, 'The Fat World of the Hutterites: Food and Fatness in the Criticism of Hutterite Anabaptists in Early Modern Moravia', *Food and History* 21 (2023), 173–200.
Floyd-Wilson, Mary, *English Ethnicity and Race in Early Modern Drama* (New York, 2003).
Flüchter, Antje, 'Weighing the Mughal: German Perception of Governmental Structures and the Staging of Power in the Early Modern Indian Mughal Empire', in Antje Flüchter and Susan Richter (eds), *Structures on the Move: Technologies of Governance in Transcultural Encounter* (Berlin and Heidelberg, 2012), 147–66.
Forth, Christopher, 'Fat, Desire and Disgust in the Colonial Imagination', *History Workshop Journal* 73 (2012), 211–39.
Forth, Christopher, 'The Qualities of Fat: Bodies, History and Materiality', *Journal of Material Culture* 18 (2013), 135–54.
Forth, Christopher, 'On Fat and Fattening: Agency, Materiality and Animality in the History of Corpulence', *Body Politics: Zeitschrift für Körpergeschichte* 3 (2015), 51–74.
Forth, Christopher, *Fat: A Cultural History of the Stuff of Life* (London, 2019).
Freedberg, David, 'Dürer's Limbs', in Stephanie Buck and Stephanie Porras (eds), *The Young Dürer: Drawing the Figure* (London, 2013), 37–56.
Fudge, Erica, 'What was it Like to Be a Cow? History and Animal Studies', in Linda Kalof (ed.), *The Oxford Handbook of Animal Studies* (Oxford, 2014), 258–78.
Fulbrook, Mary, and Ulinka Rublack, 'In Relation: The "Social Self" and Ego-Documents', *German History* 28 (2010), 263–72.
Fürbeth, Frank, 'Zur Bedeutung des Bäderwesens im Mittelalter und der frühen Neuzeit', in Heinz Dopsch and Peter F. Kramml (eds), *Paracelsus und Salzburg* (Salzburg, 1994), 463–87.
Gentilcore, David, *Food and Health in Early Modern Europe: Diet, Medicine and Society 1450–1800* (London, 2015).
Germar, Herbert, *Das Schneiderhandwerk in Leipzig bis zum Ausgange des 17. Jahrhunderts,* PhD thesis, Leipzig, 1918.
Gibbs, Frederick W., *Poison, Medicine and Disease in Later Medieval and Early Modern Europe* (Abingdon, 2019).
Gilman, Sander L., *Jewish Self-Hatred: Anti-Semitism and the Hidden Language of the Jews* (Baltimore, MD, 1986).
Gilman, Sander L., *Fat Boys: A Slim Book* (Lincoln, 2004).
Gilman, Sander L., *Diets and Dieting: A Cultural Encyclopaedia* (Abingdon, 2008).
Gilman, Sander L., *Fat: A Cultural History of Obesity* (Cambridge, 2008).
Gilman, Sander L., *Obesity: The Biography* (Oxford, 2010).
Gilman, Sander L., 'Jews and Fat: Thoughts toward a History of an Image in the Second Age of Biology', in Anat Helman (ed.), *Jews and their Foodways* (Oxford, 2016), 218–30.

Goddard, Stephen H., 'The Origin, Use and Heritage of the Small Engraving in Renaissance Germany', in Stephen H. Goddard (ed.), *The World in Miniature: Engravings by the German Little Masters, 1500–1550,* exh. cat., Spender Museum of Art (Lawrence, KS, 1988), 13–29.

Goddard, Stephen H. (ed.), *The World in Miniature: Engravings by the German Little Masters, 1500–1550,* exh. cat., Spender Museum of Art (Lawrence, KS, 1988).

Gowing, Laura, *Common Bodies: Women, Touch and Power in Seventeenth Century England* (New Haven, 2003).

Gritsch, Eric W., 'Luther as Bible Translator', in Donald K. McKim (ed.), *The Cambridge Companion to Martin Luther* (Cambridge, 2003), 62–72.

Groebner, Valentin, *Who are You? Identification, Deception, and Surveillance in Early Modern Europe,* tr. Mark Kyburz and John Peck (New York, 2007).

Hachmeister, Carl, *Der Meister des Amsterdamer Kabinetts und sein Verhältnis zu Albrecht Dürer* (Heidelberg, 1897).

Hackenberg, Michael, 'Books in Artisan Homes in Sixteenth-Century Germany', *Journal of Library History* 21 (1986), 72–91.

Hahn, Philip, *Das Haus im Buch: Konzeption, Publikationsgeschichte und Leserschaft der 'Oeconomia' Johann Colers* (Epfendorf, 2013).

Handley, Sasha, *Sleep in Early Modern England* (New Haven, 2016).

Handley, Sasha, 'Sleep-Piety and Healthy Sleep in Early Modern English Households', in Sandra Cavallo and Tessa Storey (eds), *Conserving Health in Early Modern Culture: Bodies and Environments in Italy and England* (Manchester, 2017), 185–209.

Handley, Sasha, 'Lusty Sack Possets, Nuptial Affections and the Material Communities of Early Modern Weddings', *Environment and History* 28 (2022), 375–95.

Hanß, Stefan, 'Face-Work: Making Hair Matter in Sixteenth-Century Europe', *Gender and History* 33 (2021), 314–43.

Hanß, Stefan, 'Eidechsenöl, Fledermaushirn, Bärenschmalz und Taubenkot. Haarpflege als Körper-, Medizin- und Materialwissen im 16. und 17. Jahrhundert', in Martin Mulsow (ed.), *Das Haar als Argument: Zur Wissensgeschichte von Bärten, Frisuren und Perücken* (Stuttgart, 2022), 55–80.

Hanß, Stefan, 'Gendering the Material Renaissance: Women Industriousness and the Female Body at the Court of Württemberg', *German History* 41 (2023), 367–99.

Harbison, Craig, *The Last Judgment in Sixteenth Century Northern Europe: A Study in the Relation between Art and the Reformation* (New York, 1975).

Harrington, Joel, *Reordering Marriage and Society in Reformation Germany* (Cambridge, 1995).

Hastings, Justin, 'Hic et Haec: The Feast of Corpus Christi, the Myth of Jewish Male Menstruation, and Allegoresis', *Essays in Medieval Studies* 34 (2018), 39–52.

Haude, Sigrun, *Coping with Life During the Thirty Years War (1618–1648)* (Leiden, 2021).

Havard, Lucy J., '"Preserve or Perish": Food Preservation Practices in the Early Modern Kitchen', *Royal Society Journal of the History of Science* 74 (2020), 5–33.

Hayward, Maria, *Dress at the Court of King Henry VIII* (Leeds, 2007).

Hendrix, Scott, 'Masculinity and Patriarchy in Reformation Germany', *Journal of the History of Ideas* 56 (1995), 177–93.

Heuer, Christopher, 'Dürer's Folds', *Anthropology and Aesthetics,* 59–60 (2011), 249–65.

Heydenreich, Gunnar, 'Adam and Eve in the Making', in Caroline Campbell (ed.), *Temptation in Eden: Lucas Cranach's Adam and Eve,* exh. cat., Courtauld Institute of Art, London (London, 2007), 19–33.

Heydenreich, Gunnar, *Lucas Cranach the Elder: Painting Materials, Techniques and Workshop Practice* (Amsterdam, 2007).

Hill, Kat, 'Fun and Loathing in Later Lutheran Culture', *Past and Present* 232 (2017), 67–89.

Hinz, Berthold, 'Baldung und Dürer: Nackte Figuren und ihre Bildgelegenheiten. Baldung and Dürer: Nudes and the Occasions for Depicting Them', in Bodo Brinkmann (ed.), *Hexenlust und Sündenfall: Die seltsamen Phantasien des Hans Baldung Grien. Witches' Lust and the Fall of Man: The Strange Fantasies of Hans Baldung Grien,* exh. cat., Städel Museum, Frankfurt am Main (Petersberg, 2007), 203–33.

Hirai, Hiro, *Le concept de semence dans les théories de la matière à la Renaissance: De Marsile Ficin à Pierre Gassendi* (Turnhout, 2005).
Hirschi, Caspar, *The Origins of Nationalism: An Alternative History from Ancient Rome to Early Modern Germany* (Cambridge, 2011).
Hollerbach, Teresa, 'The Weighing Chair of Sanctorius Sanctorius: A Replica', *NTM Zeitschrift für Geschichte der Wissenschaften, Technik und Medizin* 26 (2018), 121–49.
Hutchison, Jane Campbell, *Albrecht Dürer: A Biography* (Princeton, 1990).
Jancke, Gabriele, *Autobiographie als soziale Praxis: Beziehungskonzepte in Selbstzeugnissen des 15. und 16. Jahrhunderts im deutschsprachigen Raum* (Cologne, 2002).
Jancke, Gabriele, and Claudia Ulbrich, 'From the Individual to the Person: Challenging Autobiography Theory', in Claudia Ulbrich, Kaspar von Greyerz, and Lorenz Heiligensetzer (eds), *Mapping the 'I': Research on Self-Narratives in Germany and Switzerland* (Leiden, 2015), 13–33.
Jenner, Mark S. R., 'Body, Image, Text in Early Modern Europe', *Social History of Medicine* 12 (1999), 143–54.
Jerosch Herold, Bernardo, 'The Diary of the Swiss Leonhard Thurneysser and Black Africans in Renaissance Lisbon', *Renaissance Studies* 32 (2018), 463–88.
Johnson, Carina L., *Cultural Hierarchy in Sixteenth-Century Europe: The Ottomans and Mexicans* (Cambridge, 2011).
Johnson, Christine, *The German Discovery of the World: Renaissance Encounters with the Strange and Marvelous* (Charlottesville, VA, 2008).
Jütte, Robert, 'Aging and Body Image in the Sixteenth Century: Hermann Weinsberg's (1518–97) Perception of the Aging Body', *European History Quarterly* 18 (1988), 258–90.
Kantorowicz, Ernst, *The King's Two Bodies: A Study in Mediaeval Political Theology* (Princeton, 1957).
Karant-Nunn, Susan C., 'The Mitigated Fall of Humankind: Martin Luther's Reconciliation with the Body', *Past and Present* 234 (2017), 58–61.
Karant-Nunn, Susan C., *The Personal Luther: Essays on the Reformer from a Cultural Historical Perspective* (Leiden, 2017).
Katritzky, M. A., *Healing, Performance and Ceremony in the Writings of Three Early Modern Physicians: Hippolytus Guarinonius and the Brothers Felix and Thomas Platter* (Farnham, 2012).
Katz, David S., 'Shylock's Gender: Jewish Male Menstruation in Early Modern England', *Review of English Studies* 50 (1999), 440–62.
Kaufmann, Thomas, '1600: Deutungen der Jahrhundertwende im deutschen Luthertum', in Thomas Kaufmann (ed.), *Konfession und Kultur: Lutherischer Protestantismus in der zweiten Hälfte des Reformationsjahrhundert* (Tübingen, 2006), 413–64.
Kaufmann, Thomas, *Luther's Jews: A Journey into Anti-Semitism* (Oxford, 2017).
Kaufmann, Thomas, 'Luther and the Jews', *Antisemitism Studies* 3 (2019), 46–65.
Keil, Gundolf, 'Ryff, Walther Hermann', *Neue Deutsche Biographie*, 22 (2005), 310–11.
Keller, Katrin, *Kurfürstin Anna von Sachsen, 1532–1585* (Regensburg, 2010).
Kissane, Christopher, *Food, Religion, and Communities in Early Modern Europe* (London, 2018).
Klingerman, Katherine Marie, 'Binding Femininity: An Examination of the effects of Tightlacing on the Female Pelvis', MA thesis, Baton Rouge, LA, 2006.
Koerner, Joseph Leo, *The Moment of Self-Portraiture in German Renaissance Art* (Chicago, 1993).
Kolde, Theodor, 'Zum Prozess des Johann Denck und der "drei gottlosen Maler" von Nürnberg', in *Kirchengeschichtliche Studien Hermann Reuter zum 70. Geburtstag gewidmet* (Leipzig, 1888), 228–50.
Kounine, Laura, *Imagining the Witch: Emotions, Gender, and Selfhood in Early Modern Germany* (Oxford, 2018).
Krapf, Ludwig, *Germanenmythus und Reichsideologie: Frühhumanistische Rezeptionsweisen der taciteischen 'Germania'* (Tübingen, 1979).
Kratz, Henry, 'Über den Wortschatz der Erotik im spätmittelhochdeutschen und frühneuhochdeutschen', PhD thesis, Ohio, 1949.
Krause, Stefan, *Fashion in Steel: The Landsknecht Armour of Wilhelm von Rogendorf* (London, 2017).

Kümin, Beat, *Drinking Matters: Public Houses and Social Exchange in Early Modern Central Europe* (New York, 2007).

Lambert, Erin, 'New Worlds, New Images: Picturing the Resurrection of the Body in Sixteenth-Century Germany', in Anne Eusterschulte and Hannah Wälzholz (eds), *Anthropological Reformations: Anthropology in the Era of Reformation* (Göttingen, 2015), 533–40.

Lambert, Erin, 'The Reformation and the Resurrection of the Dead', *Sixteenth Century Journal* 47 (2016), 351–70.

Lambert, Erin, *Singing the Resurrection: Body, Community and Belief in Reformation Europe* (New York, 2017).

Lavin, Irving, *Past-Present: Essays on Historicism in Art from Donatello to Picasso* (Berkeley, CA, 1993).

Leitch, Stephanie, 'Burgkmair's Peoples of Africa and India (1508) and the Origins of Ethnography in Print', *Art Bulletin* 91 (2009), 134–59.

Leitch, Stephanie, *Mapping Ethnography in Early Modern Germany* (New York, 2010).

Lemire, Beverly, *Global Trade and the Transformation of Consumer Cultures: The Material World Remade, c.1500–1820* (Cambridge, 2018).

Lepp, Friedrich, *Schlagwörter des Reformationszeitalters* (Leipzig, 1908).

Leppin, Volker, *Antichrist und Jüngster Tag: Das Profil apokalyptischer Flugschriftenpublizistik im deutschen Luthertum 1548–1618* (Gütersloh, 1992).

Levine, Philippa, 'Naked Natives and Noble Savages: The Cultural Work of Nakedness in Imperial Britain', in Barry Crosbie and Mark Hampton (eds), *The Cultural Construction of the British World* (Manchester, 2015), 17–38.

Levy, Janey L., 'The Erotic Engravings of Sebald and Barthel Beham: A German Interpretation of a Renaissance Subject', in Stephen H. Goddard (ed.), *The World in Miniature: Engravings by the German Little Masters, 1500–1550*, exh. cat., Spencer Museum of Art, Lawrence, KS (Lawrence, KS, 1988), 40–53.

Levy-Navarro, Elena, *The Culture of Obesity in Early and Late Modernity: Body Image in Shakespeare, Jonson, Middleton and Skelton* (New York, 2008).

Levy-Navarro, Elena (ed.), *Historicizing Fat in Anglo-American Culture* (Columbus, OH, 2010).

Löcher, Kurt, *Barthel Beham: Ein Maler aus dem Dürerkreis* (Munich, 1999).

Lomersley, David, 'Why is Falstaff Fat?', *Review of English Studies: A Quarterly Journal of English Literature and the English Language* 47 (1996), 1–22.

Lorenz, Maren, 'Tiefe Wunden. Gewalterfahrung in den Kriegen der Frühen Neuzeit', in Ulrich Bielefeld, Heinz Bude, and Bernd Greiner (eds), *Gesellschaft—Gewalt -Vertrauen: Jan Philipp Reemtsma zum 60. Geburtstag* (Hamburg, 2012), 332–54.

Lotz-Heumann, Ute, *The German Spa in the Long Eighteenth Century: A Cultural History* (Abingdon, 2022).

Lowe, Kate, 'Visible Lives: Black Gondoliers and Other Black Africans in Renaissance Venice', *Renaissance Quarterly* 66 (2013), 412–52.

Lundin, Matthew, *Paper Memory: A Sixteenth-Century Townsman Writes his World,* Harvard Historical Studies 179 (Cambridge, 2012).

Malcolm-Davies, Jane, Caroline Johnson, and Ninya Mikhaila, '"And her Black Satin Gown must be New-Bodied": The Twenty-First Century Body in Pursuit of the Holbein Look', *Costume* 42 (2008), 21–9.

Manning Stevens, Scott, 'New World Contacts and the Trope of the "Naked Savage"', in Elizabeth D. Harvey (ed.), *Sensible Flesh: On Touch in Early Modern Culture* (Philadelphia, 2003), 125–40.

Marr, Alexander, 'Walther Ryff, Plagiarism and Imitation in Sixteenth-Century Germany', *Print Quarterly* 31 (2014), 131–43.

Martin, Andrew John, and Christof Metzger, 'Das Ideal der Antike', in Christof Metzger (ed.), *Albrecht Dürer,* exh. cat., Albertina Vienna (Munich, 2019), 192–204.

Mattern, Susan P., *Galen and the Rhetoric of Healing* (Baltimore, MD, 2008).

Medick, Hans, *Der Dreißigjährige Krieg: Zeugnisse vom Leben mit Gewalt* (Göttingen, 2018).

Melchior-Bonnet, Sabine, *The Mirror: A History* (London, 2002).

Mellinkoff, Ruth, *Outcasts: Signs of Otherness in Northern European Art of the Late Middle Ages* (Berkeley, CA, 1993).
Mentzel, Jan-David, 'Körper und Welt: Albrecht Dürers *Männerbad* in neuer Deutung', in Thomas Schauerte, Jürgen Müller, and Bertram Kaschek (eds), *Von der Freiheit der Bilder: Spott, Kritik und Subversion in der Kunst der Dürerzeit* (Petersberg, 2013), 58–73.
Merback, Mitchell B., *Perfection's Therapy: An Essay on Albrecht Dürer's Melencolia I* (New York, 2017).
Merleau-Ponty, Maurice, *The Primacy of Perception: And Other Essays on Phenomenological Psychology, the Philosophy of Art, History and Politics*, ed. James M. Edie (Evanston, IL, 1964).
Merleau-Ponty, Maurice, *The Phenomenology of* Perception (London, 1981).
Miglietti, Sara, 'Mastering the Climate: Theories of Environmental Influence in the Long Seventeenth Century', PhD thesis, Warwick, 2016.
Miles, Margaret, 'Theology, Anthropology, and the Human Body in Calvin's *Institutes of the Christian Religion*', *Harvard Theological Review* 74 (1981), 303–23.
Mol, Annemarie, *The Body Multiple: Ontology in Medical Practice* (Durham, NC, 2002).
Moore, Jason, 'Sugar and the Expansion of the Early Modern World-Economy: Commodity Frontiers, Ecological Transformation, and Industrialization', *Review: A Journal of the Fernand Braudel Center* 23 (2000), 409–33.
Morall, Andrew, 'Dürer in Venice', in Larry Silver and Jeffrey Chipps Smith (eds), *The Essential Dürer* (Philadelphia, 2010), 99–114.
Mortimer, Geoff, *Eyewitness Accounts of the Thirty-Years War 1618–1648* (Basingstoke, 2002).
Moulinier, Axel, and Sophie Vesin, 'Women's Undergarments and the Submission of the Body in the Sixteenth Century', in Denis Bruna (ed.), *Fashioning the Body: An Intimate History of the Silhouette* (New Haven, 2015), 57–66.
Moxey, Keith, *Peasants, Warrior and Wives: Popular Imagery in the Reformation* (Chicago, 1989).
Muldrew, Craig, *Food, Energy and the Creation of Industriousness: Work and Material Culture in Agrarian England, 1550–1780* (Cambridge, 2010).
Müller, Jürgen, and Thomas Schauerte (eds), *Die gottlosen Maler von Nürnberg—Konvention und Subversion in der Druckgrafik der Beham-Brüder*, exh. cat., Albrecht-Dürer-Haus, Nuremberg (Nuremberg, 2011).
Murphy, Hannah, 'Der Körper im Bad: Baden und Gesundheit im frühneuzeitlichen Deutschland', in *Stay Healthy*, exh. cat., Draiflessen Collection (Mettingen, 2021), 19–34.
Murphy, Hannah, 'Re-writing Race in Early Modern European Medicine', *History Compass* 19 (2021), e12692.
Newton, Hannah, '"She Sleeps Well and Eats an Egg": Convalescent Care in Early Modern England', in Sandra Cavallo and Tessa Storey (eds), *Conserving Health in Early Modern Culture: Bodies and Environments in Italy and England* (Manchester, 2017), 104–32.
Newton, Hannah, *Misery to Mirth: Recovery from Illness in Early Modern England* (Oxford, 2018).
Newton, Hannah, 'Inside the Sick Chamber in Early Modern England: The Experience of Illness through Six Objects', *English Historical Review* 136 (2021), 530–67.
Niekamp, Bettina, 'Das Prunkkleid des Moritz von Sachsen', in Bettina Niekamp and Agnieszka Woś Jucker (eds), with Jutta Charlotte von Bloh and Anna Jolly, *Das Prunkkleid des Kurfürsten Moritz von Sachsen (1521–1553) in der Dresdner Rüstkammer: Dokumentation—Restaurierung—Konservierung* (Riggisberg, 2008), 21–48.
Nolte, Cordula, 'Verbalerotische Kommunikation, gut schwenck oder: Worüber lachte man bei Hofe? Einige Thesen zum Briefwechsel des Kurfürstenpaares Albrecht und Anna von Brandenburg-Ansbach 1474/75', in Jan Hirschbiegel and Werner Paravicini (eds), *Das Frauenzimmer: Die Frau bei Hofe in Spätmittelalter und früher Neuzeit* (Sigmaringen, 2000), 449–61.
Orchard, Karin, *Annäherungen der Geschlechter: Androgynie in der Kunst des Cinquecento* (Münster, 1992).
Otele, Olivette, *African Europeans: An Untold History* (London, 2020).

Ott, Christine, 'Fette Körper in der Vormoderne: Überlegungen zu einer literarischen Geschichte des Dickseins', *Archiv für das Studium der neueren Sprachen und Literaturen* 256 (2019), 1–21.

Ott, Christine, 'Fat Carnival Princess in Renaissance Rome: Luigi Pulci's Political Misogyny', *Food and History* 21 (2023), 159–71.

Ott, Christine, 'Körperfülle als äesthetisches Problem in der Frühen Neuzeit', in Sofina Dembruk, Olivier Chiquet, Claudia Jacobi, and Ioana Manea (eds), *La Renaissance 'trop en corps'. Perspectives croisées sur le corps renaissant* (Heidelberg, 2023), 81–102.

Ott, Christine, 'Ein kleines dickes Mädchen. Körpernormen und -abnormitäten im 17. Jahrhundert', in Katharina Bedenbender and Julia Saviello (eds), *Dramaturgien von Bild und Raum* (Berlin, 2024), 139–49.

Ozment, Steven, *Magdalena and Balthasar: An Intimate Portrait of Life in Sixteenth-Century Europe Revealed in the Letters of a Nuremberg Husband and Wife* (New Haven, 1989).

Ozment, Steven, *Three Behaim Boys: Growing Up in Early Modern Germany* (New Haven, 1990).

Palmer Wandel, Lee, *The Eucharist in the Reformation* (Cambridge, 2006).

Panofsky, Erwin, *The Life and Art of Albrecht Dürer* (Princeton, 2005, first published 1943).

Papavramidou, Niki S., M. S., Spiros, T. Papavramidis, and Helen Christopoulou-Aletra, 'Galen on Obesity: Etiology, Effects and Treatment', *World Journal of Surgery* 28 (2004), 631–5.

Parker, Geoffrey, *Emperor: A New Life of Charles V* (New Haven, 2019).

Parker, Patricia, *Literary Fat Ladies: Rhetoric, Gender, Property* (London and New York: 1987).

Parshall, Peter, 'Imago Contrafacta: Images and Facts in the Northern Renaissance', *Art History* 16 (1993), 554–79.

Patterson, Angus. *Fashion and Armour in Renaissance Europe: Proud Lookes and Brave Attire* (London, 2009).

Peinelt, Sabine, 'Der Verleger als Vollender? Zum "Kunst und Lehrbuchlein" von Sebald Beham', in Jürgen Müller and Thomas Schauerte (eds), *Die gottlosen Maler von Nürnberg—Konvention und Subversion in der Druckgrafik der Beham-Brüder*, exh. cat., Albrecht-Dürer-Haus, Nuremberg (Nuremberg, 2011), 136–8.

Pellé, Anne-Sophie, 'Mesurer l'excès: Albrecht Dürer et la figure obèse', *Histoire de l'art* 70 (2012), 1–10.

Petrascheck-Heim, Ingeborg, 'Die Meisterstückbücher des Schneiderhandwerks in Innsbruck', *Veröffentlichungen des Tiroler Landesmuseums Ferdinandeum* 50 (1970), 159–218.

Pfisterer, Ulrich (ed.), *Die Kunstliteratur der italienischen Renaissance: Eine Geschichte in Quellen* (Stuttgart, 2002).

Phillips, Kim M., 'The Breasts of Virgins: Sexual Reputation and Young Women's Bodies in Medieval Culture and Society', *Cultural and Social History* 15 (2018), 1–19.

Pietsch, Johannes, *Zwei Schauben aus dem Bayerischen Nationalmuseum München: Ein Beitrag zur Kostümforschung* (Munich, 2004).

Pietsch, Johannes, 'Das Schneiderhandwerk im 17. Jahrhundert', in Johannes Pietsch and Karen Stolleis (eds), *Kölner Patrizier- und Bürgerkleidung des 17. Jahrhunderts: Die Kostümsammlung Hüpsch im Hessischen Landesmuseum Darmstadt* (Riggisberg, 2008). 59–125.

Pietsch, Johannes, 'Establishing Identity: Stays from Southern Germany in the Collection of the Bayerisches Nationalmuseum', in Frank Matthias Kammel and Johannes Pietsch (eds), *Structuring Fashion: Foundation Garments through History* (Munich, 2019), 73–83.

Piller, Gudrun, 'Private Body: What do Self-Narratives Bring to the History of the Body?', in Claudia Ulbrich, Kaspar von Greyerz, and Lorenz Heiligensetzer (eds), *Mapping the 'I': Research on Self-Narratives in Germany and Switzerland* (Leiden, 2015), 76–94.

Pirsig, Wolfgang, 'Dürers Mutter: aus ärztlicher Sicht', in Michael Roth (ed.), *Dürers Mutter: Schönheit, Alter und Tod im Bild der Renaissance* (Berlin, 2006), 17–22.

Pohl, Josef, 'Etymologisches über den Namen des Caspar Bruschius', *Mitteilungen des Vereins für Geschichte der Deutschen in Böhmen* 51 (1913), 404–6.

Pokorny, Erwin, 'Dürers Selbstakt', in Christof Metzger (ed.), *Albrecht Dürer* (Munich, 2019), 70–3.

Ptaszyński, Maciej, 'Theologians and their Bellies: The Erasmian Epithet *Theologaster* during the Reformation', *Erasmus Studies* 41 (2021), 200–29.

Pulz, Waltraud, *Nüchternes Kalkül—verzehrende Leidenschaft: Nahrungsabstinenz im 16. Jahrhundert* (Cologne, 2007).

Pulz, Waltraud, 'Innere Schau und/oder Nabelschau: Blicke auf die Nahrungsabstinenten der Frühen Neuzeit', in Waltraud Pulz, Jan Marco Sawilla, and Dieter R. Bauer (eds) *Zwischen Himmel und Erde: Körperliche Zeichen der Heiligkeit* (Stuttgart, 2012), 101–21.

Purnis, Jan, 'Sanctorius's Weighing Chair: Measurement, Metabolism, and Mind', in Simone Guidi and Joaquim Braga (eds), *The Quantification of Life and Health from the Sixteenth to the Nineteenth Century: Intersections of Medicine and Philosophy* (Cham, 2023), 111–32.

Pyrges, Alexander, 'Fat Knowledge: The History of Corpulence', *Curare: Zeitschrift für Medizinethnologie* 39 (2016), 126–35.

Pyrges, Alexander, 'Frühneuzeitliche Verbildlichungen von Beleibtheit: Versuch einer körper- und kunsthistorischen Einordnung', in Michael Stolberg (ed.), *Körper-Bilder in der Frühen Neuzeit* (Berlin, 2021), 103–25.

Rákóczi, Katalin, 'Die Widerspiegelung der humanistisch-reformatorischen Tendenzen der Medizin im populärwissenschaftlichen Werk von Walter Hermann Ryff', *Orvostörténeti Közlemények* 28 (1982), 9–37.

Rákóczi, Katalin, 'Walter Hermann Ryffs charakteristische Stilmittel. Ein Vergleich mit H. Brunschwyg, H. Gersdorf und O. Brunfels', *Orvostörténeti Közlemények* 30 (1984), 79–88.

Rath, Markus, *Die Gliederpuppe: Kult, Kunst, Konzept* (Berlin and Boston, 2016).

Resnick, Irven M., 'Medieval Roots of the Myth of Jewish Male Menses', *Harvard Theological Review* 93 (2000), 241–63.

Reusch, Johann J. K., 'Germans as Noble Savages and Castaways: Alter Egos and Alterity in German Collective Consciousness during the Long Eighteenth Century', *Eighteenth-Century Studies* 42 (2008), 91–129.

Ribeiro, Aileen, *Dress and Morality* (London, 1986).

Riello, Giorgio, and Ulinka Rublack (eds), *The Right to Dress: Sumptuary Laws in a Global Perspective, c.1200–1800* (Cambridge, 2019).

Riello, Giorgio, 'The World in a Book: The Creation of the Global in Sixteenth-Century European Costume Books', *Past and Present* 242 (2019), 281–317.

Rittgers, Ronald K., *The Reformation of Suffering: Pastoral Theology and Lay Piety in Late Medieval and Early Modern Germany* (Oxford, 2012).

Robisheaux, Thomas, *The Last Witch of Langenburg: Murder in a German Village* (New York, 2009).

Rogers, Clifford J., *The Oxford Encyclopedia of Medieval Warfare and Military Technology*, vol. 1 (Oxford, 2010), 19.

Roodenburg, Hermann, *The Eloquence of the Body: Perspectives on Gesture in the Dutch Republic* (Zwolle, 2004).

Roper, Lyndal, *The Holy Household: Women and Morals in Reformation Augsburg* (Oxford, 1989).

Roper, Lyndal, *Oedipus and the Devil: Witchcraft, Sexuality and Religion in Early Modern Europe* (London, 1994).

Roper, Lyndal, *Witch Craze: Terror and Fantasy in Baroque Germany* (New Haven, 2006).

Roper, Lyndal, 'Beyond Discourse Theory', *Women's History Review* 19 (2010), 307–19.

Roper, Lyndal, 'Martin Luther's Body: The "Stout Doctor" and his Biographers', *American Historical Review* 115 (2010), 351–84.

Roper, Lyndal, *Martin Luther: Renegade and Prophet* (London, 2016).

Roper, Lyndal, *Living I was your Plague: Martin Luther's World and Legacy* (Princeton, 2021).

Rosin, Robert, 'Johannes Mathesius (1504-1565)', in Hans J. Hillebrand (ed.), *The Oxford Encyclopedia of the Reformation* (Oxford, 1996), https://www.oxfordreference.com/view/10.1093/acref/9780195064933.001.0001/acref-9780195064933-e-0906.

Roth, Michael, 'Dürers Mutter in der Bildniskunst Albrecht Dürers', in Michael Roth (ed.), *Dürers Mutter: Schönheit, Alter und Tod im Bild der Renaissance* (Berlin, 2006), 129–35.

Rublack, Ulinka, 'Pregnancy, Childbirth and the Female Body in Early Modern Germany', *Past and Present* 150 (1996), 84–110.

Rublack, Ulinka, 'Fluxes: The Early Modern Body and the Emotions', *History Workshop Journal* 53 (2002), 1–16.
Rublack, Ulinka, *Dressing Up: Cultural Identity in Renaissance Europe* (Oxford, 2010).
Rublack, Ulinka, 'Matter in the Material Renaissance', *Past and Present* 219 (2013), 41–85.
Rublack, Ulinka, 'Renaissance Dress, Cultures of Making, and the Period Eye', *West 86th: A Journal of Decorative Arts, Design History and Material Culture* 23 (2016), 6–34.
Rublack, Ulinka, *Reformation Europe* (Cambridge, 2017).
Rublack, Ulinka, 'The Right to Dress: Sartorial Politics in Germany, c.1300-1750', in Giorgio Riello and Ulinka Rublack (eds), *The Right to Dress: Sumptuary Laws in a Global Perspective, c.1200–1800* (Cambridge, 2019), 37–73.
Rublack, Ulinka, 'Craft, Labour and Cabinets of Curiosities: Rethinking the Body of the Artisan', *German History* 41 (2023), 337–66.
Rublack, Ulinka, *Dürer's Lost Masterpiece: Art and Society at the Dawn of a Global World* (Oxford, 2023).
Rublack, Ulinka, *Dürer's Coats: Renaissance Men and Material Cultures of Social Recognition*, The Natalie Zemon Davis Memorial Lectures Series (Vienna, 2025).
Ruvoldt, Maria, *The Italian Renaissance Imagery of Inspiration: Metaphors of Sex, Sleep and Dreams* (Cambridge, 2004).
Sabean, David, *Power in the Blood: Popular Culture and Village Discourse in Early Modern Germany* (Cambridge, 1984).
Sandnes, Karl Olav, *Belly and Body in the Pauline Epistles* (Cambridge, 2002).
Scales, Len, 'German Militiae: War and German Identity in the Later Middle Ages', *Past and Present* 180 (2003), 41–82.
Scales, Len, *The Shaping of German Identity: Authority and Crisis, 1245–1414* (Cambridge, 2012).
Schauerte, Thomas, *Dürer und Celtis. Die Nürnberger Poetenschule im Aufbruch* (Leipzig, 2015).
Schleif, Corine, 'Albrecht Dürer between Agnes Frey and Willibald Pirckheimer', in Larry Silver and Jeffrey Chipps Smith (eds), *The Essential Dürer* (Philadelphia, 2010), 185–205, 267–71.
Schleif, Corine, and Volker Schier, *Katerina's Windows: Donation and Devotion, Art and Music, as Heard and Seen in the Writings of a Birgittine Nun* (University Park, PA, 2008).
Schmeidler, Bernhard, 'Anti-asketische Äusserungen aus Deutschland im 11. und beginnenden 12. Jahrhundert', in *Kultur und Universalgeschichte: Walter Goetz zu seinem 60. Geburtstag* (Leipzig and Berlin, 1927), 35–52.
Schmidt, Alexander, *Vaterlandsliebe und Religionskonflikt: Politische Diskurse im Alten Reich (1555–1648)* (Leiden, 2007).
Schober, Sarah Maria, *Gesellschaft im Exzess: Mediziner in Basel um 1600* (Frankfurt, 2019).
Schoen, Christian, *Albrecht Dürer: Adam und Eva. Die Gemälde, ihre Geschichte und Rezeption bei Lucas Cranach d. Ä. und Hans Baldung Grien* (Berlin, 2001).
Schoenholzer Nichols, Thessy, 'It does Not Need to be Hard to Hold', in Frank Matthias Kammel and Johannes Pietsch (eds), *Structuring Fashion: Foundation Garments through History* (Munich, 2019), 29–38.
Schubert, Ernst, 'Albrecht Achilles, Markgraf und Kurfürst von Brandenburg 1414-1486', *Fränkische Lebensbilder* 4 (1971), 130–72.
Schwartz, Hillel, *Never Satisfied: A Cultural History of Diets, Fantasies and Fat* (New York, 1986).
Schwerhoff, Gerd, 'Wie gottlos waren die "gottlosen Maler"? Zur Rekonstruktion des Nürnberger Verfahrens von 1525 und seiner Hintergründe', in Jürgen Müller and Thomas Schauerte (eds), *Die gottlosen Maler von Nürnberg—Konvention und Subversion in der Druckgrafik der Beham-Brüder*, exh. cat., Albrecht-Dürer-Haus, Nuremberg (Nuremberg, 2011), 33–48.
Scribner, Robert, *Religion and Culture in Germany (1400–1800)*, ed. Lyndal Roper (Leiden, 2001).
Silver, Larry, 'Germanic Patriotism in the Age of Dürer', in Dagmar Eichberger and Charles Zika (eds), *Dürer and his Culture* (Cambridge, 1998), 38–68.
Siraisi, Nancy, *History, Medicine, and the Traditions of Renaissance Learning* (Ann Arbor, MI, 2007).
Smith, Pamela, *The Body of the Artisan: Art and Experience in the Scientific Revolution* (Chicago, 2004).

Smith, Pamela, *From Lived Experience to the Written Word* (Chicago, 2022).

Smith, Steven R., 'The London Apprentices as Seventeenth-Century Adolescents', *Past and Present* 61 (1973), 149–61.

Soergel, Philip M., *Miracles and the Protestant Imagination: The Evangelical Wonder Book in Reformation Germany* (Oxford, 2012).

Spinks, Jennifer, *Monstrous Births and Visual Culture in Sixteenth-Century Germany* (London, 2009).

Spinks, Jennifer, 'Objects in Motion: Albrecht Dürer's *Nemesis*', in Edward H. Wouk and Jennifer Spinks (eds), *Albrecht Dürer's Material World* (Manchester, 2023), 35–47.

Stayer, James, *The German Peasant's War and Anabaptist Community of Goods* (Montreal, 1991).

Stearns, Peter N., *Fat History: Bodies and Beauty in the Modern West* (New York, 1997).

Steiger, Johann Anselm, 'Strigenitz, Gregor', *Neue Deutsche Biographie* 25 (2013), 556–7.

Stewart, Alison, 'Sebald Beham and Barthel Beham', in Jane Turner (ed.), *The Dictionary of Art*, vol. 3 (New York, 1996), 505–8.

Stewart, Alison, *Before Bruegel: Sebald Beham and the Origins of Peasant Festival Imagery* (Aldershot, 2008).

Stewart, Alison, 'Sebald Beham: Entrepreneur, Printmaker, Painter', *Journal of Historians of Netherlandish Art* 4 (2012), 1–25.

Stewart, Alison, 'Man's Best Friend? Dogs and Pigs in Early Modern Germany', in Pia F. Cuneo (ed.), *Animals and Early Modern Identity* (Farnham, 2014), 19–44.

Stielau, Allison, 'The Weight of Plate in Early Modern Inventories and Secularization Lists', *Journal of Art Historiography* 11 (2014), 1–24.

Stolberg, Michael, '"Abhorreas pinguedinem": Fat and Obesity in Early Modern Medicine (c.1500–1750)', *Studies in History and Philosophy of Science* 43 (2012), 370–8.

Stolleis, Karen, 'Die Kleider der Maria Jacobäa Fugger (1562–1588)', in Mechthild Flury-Lemberg and Karen Stolleis (eds), *Documenta Textilia: Festschrift für Sigrid Müller-Christensen* (Munich, 1981), 357–70.

Stolleis, Karen, 'Kölner Patrizier- und Bürgerkleidung in der frühen Neuzeit', in Johannes Pietsch and Karen Stolleis (eds), *Kölner Patrizier- und Bürgerkleidung des 17. Jahrhunderts: Die Kostümsammlung Hüpsch im Hessischen Landesmuseum Darmstadt* (Riggisberg, 2008), 19–57.

Storey, Tessa, 'English and Italian Health Advice: Protestant and Catholic Bodies', in Sandra Cavallo and Tessa Storey (eds), *Conserving Health in Early Modern Culture: Bodies and Environments in Italy and England* (Manchester, 2017), 210–34.

Strings, Sabrina, *Fearing the Black Body: The Racial Origins of Fat Phobia* (New York, 2019).

Stuart, Kathy, *Defiled Trades and Social Outcasts: Honor and Ritual Pollution in Early Modern Germany* (Cambridge, 2009).

Studt, Birgit, 'Die Badenfahrt: Ein neues Muster der Badepraxis und Badegeselligkeit im deutschen Spätmittelalter', in Michael Matheus (ed.), *Badeorte und Bäderreisen in Antike, Mittelalter und Neuzeit* (Stuttgart, 2001), 33–52.

Swann, Elizabeth, *Taste and Knowledge in Early Modern England* (Cambridge, 2020).

Tacke, Andreas, 'Winners and Losers: The Impact of the Reformation on the Art Market', in Kayo Hirakawa (ed.), *Sacred and Profane in Early Modern Art* (Kyoto, 2016), 37–58.

Tara, Sylvia, *The Secret Life of Fat* (New York, 2017).

Tarrant, Naomi, *The Development of Costume* (Edinburgh, 1994).

Telle, Joachim (ed.), *Pharmazie und der gemeine Mann: Hausarznei und Apotheke in der frühen Neuzeit* (Weinheim, 1988).

Timken-Zinkann, R. F., 'Medical Aspects of the Art and Life of Albrecht Dürer (1471–1528)', *Proceedings of the XXIII International Congress of the History of Medicine, London, 2–9 September 1972* (London, 1974), 870–5.

Tlusty, B. Ann, *Bacchus and Civic Order: The Culture of Drink in Early Modern Germany* (Charlottesville, VA, and London, 2001).

Toulalan, Sarah, '"To[o] Much Eating Stifles the Child": Fat Bodies and Reproduction in Early Modern England', *Historical Research* 87 (2014), 65–93.

Toulalan, Sarah, '"If Slendernesse be the Cause of Unfruitfulnesse; you must Nourish and Fatten the Body": Thin Bodies and Infertility in Early Modern England', in Gayle Davis and

Tracey Loughran (eds), *A Handbook of Infertility in History: Approaches, Contexts and Perspectives* (London, 2017), 171–97.

Ulbrich, Claudia, 'Schreibsucht? Zu den Leidenschaften eines gelehrten Bauern', in Alf Lüdtke and Reiner Prass (eds), *Gelehrtenleben: Wissenschaftspraxis in der Neuzeit,* (Cologne, 2008), 101–12.

van Putten, Jasper, *Networked Nation: Mapping German Cities in Sebastian Münster's Cosmographia* (Leiden, 2018).

Varriano John, *Wine a Cultural History* (London, 2011).

Vaughan, Theresa A., *Women, Food and Diet in the Middle Ages: Balancing the Humours* (Amsterdam, 2020).

Vigarello, Georges, *Concepts of Cleanliness: Changing Attitudes in France since the Middle Ages,* tr. Jean Birrell (Cambridge, 1988).

Vigarello, Georges, *The Metamorphoses of Fat: A History of Obesity,* tr. Christopher Jon Delogu (New York, 2013).

Vincent, Susan, *The Anatomy of Fashion: Dressing the Body from the Renaissance to Today* (Oxford and New York, 2009).

von Borries, Johann Eckart, *Albrecht Dürer: Christus als Schmerzensmann* (Karlsruhe, 1972).

von Greyerz, Kaspar, *Passagen und Stationen: Lebensstufen zwischen Mittelalter und Moderne* (Göttingen, 2010).

von Schlachta, Astrid, *Hutterische Konfession und Tradition (1578–1619): Etabliertes Leben zwischen Ordnung und Ambivalenz* (Göttingen, 2009).

Walkden, Michael, '"You are What you Eat": Historical Changes in Ideas about Food and Identity', *Historical Research* 87 (2014), 377–92.

Walker Bynum, Caroline, *Holy Feast and Holy Fast: The Religious Significance of Food to Medieval Women* (Berkeley-Los Angeles, 1987).

Walker Bynum, Caroline, 'Material Continuity, Personal Survival, and the Resurrection of the Body: A Scholastic Discussion in its Medieval and Modern Contexts', *History of Religions* 30 (1990), 51–85.

Walker Bynum, Caroline, *Fragmentation and Redemption: Essays on Gender and the Human Body in Medieval Religion* (New York, 1992).

Walker Bynum, Caroline, *The Resurrection of the Body in Western Christianity, 200–1336* (New York, 1995).

Walker Bynum, Caroline, 'Why All the Fuss about the Body? A Medievalist's Perspective', *Critical Inquiry* 12 (1995), 1–33.

Wall, Wendy, 'Just a Spoonful of Sugar: Syrup and Domesticity in Early Modern England', *Modern Philology* 104 (2006), 149–72.

Warburg, Aby, *The Renewal of Pagan Antiquity: Contributions to the Cultural History of the European Renaissance,* introduction by Kurt W. Forster, tr. David Britt (Los Angeles, 1999).

Warr, Tracey, and Amelia Jones (eds), *The Artist's Body* (London, 2000).

Weixlgärtner, Arpad, 'Dürer und die Gliederpuppe', *Beiträge zur Kunstgeschichte: Franz Wickhoff gewidmet* (1903), 80–90.

West, Candace, and Don H. Zimmerman, 'Doing Gender', *Gender and Society* 1 (1987), 125–51.

Wiesner, Merry E., 'Beyond Women and the Family: Towards a Gender Analysis of the Reformation', *Sixteenth Century Journal* 18 (1987), 311–21.

Winchcombe, Rachel, *Encountering Early America* (Manchester, 2021).

Winchcombe, Rachel, 'Comfort Eating: Food, Drink and Emotional Health in Early Modern England', *English Historical Review* 138 (2023), 61–91.

Winchcombe, Rachel, 'The Limits of Disgust: Eating the Inedible During Jamestown's "Starving Time"', *Global Food History* 11 (2023), 7–293.

Wind, Edgar, 'Dürer's "Männerbad": A Dionysian Mystery', *Journal of the Warburg Institute* 2 (1939), 269–71.

Woods, Kathryn, 'Dismembering Appearances: The Cultural Meaning of the Body and its Parts in Eighteenth-Century Understanding', PhD thesis, Warwick, 2014.

Wouk, Edward H., and Jennifer Spinks (eds), *Albrecht Dürer's Material World.* exh. cat., Whitworth Art Gallery, Manchester (Manchester, 2023).

Wriedt, Markus, 'Invectives as a Stylistic Device in Martin Luther's Reformation Rhetoric', *Journal of Early Modern Christianity* 10 (2023), 43–71.
Wunder, Heide, *He is the Sun, She is the Moon: Women in Early Modern Germany,* tr. Thomas Dunlap (Cambridge, 1998).
Zander-Seidel, Jutta *Textiler Hausrat: Kleidung und Haustextilien in Nürnberg von 1500–1650* (Munich, 1990).
Zander-Seidel, Jutta (ed.), *In Mode: Kleider und Bilder aus Renaissance und Frühbarock,* exh. cat., Germanisches Nationalmuseum, Nuremberg (Nuremberg, 2015).
Zemon Davis, Natalie, 'Women on Top', in *Society and Culture in Early Modern France* (Stanford, CA, 1975), 124–51.
Zemon Davis, Natalie, '"Women's History" in Transition: The European Case', *Feminist Studies* 3 (1976), 83–103.
Zika, Charles, *The Appearance of Witchcraft* (London, 2007).
Zimmermann, Gerd, *Ordensleben und Lebensstandard: Die Cura corporis in den Ordensvorschriften des abendländischen Hochmittelalters* (Münster, 1973).
Zitzlsperger, Philipp, *Dürers Pelz und das Recht im Bild: Kleiderkunde als Methode der Kunstgeschichte* (Berlin, 2012).
Zschelletzschky, Herbert, *Die 'Drei gottlosen Maler' von Nürnberg* (Leipzig, 1975).

Index

For the benefit of digital users, indexed terms that span two pages (e.g., 52–53) may, on occasion, appear on only one of those pages.